Public Health Law Research

D1501160

Public Health Law Research

Theory and Methods

Alexander C. Wagenaar
Scott Burris

EDITORS

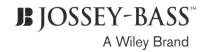

Cover design by JPuda
Cover images: sign © Kameleon007/istockphoto; hand drawing © BrianAJackson/istockphoto;
texting © monkeypics/istockphoto; arches © Kameleon007/istockphoto

Copyright © 2013 by John Wiley & Sons, Inc. All rights reserved.

Published by Jossey-Bass
A Wiley Imprint
One Montgomery Street, Suite 1200, San Francisco, CA 94104-4594—www.josseybass.com

No part of this publication may be reproduced, stored in a retrieval system, or transmitted in any
form or by any means, electronic, mechanical, photocopying, recording, scanning, or otherwise,
except as permitted under Section 107 or 108 of the 1976 United States Copyright Act, without either
the prior written permission of the publisher, or authorization through payment of the appropriate
per-copy fee to the Copyright Clearance Center, Inc., 222 Rosewood Drive, Danvers, MA 01923,
978-750-8400, fax 978-646-8600, or on the Web at www.copyright.com. Requests to the publisher
for permission should be addressed to the Permissions Department, John Wiley & Sons, Inc.,
111 River Street, Hoboken, NJ 07030, 201-748-6011, fax 201-748-6008, or online at
www.wiley.com/go/permissions.

Limit of Liability/Disclaimer of Warranty: While the publisher and author have used their best
efforts in preparing this book, they make no representations or warranties with respect to the
accuracy or completeness of the contents of this book and specifically disclaim any implied
warranties of merchantability or fitness for a particular purpose. No warranty may be created or
extended by sales representatives or written sales materials. The advice and strategies contained
herein may not be suitable for your situation. You should consult with a professional where
appropriate. Neither the publisher nor author shall be liable for any loss of profit or any other
commercial damages, including but not limited to special, incidental, consequential, or other
damages. Readers should be aware that Internet Web sites offered as citations and/or sources
for further information may have changed or disappeared between the time this was written and
when it is read.

Jossey-Bass books and products are available through most bookstores. To contact Jossey-Bass
directly call our Customer Care Department within the U.S. at 800-956-7739, outside the U.S. at
317-572-3986, or fax 317-572-4002.

Wiley publishes in a variety of print and electronic formats and by print-on-demand. Some material
included with standard print versions of this book may not be included in e-books or in print-on-
demand. If this book refers to media such as a CD or DVD that is not included in the version you
purchased, you may download this material at http://booksupport.wiley.com. For more information
about Wiley products, visit www.wiley.com.

Library of Congress Cataloging-in-Publication Data

    Public health law research : theory and methods / Alexander C. Wagenaar, Scott Burris,
editors. — 1st ed.
      p.   cm.
    Includes bibliographical references and index.
    ISBN 978-1-118-13762-8 (pbk.); ISBN 978-1-118-41923-6 (ebk.); ISBN 978-1-118-42088-1 (ebk.);
    ISBN 978-1-118-59118-5 (ebk.)
      I. Wagenaar, Alexander C.   II. Burris, Scott.
      [DNLM: 1. Health Services Research.   2. Public Health—legislation & jurisprudence.
    WA 33.1]
    KF3821
    344.7304'1—dc23

                               2013012424

Printed in the United States of America
FIRST EDITION
PB Printing 10 9 8 7 6 5 4 3 2 1

Contents

PART THREE

Identifying and Measuring Legal Variables

PART FOUR

Designing Public Health Law Evaluations

Figures and Tables

Tables

Foreword

This book represents a major milestone in the development of public health law research, both as a field of study and as a tool for using law and policy to improve health. A vibrant community of innovative scientists engaged in rigorous public health law research is essential for making informed decisions on the laws and policies that will lead to better health.

For the Robert Wood Johnson Foundation, this book represents a unique and lasting contribution to the field of public health law. The Foundation conceived and funded a national program for public health law research to make the case for laws that improve health. At this writing, the Public Health Law Research program has funded sixty studies in its first four years. Many of those studies have already had an impact at the local, state, and national levels. For example, a program study has shown how local laws in Rochester, New York, have made a difference in children's exposure to lead. Another program study on New Jersey's graduated driver licensing laws has shown how the law reduced teen car crashes and saved lives. And yet another program study on drug patent laws and their impact on public health has already been cited by the United States Solicitor General in documents filed before the U.S. Supreme Court.

Some of the studies funded by the Public Health Law Research program raised new questions. Others provided new insights. Collectively, they point to a need for a critical review of the basic concepts, theories, mechanisms, and measurement techniques of public health law research. That this need has been recognized and acted on is a tribute to the leadership of the Public Health Law Research program and the authors who have contributed to this book.

The intersection of law, policy, advocacy, and health is complex. Applied at the right time, in the right places, with the right partners, laws and policies have the potential to create lasting positive changes in the lives of people. I am confident that this book will enhance the quality of public health law research. It will strengthen the role of research in policy deliberations. And that will heighten the ability of policy makers, advocates, and leaders to craft and implement effective laws and policies to improve health for years to come.

I want to express my gratitude to the authors, editors, and all who have made this book possible. To the reader, I invite you to take full advantage of the insights and wisdom herein and apply them to your work to improve health.

Michelle A. Larkin, JD, MS, RN
Assistant Vice President, Health Group
Robert Wood Johnson Foundation
April 2013

Preface

"Each individual in society has a right to be protected in the enjoyment of his life. . . . And it is the duty of the State to extend over the
people its guardian care, that those who cannot or will not protect
themselves, may nevertheless be protected; and that those who can
and desire to do it, may have the means of doing it more easily. This
right and authority should be exercised by wise laws, wisely administered; and when this is neglected the State should be held answerable
for the consequences of this neglect. If legislators and public officers
knew the number of lives unnecessarily destroyed, and the suffering
unnecessarily occasioned by a wrong movement or by no movement
at all, this great matter would be more carefully studied, and errors
would not be so frequently committed."

> —Lemuel Shattuck, *Report of a General Plan for the
> Promotion of Public and Personal Health*, 1850 (p. 304).

Modern public health practice began with counting. The idea that disease
and injury could be prevented started with what became the science of
epidemiology—people counting cases and documenting their distribution. The idea of preventable disease led directly to the idea that society has the
opportunity and indeed the obligation to take a strong hand in doing the preventing. When we take collective action, we usually do it through government,
acting on behalf of the community. Once government is in the picture, law is
there, too.

Law matters to public health. It is a tool for intervention to promote healthier places and people. It sets the powers, duties, and limitations of health agencies.
Sometimes laws and legal practices with no deliberate relation to health have
positive or negative effects on our health. Yet if we go back to the roots of
modern public health practice—to epidemiology—and we look at public health
as it is practiced today, we can see why it is not enough to assert the important
roles of law in public health. Science is the lifeblood of public health, the source
of much of its effectiveness and legitimacy. Effective public health work begins
with understanding the nature, effects, and distribution of the threats to our
health and the facilitators of our well-being, and extends to carefully evaluating
the interventions designed to support our thriving. So it must also be with law.

If law matters to public health, we have to be able to show how, under what circumstances, to what degree. We have to produce *evidence*. Public health law research (PHLR) is the field devoted to creating and disseminating that evidence.

This book describes scientific theory and methods for investigating the development, implementation, and effects of public health law. The empirical study of law can be conducted in many disciplines, or in collaboration between disciplines. Either way, it is an exercise applying normal scientific methods. There is no special science of public health law research. Epidemiology, economics, physiology, and sociology do not change when law is the topic of investigation. That said, there are unique challenges to studying law, and a set of theory, measurement, and research design tools that specifically help to meet those challenges. *Public Health Law Research* is not a general primer on scientific research methods. Its focus is on the problems that tend to arise in public health law research—and their solutions. And so it is intended for many kinds of readers: experienced social science researchers who are interested in adding public health law research to their repertoire; experienced health scientists who wish to expand their research from interventions at the individual or small-group levels to community or society-wide "treatments" operating through law; legal scholars interested in how scientists approach the study of law; policy analysts seeking improved ability to assess the methods behind empirical evaluations of laws and policies; students and novice scientists who can hone their general skills through the study of public health law; and non-scientists who are seeking a general orientation to PHLR.

The book is presented in four parts, each beginning with an introduction delineating the topics to be covered. Part One is an introduction to the basic concepts of the field of PHLR. Part Two presents a rich collection of theories that researchers have used to study *how* law influences behavior—the mechanisms or processes through which a rule manages to have measurable effects on what people do and how they fare. Part Three is devoted to special questions of measurement that arise when law is the independent variable. Finally, with this grounding in how law works and how it can be measured, Part Four considers the various study designs for public health law research.

Lemuel Shattuck's words were true when he wrote them of Massachusetts in 1850, and they are true of every state today. We all lose when lives are unnecessarily lost or reduced by preventable ills. None of us can, alone, create the conditions in which we can be healthy. Through careful scientific study, researchers can help society use its resources for health effectively and efficiently, and avoid errors in the deployment of law.

A.C.W.
S. B.

Acknowledgments

The editors and authors acknowledge the invaluable support of the Robert Wood Johnson Foundation through their financial and programmatic support for the Public Health Law Research program, based at the Temple University Beasley School of Law. Opinions expressed herein are the responsibility of the editors and authors and do not necessarily represent the view of the Robert Wood Johnson Foundation. The editors thank the Public Health Law Research Program Methods Core members, Jennifer K. Ibrahim, Michelle M. Mello, Jeffrey W. Swanson, and Jennifer Wood for their assistance in devising the plan for the book. We also thank those who reviewed and commented on individual chapters, including the members of the Methods Core, Evan Anderson, Philip Cook, Thomas Getzen, Eleanor Kinney, Angie McGowan, Anthony Moulton, Prabhu Ponkshe, F. Douglas Scutchfield, Jonathan Shuster, and *The Milbank Quarterly*'s anonymous reviewers. Tim Akers, Marice Ashe, Dhrubajyoti Bhattacharya, Michelle Larkin, and Roberto Potter provided valuable feedback in the early stages of the manuscript's development. Marice Ashe, Anne Barry, Lisa Ikemoto, and Jean O'Connor provided thoughtful and constructive comments on the complete draft manuscript. Finally, we thank Jillian Penrod for her careful and sure management of the complicated process of assembling a book like this, and Heidi Grunwald for her careful and sure management of everything else we do at Public Health Law Research.

*This book is dedicated to everyone who uses science
to make the case for laws that improve health.*

The Editors

Alexander C. Wagenaar, Ph.D., is professor of health outcomes and policy and a professor in the Institute for Child Health Policy at the University of Florida, College of Medicine. He has published one previous book, numerous book chapters, and over 170 scientific articles on social epidemiology, public health policy, legal evaluations, community intervention trials, alcohol and tobacco studies, violence prevention, traffic safety, and injury control. He currently serves as associate director of the Robert Wood Johnson Foundation's Public Health Law Research Program, based at Temple University Beasley School of Law. He is a scientific reviewer for dozens of journals, and serves on the editorial boards of *Prevention Science* and the *Journal of Safety Research*. In 1999, Dr. Wagenaar received the Jellinek award for lifetime achievement in research on alcohol. In 2001 he received the Innovator's Award from the Robert Wood Johnson Foundation, and in 2004 was named by the Institute for Scientific Information as a Highly Cited Researcher, an honor limited to less than one-half of one percent of published scientists worldwide. In 2009 he received the Prevention Science Award from the Society for Prevention Research for contributions of his three decades of research in advancing the methods and outcomes of prevention research. In 2010 he received an honorary Research Professorship award from the University of Florida Foundation.

Scott Burris, J.D., is a professor of law at Temple Law School, where he directs the Center for Health Law, Policy and Practice and the Robert Wood Johnson Foundation's Public Health Law Research program. He is the author of over one hundred books, book chapters, articles, and reports on issues including discrimination against people with HIV and other disabilities; HIV policy; research ethics; and the health effects of criminal law and drug policy. His work has been supported by organizations including the Robert Wood Johnson Foundation, the Open Society Institute, the National Institutes of Health, and the Centers for Disease Control and Prevention. He has served as a consultant on public health law with organizations ranging from the United Nations Development Programme and the American Psychological Association to the Institute of Medicine and the producers of the Oscar-winning film *Philadelphia*. Burris is a graduate of Washington University in St. Louis and the Yale Law School.

The Contributors

Evan D. Anderson, J.D., was formerly the Senior Legal Fellow at the Robert Wood Johnson's Public Health Law Research program. His work focuses on empirical legal studies, with an emphasis on the measurement of law for policy evaluation. His education training includes economics, epidemiology, and law. Prior to joining the Public Health Law Research program, Mr. Anderson was a research associate at the Johns Hopkins Bloomberg School of Public Health and a fellow at the Center for Law and the Public's Health: A Collaborative at Johns Hopkins and Georgetown Universities.

Allison J. Carnegie, Ph.D., received a joint degree in the Department of Political Science and the Department of Economics at Yale University. Her research interests include international relations, political economy, quantitative methods, and formal theory. Her work has been published in the *American Journal of Political Science* and the *Election Law Journal*. She has been awarded the Falk, Ethel Boies Morgan, Kaufman, and Yale University Dissertation fellowships.

Frank J. Chaloupka, Ph.D., is a distinguished professor at the University of Illinois at Chicago, where he has been on the faculty since 1988. He is director of the UIC Health Policy Center and director of the new WHO Collaborating Centre on the Economics of Tobacco and Tobacco Control. Dr. Chaloupka holds appointments in the College of Liberal Arts and Sciences' Department of Economics and the School of Public Health's Division of Health Policy and Administration. He is a fellow at the University of Illinois' Institute for Government and Public Affairs, and is a research associate in the National Bureau of Economic Research's Health Economics Program and Children's Program. Dr. Chaloupka is codirector of Bridging the Gap: Research Informing Policy and Practice for Healthy Youth Behavior and director of BTG's ImpacTeen Project. He is also codirector of the International Tobacco Evidence Network.

Brian R. Flay, D.Phil., is professor of public health at Oregon State University, where he also directs the Youth Core of the Hallie Ford Center for Healthy Children and Families. Prior to moving to OSU, he was distinguished professor of Community Health Sciences (Public Health) and Psychology at the University of Illinois at Chicago (UIC). He received his D.Phil. degree in social psychology from Waikato University (New Zealand) in 1976. After receiving postdoctoral training in evaluation research and social psychology at Northwestern University under a Fulbright/Hays Fellowship, he started research on health promotion and disease prevention at the University of Waterloo (Canada). He was then at the University of Southern California for eight years. He was at UIC from 1987 to 2005, where he started the Prevention Research Center, now the Institute for Health Research and Policy (IHRP), a cluster of university-wide centers focusing on health behavior, health promotion and disease prevention, health in the elderly, health services, and health policy.

Alan S. Gerber, Ph.D., is the Charles C. and Dorathea S. Dilley Professor of Political Science at Yale and founding director of the Yale Center for the Study of American Politics. He was an undergraduate at Yale and received his Ph.D. degree in economics from MIT. He is the author of two books and dozens of articles, and his research interests include experimental research methods, research design, campaigns and elections, political psychology, and public opinion. Gerber is a National Bureau of Economic Research faculty research fellow in political economy and was elected to the American Academy of Arts and Sciences in 2009. He spent 2004–2005 as a fellow at the Center for Advanced Studies in the Behavioral Sciences at Stanford University. In 2003, Gerber received the Heinz I. Eulau Award for best article published in the *American Political Science Review* during 2002.

Donald P. Green, Ph.D., is professor of political science at Columbia University. The author of four books and more than one hundred essays, Green's research interests span a wide array of topics: voting behavior, partisanship, campaign finance, hate crime, and research methods. With Alan Gerber, he recently coauthored a textbook on this research method titled *Field Experiments: Design, Analysis, and Interpretation* (2012). As director of the Institution for Social and Policy Studies at Yale University (1996–2011), Green launched its field experimental initiative and founded an experimental data archive. He was elected to the American Academy of Arts and Sciences in 2003 and was awarded the Heinz I. Eulau Award for best article published in the *American Political Science Review* during 2009.

Mark Hall, J.D., is one of the nation's leading scholars in the areas of health care law and policy and bio- and medical ethics. The author or editor of fifteen books, including *Making Medical Spending Decisions* (Oxford University Press), and *Health Care Law and Ethics* (Aspen), he is currently engaged in research in the areas of consumer-driven health care, doctor-patient trust, insurance regulation, and genetics. He has published scholarship in the law reviews at

Berkeley, Chicago, Duke, Michigan, Pennsylvania, and Stanford, and his articles have been reprinted in a dozen casebooks and anthologies. Mark also teaches in the M.B.A. program at the Babcock School and is on the research faculty at Wake Forest's Medical School. He regularly consults with government officials, foundations, and think tanks about health care public policy issues.

Delia Hendrie, M.A., is a senior research fellow at Curtin University Health Innovation Research Institute in Perth, Western Australia. She teaches health economics and financial management in postgraduate programs in health policy and management. Delia is also a lecturer in the School of Population Health at the University of Western Australia and has a role in research in the Road Accident Prevention Research Unit, where she utilizes her wide experience in economics and health economics research, in both Australia and South Africa. She has published articles in such journals as *Australian Health Review*, *Journal of Burn Care & Research*, and *Injury Prevention* and contributed a chapter on cost-benefit analysis to *Neurotrauma and Critical Care of the Brain*.

Jennifer K. Ibrahim, Ph.D., M.P.H., M.A., is an associate professor in the Department of Public Health at Temple University. She earned a B.S. degree from Boston College in 1997, an M.P.H. degree from the University of Massachusetts Amherst in 1999, and a Ph.D. degree in health services and policy analysis and an M.A. in political science from the University of California, Berkeley, in 2002. Prior to joining the faculty at Temple University, she was an American Legacy Foundation postdoctoral fellow at the University of California, San Francisco. Ibrahim's area of research interest is in health policy development and implementation, particularly at the state and local levels. Most recently, she has been investigating means to address tobacco use through policy modifications and integration within existing public health systems. In addition, Ibrahim is beginning new projects exploring the infrastructure, communications, and policies regarding domestic food safety.

Wesley G. Jennings, Ph.D., is an assistant professor in the Department of Criminology and has a Courtesy Assistant Professor Appointment in the Department of Mental Health Law and Policy at the University of South Florida College of Behavioral and Community Sciences. He received his doctorate degree in criminology from the University of Florida in 2007. He has published over sixty peer-reviewed articles, and his major research interests include longitudinal data analysis, semi-parametric group-based modeling, sex offending, gender, and race and ethnicity. He is also currently a co-investigator on a National Institute of Justice–funded project examining sex offender recidivism and collateral consequences. In addition, he is the current editor of the *American Journal of Criminal Justice* and a recent recipient of the 2011 William S. Simon/Anderson Publishing Outstanding Paper Award from the Academy of Criminal Justice Sciences.

Kelli A. Komro, Ph.D., M.P.H., is a professor of health outcomes and policy in the College of Medicine, associate director of the Institute for Child Health Policy, and research foundation professor at the University of Florida. Her work has focused on developing complex community-wide preventive interventions to reduce child health disparities, both in the United States and internationally. Her large NIH-funded trials have focused on specific underserved populations of youth, including urban central-city African Americans; urban central-city Hispanics and Latinos; Native Americans, specifically Cherokee Indians; and rural, largely white, poor populations. She is the author of over eighty publications on child health disparities, theory and intervention design, community trial and longitudinal research designs, and measurement. NIH has continually funded her research since the 1990s. She is the recipient of two national mentoring awards and a University of Florida College of Medicine teaching award. Professor Komro is an epidemiologist and a graduate of the University of Minnesota School of Public Health.

Glen P. Mays, Ph.D., serves as the F. Douglas Scutchfield Endowed Professor of Health Services and Systems Research at the University of Kentucky College of Public Health. Prior to joining the University of Kentucky in August 2011, he served as professor and chairman of the Department of Health Policy and Management in the Fay W. Boozman College of Public Health at the University of Arkansas for Medical Sciences, where he also directed the Ph.D. program in Health Systems Research. Dr. Mays's research focuses on strategies for organizing and financing public health services, preventive care, and chronic disease management for underserved populations. Currently, he directs the Public Health Practice-Based Research Networks Program funded by the Robert Wood Johnson Foundation, which brings together public health agencies and researchers from around the nation to study innovations in public health practice. Mays also serves as co-principal-investigator of the Robert Wood Johnson Foundation–funded National Coordinating Center for Public Health Services and Systems Research at the University of Kentucky. Mays earned an undergraduate degree in political science from Brown University, earned M.P.H. and Ph.D. degrees in health policy and administration from UNC-Chapel Hill, and completed a postdoctoral fellowship in health economics at Harvard Medical School.

Michelle M. Mello, J.D., Ph.D., is professor of law and public health in the Department of Health Policy and Management at the Harvard School of Public Health. Dr. Mello conducts empirical research into issues at the intersection of law, ethics, and health policy. She is the author of more than a hundred articles and book chapters on the medical malpractice system, medical errors and patient safety, research ethics, the obesity epidemic, pharmaceuticals, clinical ethics, and other topics. Among other current projects, Dr. Mello is studying disclosure and compensation of medical injuries as the recipient of a Robert Wood Johnson Foundation (RWJF) Investigator Award in Health Policy Research. In 2006, she received the Alice S. Hersh New Investigator Award from AcademyHealth for exceptional promise for contributions to the field of health services research. Dr. Mello is director of the Program in Law and Public Health at the Harvard School of Public Health and chair of the school's Institutional Review Board. She teaches courses in public health law and public health ethics. Dr. Mello currently serves as a key consultant to the National Program Office of RWJF's Public Health Law Research program and a member of the Institute of Medicine's Committee on Ethical and Scientific Issues in Studying the Safety of Approved Drugs. She holds a J.D. degree from the Yale Law School; a Ph.D. degree in health policy and administration from the University of North Carolina at Chapel Hill; an M.Phil. degree from Oxford University, where she was a Marshall Scholar; and a B.A. degree from Stanford University.

Avital Mentovich, Ph.D.c, received B.A. degrees in psychology, philosophy, and law, and practiced law for several years as a criminal and constitutional lawyer. She is pursuing a Ph.D. degree in social psychology at New York University.

Tom Mieczkowski, Ph.D., is professor and chair of the Department of Criminology in the College of Behavioral and Community Sciences at the University of South Florida. He is a researcher and academic whose interests have included drug smuggling, theories of syndicated crime organizations, street gangs, drug distribution organizations and methods, drug epidemiology, validation of various drug detection technologies, and estimation of drug prevalence and incidence using bioassays and survey methods. Dr. Mieczkowski has published over a hundred scholarly articles and book chapters, and three books. Since receiving his Ph.D. degree from Detroit's Wayne State University in 1985, he has received more than $1 million in research funding. He is a member of the International Association of Forensic Toxicology, The British Academy of Forensic Sciences, The European Hair Research Society, and The American Society of Criminology.

Ted R. Miller, Ph.D., is a principal research scientist at the Pacific Institute for Research and Evaluation's Center for Public Health Improvement and Innovation. He has led more than 150 studies, including 25 surveys, dozens of statistical analyses of large data bases, and more than 50 economic analyses. His primary emphasis areas include health economics, injury prevention, substance abuse prevention, and, in earlier years, housing, economic development, environmental, and public finance analyses. He founded the Children's Safety Network Economics and Insurance Resource Center, which has worked since 1992 to forge child safety partnerships between insurers and advocates. His cost estimates are used by the U.S. Department of Transportation, the U.S. Consumer Product Safety Commission, the Justice Department, and several foreign governments. Increasingly, Dr. Miller has extended his costing methods to analyze other health problems and societal ills. Dr. Miller is a fellow in the Association for the Advancement of Automotive Medicine. He was the 1999 recipient of the Excellence in Science Award from the American Public Health Association's Injury Control and Emergency Health Services Section and received the Vision Award from the State and Territorial Injury Prevention Directors Association in 2005.

Ryan J. O'Mara is an M.D.-Ph.D. student and Institute for Child Health Policy research fellow at the University of Florida, College of Medicine. Currently training at the intersection of medicine, public health, and social policy, he is working to identify behavioral and social determinants of health, to develop and evaluate social policies and interventions to improve population health and well-being, and to prepare to fill leadership positions in advocacy and public service. To date, he has authored over a dozen papers on youth risk behavior with relevance to public health laws and policies. He has served on numerous local government boards, coalitions, and task forces to assist translating empirical research into policy strategies to address community public health and safety issues. Mr. O'Mara received his B.S. and M.S. degrees in health behavior at the University of Florida.

Marc B. Schure holds master's degrees in adult education and health promotion. He has worked with community members on a variety of public health promotion research projects ranging from community-based obesity prevention to environmental health in family residences to measuring community health. Currently, Mr. Schure is working as a research assistant at Oregon State University while pursuing a doctoral degree in public health, with an emphasis on healthy aging. His research interests include resilience in older adults, the role of depression on physical functioning and disability, and community-based health promotion programs aimed at improving the quality of life for older adults. He is expected to graduate with a Ph.D. degree in public health in spring of 2013.

F. Douglas Scutchfield, M.D., Sc.D., received his M.D. degree from the University of Kentucky, where he was selected as a member of Alpha Omega Alpha. He completed internship and residency training at Northwestern University, the Centers for Disease Control and Prevention, and the University of Kentucky. At the University of Kentucky, Dr. Scutchfield held administrative responsibilities of founding director of the School of Public Health and founding director of the Center for Health Services Research and Management. He holds faculty appointments in the Department of Preventive Medicine and Environmental Health, the Department of Family Practice, the Department of Health Services, and the Martin School of Public Policy and Administration. Dr. Scutchfield was also the founder of the Graduate School of Public Health at San Diego State University. His current research focuses on community health, public health organization and delivery, quality of care issues, and democracy in health care decision making. He currently serves as editor of the *American Journal of Preventive Medicine*.

Robin Stryker, J.D., is professor of sociology and an affiliated professor of law at the University of Arizona. She has two interrelated research programs, one in American regulatory law and politics, the other in cross-national study of the welfare state and labor markets. She has written on sociological theory and methods, and on a variety of substantive topics, including organizations and institutional change, law's legitimacy, globalization and the welfare state; cross-national family policy and gendered labor markets; law, science, and public policy; the political economy and culture of labor, antitrust, and employment regulation; affirmative action and pay equity; and U.S. political culture and welfare reform. Supported by National Science Foundation grants (2005–2009; 2010–2012) and a John Simon Guggenheim Foundation Fellowship (2008–2009), she is writing a book on the role of economic, sociological, psychological, and statistical expertise in equal employment opportunity law and politics, 1965 to the present, and she is coediting a book on domestic and global legal rights and their translation into practice.

Jeffrey W. Swanson, Ph.D., is professor of psychiatry and behavioral sciences at Duke University School of Medicine. He is a medical sociologist (Ph.D., Yale, 1985) with expertise in psychiatric epidemiology and mental health law and policy studies. Swanson is author or coauthor of more than 175 research publications on topics including violence and severe mental illness, effects of involuntary outpatient commitment law, and psychiatric advance directives. Swanson was principal investigator of the first major study of the implementation of psychiatric advance directive laws for adults with severe mental illness in the United States, funded by a grant from the National Institute of Mental Health and the John D. and Catherine T. MacArthur Foundation. He is the recipient of an Independent Research Scientist Career Award from the National Institute of Mental Health in support of his research program on violence and severe mental illness. He is a member of the John D. and Catherine T.

MacArthur Foundation Research Network on Mandated Community Treatment. He directs research for the National Resource Center on Psychiatric Advance Directives. He formerly served as associate editor of *Administration and Policy in Mental Health* and *Mental Health Services Research*. Swanson received the 2011 Carl Taube Award from the American Public Health Association and the 2010 Eugene C. Hargrove, M.D. Award from the North Carolina Psychiatric Foundation, both for outstanding career contributions to mental health research.

Sue Thomas, Ph.D., is senior research scientist and director of the Pacific Institute for Research and Evaluation (PIRE)-Santa Cruz. Reflecting the PIRE-Santa Cruz office specialty in measuring law for social science research, Dr. Thomas has published five books and dozens of journal articles, book chapters, encyclopedia entries, and book reviews on women, politics, and policy. Among her publications are two widely recognized books published by Oxford University Press: *How Women Legislate* and *Women and Elective Office: Past, Present and Future*. She is also coauthor of an award-winning text on American government, now in its thirteenth edition. Dr. Thomas's published work has been recognized with two awards: the top-cited article in *Political Research Quarterly* in its first sixty years, and the Jeffrey Pressman Award for the best article published in *Policy Studies Review* in 1995. In addition to her work at PIRE, Dr. Thomas has taught courses at University of California, Santa Cruz, and has served as an associate editor and book editor of *Politics & Gender*. Before joining PIRE, Dr. Thomas was associate professor of government and director of women's studies at Georgetown University.

Charles Tremper, J.D., Ph.D., is a principal with Perutilis Research & Consulting. He has been a professor of law and psychology at the University of Nebraska, and a visiting scholar at Yale University. His recent work focuses on issues at the intersections of law, policy, social science, and technology. He has published in each of these fields as well as in privacy, evaluation, criminology, education, risk management, mental health, and the environment. Dr. Tremper received his B.A., J.D., and Ph.D. degrees from UCLA.

Tom R. Tyler, Ph.D., is the Macklin Fleming Professor of Law and Professor of Psychology at Yale Law School. He is also a professor (by courtesy) at the Yale School of Management. Dr. Tyler's research explores the role of justice in shaping people's relationships with groups, organizations, communities, and societies. In particular, he examines the role of judgments about the justice or injustice of group procedures in shaping legitimacy, compliance, and cooperation. He is the author of several books, including *Why People Cooperate* (2011); *Legitimacy and Criminal Justice* (2007); *Why People Obey the Law* (2006); *Trust* *in the Law* (2002); and *Cooperation in Groups* (2000). He was awarded the Harry Kalven prize for "paradigm shifting scholarship in the study of law and society" by the Law and Society Association in 2000, and in 2012 was honored by the International Society for Justice Research with its Lifetime Achievement Award for innovative research on social justice. He holds a B.A. degree in psychology from Columbia and M.A. and Ph.D. degrees in social psychology from the University of California at Los Angeles.

Jennifer Wood, Ph.D., is an associate professor of criminal justice at Temple University and is a Methods Core member of Robert Wood Johnson's Public Health Law Research program. Her work focuses on the delivery of policing and security in the context of wider shifts in regulation and governance. Her current research examines the nexus between security and public health, and is exploring more effective ways for local policing and crime prevention initiatives to contribute to health outcomes, with an emphasis on mental health as well as violence-related injury. She teaches courses on qualitative research, criminal behavior, crime and social policy, and policing. She is coauthor of *Imagining Security* (2007, with Clifford Shearing); coeditor of *Democracy, Society and the Governance of Security* (2006, with Benoît Dupont); and coeditor of *Fighting Crime Together: The Challenges of Policing and Security Networks* (2006, with Jenny Fleming). Prior to joining Temple University in 2007, Dr. Wood was a fellow at the Regulatory Institutions Network, Australian National University.

Public Health Law Research

Part One

Framing Public Health Law Research

P art One focuses on the position of public health law research (PHLR) in the broader context of public health science and the study of law. Chapter 1 defines public health law research as the scientific study of the relation of law and legal practices to population health, and presents a framework for understanding this emerging field. Law is broadly defined in PHLR, including both "law on the books"—constitutions, statutes, regulations—and "law on the streets"—the rules as put into action by law enforcement agents and people and organizations subject to law. Three kinds of public health law are differentiated: interventional public health law (in which the objective is to address a public health problem), incidental public health law (all law without public health aims but with public health effects), and infrastructural public health law (which shapes public health agencies and systems). The third category, infrastructural law, is a point of intersection between PHLR and public health systems and services research; Chapter 2 explores this relationship and its research needs. The breath of law with possible public health effects, combined with the breath of health problems of concern to public health scientists and practitioners, highlights the size and scope of the field and the tremendous untapped opportunities for scientific research to advance the effective use of law to promote the health of the population.

1

A Framework for Public Health Law Research

Scott Burris   Alexander C. Wagenaar   Jeffrey W. Swanson

Jennifer K. Ibrahim   Jennifer Wood   Michelle M. Mello

Learning Objectives

- Describe the field of public health law research.
- Differentiate three types of public health law.
- Identify principle types of public health law research.

Law is an important discipline within public health (Gostin, Burris, & Lazzarini, 1999). Legal "powers, duties and restraints" structure the mission of public health agencies and shape how it is carried out (Gostin, 2008). Law is a prominent intervention tool to achieve particular public health goals. Laws and their implementation also have important unintended effects, both positive and negative, on population health. Although public health law has a long pedigree in the United States (Tobey, 1939), it was one of the fields of public health that fell into neglect during the time that public health was thought to have conquered infectious disease. Over the past two decades, though, the reemergence of infectious disease as a major public health concern and a growing awareness of the complexity of health regulation at the local, national, and global levels have restored law to an important place within public health and academic law. No longer confined to end-of-the-day conference panels on "legal and ethical issues," public health law now has its own office at the Centers for Disease Control and Prevention, academic centers, journals, national and international professional societies, and a shelf of important treatises (Larkin & McGowan, 2008).

Notwithstanding these developments, there has been little discussion of empirical public health law *research* and its place within the fields of law and public health. Evidence produced by empirical research has an important role in public health law practice and scholarship. It constitutes the "facts" justifying regulatory action and supporting normative arguments about which policies are most desirable, most effective, or most consistent with human rights or other legal standards. To be sure, law legitimately serves as a site for the articulation and clash of values, and lawmaking often necessitates decisions that cannot await full information. Not all law is or can be "evidence-based," even in public health. At the same time, empirical research is not just an ammunition dump for adversarial legal battle. The responsible use of law as a tool for improving public health requires a commitment to the pursuit and consideration of scientific evidence when possible. In public health, just as in health care (Sox & Greenfield, 2009), evidence should inform the investment in and implementation of policy, and a consciousness of data and the scientific method can improve the decisions of policy makers and practitioners even in the absence of data. This is the promise of public health law research.

Defining Public Health Law Research

We define public health law research (PHLR) as *the scientific study of the relation of law and legal practices to population health*. This includes direct relationships between law and health and relationships mediated through effects of law on health behaviors and other processes and structures that affect population health. In this section, we elaborate on this definition to distinguish PHLR from other fields and forms of public health law knowledge.

Distinguishing PHLR from Public Health Law

Lawrence Gostin's widely cited definition of public health law is "the study of the legal powers and duties of the state to ensure the conditions for people to be healthy (for example, to identify, prevent, and ameliorate risks to health and safety in the population), and the limitations on the power of the state to constrain the autonomy, privacy, liberty, proprietary, or other legally protected interests of individuals for protection or promotion of community health" (Gostin, 2000). Using this power-duty-restraint formula, Gostin succeeds in focusing the field on the state's role in managing collective action to protect population health, while still encompassing a diverse range of cooperating actors and related functions, including private actors and the health care system. Some scholars have argued from diverse standpoints that Gostin and his colleagues in public health are expanding the jurisdiction of public health beyond its legitimate mission and into a realm of wrongful—and counterproductive—meddling in the autonomy of citizens (Epstein, 2003; Hall, 2003; Rothstein, 2002). Yet for others this definition may be too narrow. Regulatory researchers, for example, question the importance of the distinction between public and private actors in health governance (Black, 2008; Lobel, 2004; Trubek, 2006). Other commentators insist that public health law should be treated as one of the social determinants of health (Burris, Kawachi, & Sarat, 2002; Magnusson, 2007; Mariner, 2009).

Debate over the boundaries of public health law plays out differently in the realm of public health law *research*. In defining PHLR, we are concerned not with what is right, proper, or legitimate to include within the jurisdiction of public health law, but with whether law can empirically be shown to affect the health of the population. Commentators might disagree upon whether equality, for example, ought to be considered a public health issue, but that is a different question from whether it is possible to empirically identify ways in which law affects health inequalities. Empirical data can be highly salient to disputes about normative concepts and positions, but do not in and of themselves resolve disputes about the legitimate scope of public health or public health law or the extent to which health promotion should be traded off against other social goods, such as civil liberties. PHLR, then, is distinguished from public health law by its focus on description, explanation, and prediction—that is, its focus on empirical investigation.

Research Versus Scholarship

When we refer to "research," we intend a particular meaning: the use of systematic methods within an explicit theoretical framework to collect and analyze data. PHLR includes both qualitative and quantitative studies using experimental, quasi-experimental, observational, and participatory designs. It ranges from health impact assessments gathering limited data on legal effects in order to inform policy making in real time, on the one hand, to complex experiments and quasi-experiments studying the effects of law on health over extended periods of time, on the other. Formal decision analyses; simulations; econometric analyses; laboratory and field experiments; survey, interview, and focus group studies; systematic reviews; and meta-analyses are included, as is legal research to systematically and reproducibly collect, classify, and quantify laws and judicial decisions for analytic purposes (Hall & Wright, 2008; Tremper, Thomas, & Wagenaar, 2010).

Theory and methods may be drawn from a variety of disciplines in the social sciences, including epidemiology, biostatistics, law, sociology, history, political science, economics, anthropology, and psychology. From the natural sciences, PHLR imports the scientific method, approaching research questions with a hypothesis to be tested rather than a position to be defended; gathering data for the purpose of testing whether the world is actually consistent or inconsistent with the hypothesis; and reaching conclusions on the basis of a careful and restrained analysis and interpretation of all relevant data.

Public health law research as we define it is thus distinguishable from public health law scholarship. *Scholarship* embraces a range of non-empirical work about public health law, from work grounded in philosophy or ethics (Ruger, 2006) to doctrinal exegesis (Lazzarini & Rosales, 2002) to the crafting of model laws to legal analysis arguing how the law ought to be applied in various situations (Ruhl, Stephens, & Locke, 2003). What we call PHLR does not exhaust all forms of knowledge gathering or analysis concerning public health law. Public health law scholarship includes many outstanding and influential works that have shaped the field of public health law, but do not fall within our definition of PHLR.

Law and *Public Health*

A key challenge in defining PHLR arises from the potential breadth of the definitions of *law* and *public health* (Magnusson, 2007). In linking the two in PHLR, we take a broad sociological stance, encompassing not simply written laws on one side and morbidity and mortality on the other, but the whole range of institutions, practices, and beliefs through which laws influence health and the determinants of health. This is particularly important given that the timelines for law to influence health may be long and data on key outcome variables scarce; it may be important to examine effects of law on mediating factors such as organizational practices or health behaviors. The key aspect of such a study, from the perspective of whether it is properly classified as PHLR, is that it examines the relationship between a law variable and a public health variable.

Social epidemiology, the branch of epidemiology aimed at understanding social determinants of health (Berkman & Kawachi, 2000), provides a theoretical framework into which PHLR can readily fit (Burris, Kawachi, & Sarat, 2002). Most things human beings do, and most characteristics of our environments, have some effect on the level and distribution of health in a population. Whether styled as health inequities or health disparities, differences in health among identifiable subpopulations have become a major concern in health and policy (Commission on Social Determinants of Health, 2008). Health law scholars, too, increasingly recognize the need to examine individual interests and choices through the lens of population health, recognizing that "the choices individuals exercise and the health risks they face are determined, to a large degree, by the environments they experience and the populations they comprise" (Parmet, 2009, p. 268; see also Sage, 2008).

Our conception of *law* is not confined to "law on the books"—constitutions, statutes, judicial opinions, and so on. The mainstream of empirical legal research over the past thirty years has acknowledged the salience of law as it is implemented in practice and experienced by those it targets. Studies of legality or legal consciousness (Ewick & Silbey, 1998), behavioral law and economics research (Jolls, 2006), scholarship on compliance theory (Tyler, 1990), scholarship on deterrence theory and tort law (Mello & Brennan, 2002), and regulation and governance studies (Braithwaite, Coglianese, & Levi-Faur, 2007) all explore this theme. PHLR is necessarily interested in the psychosocial mechanisms through which compliance is achieved (Tyler, 1990), the range of regulatory techniques that may be deployed (Braithwaite, Coglianese, & Levi-Faur, 2007), and how law "operates through social life as persons and groups deliberately interpret and invoke law's language, authority and procedures to organize their lives and manage their relationships" (Ewick & Silbey, 1998, p. 20). Law is fundamentally a social practice embedded in institutions and implemented by agents. It is part of, not distinct from, the social environment whose influence on health is the focus of social epidemiology.

PHLR also properly encompasses laws that were intended to affect population health as well as laws that have unintended health effects. "Interventional public health law" is law or legal practices that are intended to influence health outcomes or health-related mediators directly. "Infrastructural public health law" establishes the powers, duties, and institutions of public health (Moulton, Mercer, Popovic, et al., 2009). But much of the law that influences population health was not adopted for that purpose, and may on its face seem to have no connection to health at all. For example, criminal laws aimed at controlling illicit drug use may increase the risk of users acquiring HIV (Friedman, Cooper, Tempalski, et al., 2006). Research that investigates the relationship of law and legal practices to population health falls within PHLR when it investigates health effects or otherwise deploys an explicit population health framework, whether or not the law itself is health-oriented on its face. We label this important category of PHLR "incidental public health law."

Finally, PHLR is distinguishable from other kinds of public health research in that it evaluates not merely the effectiveness of a public health intervention but the effectiveness of *law* as the tool used to implement or facilitate the intervention. For example, research on whether abstinence-only education reduces teenage pregnancy is not PHLR merely because abstinence-only education happens to be required by law, but PHLR does encompass research on how abstinence-only education rules are implemented (Sonfield & Gold, 2001) and whether the existence of state-level, abstinence-only legal mandates is associated with differences in state reproductive health outcomes.

Health Services Research and Public Health Systems and Services Research

Access to health care is an important determinant of population health, and health care is widely acknowledged to be a key component of the public health system (Institute of Medicine, 2002). The study of how law affects population health through the mediating structure of the health care system falls squarely within the definition of PHLR. PHLR therefore overlaps with the field of health services research, "the multidisciplinary field of scientific investigation that studies how social factors, financing systems, organizational structures and processes, health technologies, and personal behaviors affect access to health care, the quality and cost of health care, and ultimately our health and well-being" (AcademyHealth, 2009). Effects of law on racial disparities in cardiac care outcomes, for example, is an important subject for both health services research and PHLR.

The area of overlap, however, is limited to research that focuses on *law* as an independent variable and population health (or an intermediate outcome with a well-demonstrated relationship to population health) as the outcome of interest. Research is not PHLR if it merely examines effects of some element of health care organization, financing, or delivery on health, without an important connection to law—for example, a study of the effect of capitated reimbursement in private managed care plans on utilization of branded drugs.

Public health systems and services research "examines the organization, financing, and delivery of public health services within communities and the impact of those services on public health" (Scutchfield, 2009). Its relationship with PHLR is discussed in Chapter 2.

A Causal Diagram for PHLR

A wide range of laws and legal practices affects the health of the population in cities, counties, states, and nations. Cataloging all possible effects of law is impossible, and any schema for organizing such effects is characterized by tradeoffs and simplifications. Nevertheless, the field of PHLR is advanced by a shared understanding of the range of possible effects of laws, and potential mechanisms for such effects, encompassed within the field.

The way that law influences population health at the most general level is illustrated in Figure 1.1. In general, the independent variable in PHLR will be some aspect of lawmaking, laws, or the activities of legal agents. These will be studied in relation to dependent variables that can be arrayed along the presumed causal chain that includes key mediators as well as the distal or ultimate outcomes of interest—population morbidity and mortality.

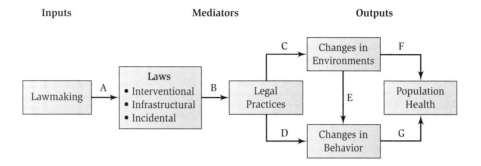

Figure 1.1. Influence of Public Health Law.

First are studies of policy making—the factors that influence which laws are enacted and that shape the specific characteristics of the statutes and regulations adopted (path A in Figure 1.1). In these studies, public health laws (or judicial decisions) themselves are the outcome variable, and political and other jurisdictional characteristics are often the key explanatory variables tested.

Paths B and C examine key mediators in the causal chain linking laws and health outcomes. Studies of how law affects legal practices (path B) focus on the implementation or enforcement of the law on the books, including how the law affects the structure or operation of various regulatory systems. Laws may vary considerably in the degree to which they are effectively implemented; for example, whether a legal mandate for health education in schools translates into all pupils receiving the education that legislators envisioned may depend critically on the appropriation attached to the bill. There are opportunities and resources for litigation in some matters and not others. Unfunded mandates, unclear statutory provisions, failure to identify an administrative agency responsible for issuing implementing guidelines and overseeing rollout of the new legal provisions, lack of political commitment, and many other factors may undermine implementation. Similarly, laws may induce varying levels of compliance on the part of the regulated entities or population, depending on the degree of political resistance, the extent to which the administering agency is armed with effective enforcement mechanisms, the litigation environment, and many other factors. Completeness of implementation and effectiveness of mechanisms for ensuring compliance with the law are critical elements influencing the law's effect on health outcomes. Legal practices studies explore these influences as mediators of the statute or regulation's effect on health.

Paths C and D involve studying the effect of law (as implemented through legal practices) on environments and health behaviors. We use the term *environment* broadly to refer not only to the physical environment, but also to social structures and institutions. Even private institutions, such as corporations or the family, are influenced by law. Laws and their implementation affect social institutions and environments by creating or reducing opportunities, increasing or decreasing available resources, expanding or reducing rights and obligations, and creating incentives and penalties. Research in this area examines these mechanisms of influence and how they shape the conditions for people to be healthy.

Law may affect health behaviors both directly (path D) and by shifting the environmental conditions that make particular behavioral choices more or less attractive (path C-E). For example, land use laws may influence where supermarkets and restaurants are located, affecting the availability of healthy food options and the healthfulness of the diet of local residents. Ultimately, changes in environments and behaviors lead to changes in population-level morbidity and mortality (paths F and G).

PHLR examines health outcomes directly or may use mediating environmental and behavioral changes as proxy outcome variables. While directly measuring health effects generally is desirable because it provides more information to policy makers about the public health returns to lawmaking, a focus on intermediate outcomes is often appropriate. For example, laws designed to improve rates of immunization with the human papillomavirus vaccine might best be evaluated in terms of their effects on the prevalence and burden of cervical cancer, but the time horizon for observing such effects is on the order of decades. Consequently, measuring rates of vaccinations is a reasonable intermediate measure.

PHLR in Practice

The contours of PHLR as a distinct field are only beginning to emerge. Table 1.1, based on extant scholarship in the field and the conceptual model we have described, offers a typology of the principal forms of PHLR studies. In this section, we describe the primary methods for studying each of the paths described earlier.

Policy-Making Studies

Studies of policy-making processes are a mainstay of political science and sociology. They explore issues such as the determinants of legislative, administrative, and judicial lawmaking (Law, 2005; McDougall, 1997; Waters & Moore, 1990); lawmaking processes (Rosenberg, 1991); and stakeholders' use of law to achieve their goals (McCann, 1994). Although in broad terms the policy process does not vary by topic area, health policy making has generated a substantial research literature focusing on how generic policy-making processes unfold in a health context. This literature treats policy-making processes as among the legal practices that affect the potential for law to promote health.

Table 1.1. Typology of Public Health Law Research Studies.

Study Type	Purpose	Methods Examples
Policy-making Studies	Identify factors influencing the likelihood that public health laws will be adopted, the nature of laws adopted, and the process through which they are adopted	Multivariate regression Key informant interviews Content analysis of transcripts, rulemaking notices, memos, and other policy materials Surveys of policy makers
Mapping Studies	Analyze the state of the law or the legal terrain currently or over time and the application of laws surrounding a particular public health topic	Content analysis of statutes, administrative regulations, and formal policy statements Key informant interviews Surveys of state and local policy makers
Implementation Studies	Examine how and to what extent the "law on the books" is implemented and enforced through legal practices	Content analysis of administrative agency documents, including public communications Key informant interviews Direct observation of enforcement actions Examination of business records of regulated entities Surveys of regulators, regulated entities, and the public
Intervention Studies	Assess the effect of a legal intervention on health outcomes or mediating factors that influence health outcomes	Descriptive analysis of outcomes data Multivariate regression Case-control designs Controlled experiments; natural experiments Simulations Surveys of persons targeted by the law
Mechanism Studies	Examine the specific mechanisms through which the law affects environments, behaviors, or health outcomes	Controlled experiments Surveys, focus groups, or interviews of persons targeted by the law

Advocacy groups traditionally have been crucial instigators of health law, and researchers of "legal mobilization" have studied how advocates have integrated legislation and litigation into their strategies (Ashe, Jernigan, Kline, & Galaz, 2003; Mamudu & Glantz, 2009). The relative advantages of litigation versus legislative approaches have been investigated empirically and debated in public health law scholarship (Jacobson & Soliman, 2002; Jacobson & Warner, 1999; Parmet & Daynard, 2000; Wagenaar, 2007), as have the factors influencing legislative outcomes and the legislative process (Backstrom & Robins, 1995; Corrigan, Watson, Heyrman, et al., 2005). Of particular interest for PHLR are studies that examine how research evidence influences policy makers (Chalkidou, Tunis, Lopert, et al., 2009; Cochrane Collaboration, 2009; Innvaer, Vist, Trommald, & Oxman, 2002; Jewell & Bero, 2008; Lavis, Oxman, Moynihan, & Paulsen, 2008). Other work has examined the behavior and strategies of policy actors; for example, how they use devices such as preemption and litigation to shift policy battles into fora where they have a greater expectation of success (Jacobson & Wasserman, 1999), how community organizations may be brought more effectively into the lawmaking or law enforcement process (Tyler & Markell, 2008), or how consulting can be used to more effectively translate research knowledge for policy makers (Jacobson, Butterill, & Goering, 2005). There has been growing interest in the question of how model laws are developed for public health purposes, and whether and under what circumstances model legislation is more likely than other proposals to be enacted (Hartsfield, Moulton, & McKie, 2007).

Both quantitative and qualitative methods are appropriate for policy-making studies. Statistical analyses are useful for examining the extent to which various observable characteristics of a state or local government—such as the political party in control of the legislature and the health status of the population—predict the likelihood that a particular kind of law will pass. For example, researchers have used multivariate regression to examine predictors of state legislative action on childhood obesity (Boehmer, Luke, Haire-Joshu, Bates, & Brownson, 2008; Cawley & Liu, 2008). Such research may make important contributions by identifying "friendly" venues for experimentation with new public health law approaches and suggesting strategies for spreading successful strategies to other jurisdictions.

Qualitative methods are appropriate for obtaining a rich understanding of the policy-making process. (Chapter 15 in this volume describes qualitative methods.) Interviews are commonly and effectively used to understand the factors that lead policy makers to take or fail to take particular actions. Researchers have, for instance, conducted key informant interviews with state legislators and their staff to examine factors enabling and inhibiting the passage of obesity prevention laws (Dodson, Fleming, Boehmer, et al., 2009). Content analysis is another useful method of exploring political deliberations that occur "on the record"—for example, legislative hearings and debate concerning particular public health issues or legislation, and the notice-and-comment process of administrative agency rulemaking. Researchers have used content analysis to explore, for example, the use of evidence and argumentation in debates over workplace smoking legislation (Apollonio & Bero, 2009; Bero, Montini, Bryan-Jones, & Mangurian, 2001). Although it may be difficult to generalize the results of qualitative studies across jurisdictions, the high-resolution picture of the policy-making environment that they provide can have great value in formulating strategies for advancing evidence-based public health law.

Mapping Studies

PHLR includes studies that gather purely legal data for empirical purposes: information about the prevalence and distribution of specific laws (Gostin, Lazzarini, Neslund, & Osterholm, 1996; Hodge, Pulver, Hogben, Bhattacharya, & Brown, 2008), what levels of government have relevant authority (Horlick, Beeler, & Linkins, 2001), and variation in characteristics of the law across jurisdictions and over time (Centers for Disease Control and Prevention, 1999f; Chriqui, Ribisl, Wallace, et al., 2008; Shaw, McKie, Liveoak, & Goodman, 2007; Wells, Williams, & Fields, 1989). Methods may include content analysis of legal texts (laws, regulations, court decisions, and so on), qualitative research designed to elicit information from officials and others who are knowledgeable about the state of the law, or a combination of the two approaches (Horlick, Beeler, & Linkins, 2001). Although no independent-dependent variable relationship is studied, these studies can be scientific—and therefore fall within the field of PHLR—if they involve the systematic collection and analysis of data using replicable methods. Methods for mapping law are the focus of two chapters in this volume (Chapters 11 and 12).

Mapping studies often contribute information that is useful in its own right—state and local policy makers are keen to know what other jurisdictions are doing and what they might consider borrowing or learning from policy experiments in other jurisdictions. Mapping studies facilitate "policy surveillance," the "ongoing, systematic collection, analysis, interpretation, and dissemination of data" about law (Chriqui, O'Connor, & Chaloupka, 2011, p. 21). However, mapping studies are typically an early phase of larger projects designed to evaluate the magnitude and nature of effects of laws on health. Properly conducted, they provide reliable and valid measurement of the key explanatory variable(s) in such studies. Thus a rigorously conducted mapping study requires consistent implementation of a clearly defined protocol for identifying and classifying laws. It will specify a definition of the type of law being investigated, perhaps with explicit inclusion and exclusion criteria; search methods that acknowledge strengths and weaknesses of extant databases; and a coding scheme identifying key features of the laws, such as population covered and enforcement mechanisms specified (Tremper, Thomas, & Wagenaar, 2010). They may also characterize laws according to some overall scale of stringency, scope, or strength through transparent and reproducible means. For example, a recent mapping study of state laws regulating sales of sugar-sweetened beverages in schools coded laws according to seven substantive features and eight process features and then grouped laws into "strong," "moderate," and "weak" categories (Mello, Pomeranz, & Moran, 2008).

Implementation Studies

For a law to be effective, its implementation must be such that it actually influences the behavior of its targets. The process of putting a law into practice can be understood in terms of a series of mediating factors, including attitudes, management methods, capacities, and resources of implementing agencies and their agents; methods and extent of enforcement; the relationship between legal rules and broader community norms; and attitudes and other relevant characteristics of the population whose behavior is targeted for influence. Text of the law and resources appropriated for its enforcement constrain, but do not eliminate, discretion of bureaucratic entities to reshape rules to fit their existing culture and mission (Deflem, 2004).

Implementation research classically starts with investigating the "transformation process" that occurs along path B in Figure 1.1, the differences between the goals and methods of the law as explicitly or implicitly contemplated in the "law on the books" and the "law on the streets" actually put into practice by legal agents charged with enforcing the law (Percy, 1989). Case studies or other analyses of how health agencies organize their mission or perform in a given mission are a common form of implementation research (Buehler, Whitney, & Berkelman, 2006) and often look at the question of what legal powers an agency has or how it uses them (Lawson & Xu, 2007). Creative compliance and outright resistance on the part of targets of regulation are also studied (Nakkash & Lee, 2009). Implementation research in PHLR includes studies of the relationship between "legal infrastructure," legal or other competencies, and agency function (Kimball, Moore, French, et al., 2008). Such studies may examine effects of law on private agencies operating under a legal authorization, such as the effect of legal authorization on syringe exchange programs (Bluthenthal, Heinzerling, Anderson, Flynn, & Kral, 2007). Implementation researchers also measure proximate outcomes of new rules that may provide an early indication of health-relevant effects—for instance, the actual speeds observed on highways after a change in the nominal speed limit (Retting & Cheung, 2008).

Research on legal practices in PHLR may investigate the means through which systems can be better governed or regulation better designed in order to achieve their goals. Although it has as yet had little influence specifically on PHLR, the study of techniques of regulation and governance has become an important part of broader empirical legal research and scholarship (Ayres & Braithwaite, 1995; Croley, 2008; Moran, 2002; Rhodes, 1997). For nearly three decades, regulation in the United States and many other developed countries has exhibited an increasing pluralism, not just in spreading of regulatory functions beyond government to private parties and public-private hybrids (Burris, Kempa, & Shearing, 2008; Lobel, 2004; Osborne & Gaebler, 1993) but also in the use of a wide range of strategies beyond detailed rules backed by carrots and sticks (Parker & Braithwaite, 2003). Contemporary regulators use cooperation, deliberation, education, competition, and other "soft" strategies that can be more effective than traditional command-and-control bureaucracy (Lobel, 2004). Theory and research in governance have highlighted the importance of actors outside of government—such as advocacy groups, corporations, and gangs—in managing the course of events in social systems, and have investigated how these actors regulate governments and each other (Buse & Lee, 2005; Scott, 2002).

New regulatory and governance approaches have raised a fascinating range of empirical questions, from the role of audit as a compliance tool (Power, 1997) to the design and effectiveness of public-private and self-governing regulatory structures (Gunningham, 2009a; Ostrom, 2005). This work resonates with research in behavioral law and economics, captured in Sunstein and Thaler's book *Nudge*, which describes how regulators can creatively structure options to systematically influence behavior by means other than simple legal rules (Sunstein & Thaler, 2008).

Because so much regulation is now conducted outside of traditional bureaucratic frameworks (and indeed outside of the government), scholars working in this area begin with a generic definition of regulation and its constituent elements. *Regulation* is the "sustained and focused attempt to alter the behaviour of others according to defined standards or purposes in order to address a collective issue or resolve a collective problem" (Black, 2008, p. 139). It uses a combination of basic strategies of control, including standard setting, monitoring, and enforcement (Scott, 2001). The use of these strategies can be studied regardless of the particular mode through which the regulatory task is accomplished, and without regard to what sort of entity is performing it (Braithwaite & Drahos, 2000). This analytic approach allows researchers both to better capture the regulatory role of actors outside of traditional regulatory agencies—for example, the role of Mothers Against Drunk Driving in fostering stronger social norms condemning drunk driving—and to offer more creative approaches to regulation, as exemplified by *Nudge* and other works in behavioral law and economics (Lobel & Amir, 2009).

Although research in regulation and governance has been limited in public health law (Biradavolu, Burris, George, Jena, & Blankenship, 2009; Burris, 2008; Trubek, 2006), its applicability is plain (Magnusson, 2009). Public health services are provided by a diversity of public and private actors (Institute of Medicine, 2002). It is widely recognized that complex systems such as health care cannot be managed solely or even primarily by top-down rules, but require use of a range of flexible tools, such as professional self-regulation, ethics, accreditation, collaborative and deliberative decision making, continuous quality improvement, and market incentives (Berwick & Brennan, 1995; Braithwaite, Healy, & Dwan, 2005; Lobel, 2004; Trubek, 2006). Internationally, health governance has been dramatically altered by the rise of new public-private hybrid institutions, such as the Global Fund to Fight AIDS, Tuberculosis, and Malaria; the enormous wealth of the Gates Foundation; and the consolidation of authority over national health, safety, and intellectual property law in the World Trade Organization (Hein, Burris, & Shearing, 2009; McCoy & Hilson, 2009). The Framework Convention on Tobacco Control is a typical instance of the "soft law" approach, setting broad goals for national action but minimizing binding rules in favor of deliberation and flexibility. Legal scholarship has begun to explore the "constitutional" implications of these structural changes (Fidler, 2004), but they have not been extensively investigated in PHLR.

Intervention Studies

Intervention studies evaluate the intended and incidental effects of legal interventions on health outcomes or key mediating factors that drive health outcomes. They may focus on "law on the books"—for example, examining the effect of states' passage of graduated driver's license statutes on rates of injury-causing crashes (Foss, Feaganes, & Rodgman, 2001)—or on legal practices, such as the effect of issuing restraining orders against perpetrators of domestic violence on future victimization (Harrell & Smith, 1996). Intervention studies can be deployed to evaluate interventional health law, but also to investigate the health effects of public health's legal infrastructure and the unplanned effects of what we have called incidental public health law. Intervention studies lie at the heart of PHLR, as they most directly address the core question of the field: When it comes to using legal tools to promote health, what works?

Intervention studies can draw from an extensive methodological toolkit (Table 1.1). The strongest are experimental or quasi-experimental designs employing careful controls and comparisons. These designs are discussed in two chapters in this volume (Chapters 13 and 14). Variation in how and when laws are implemented from jurisdiction to jurisdiction provide a rich set of opportunities for quasi-experimental studies, although sophisticated methods may be required to account for other ways in which jurisdictions differ from one another, and extensive longitudinal data are required. Useful study designs and analytical methods can be borrowed from the fields of econometrics and epidemiology (Ludwig & Cook, 2000). Real-world, randomized experiments are rare, but have been employed to study judicial-branch reforms such as specialized courts (Gottfredson, Najaka, & Kearley, 2003). Experimental studies can also be carried out using simulations, such as tabletop exercises (Dausey, Buehler, & Lurie, 2007; Hodge, Lant, Arias, & Jehn, 2011; Hupert, Mushlin, & Callahan, 2002; Lurie, Wasserman, Stoto, et al., 2004).

There is already a substantial evidence base on the effectiveness of interventional public health law, ranging from single studies through literature reviews to meta-analyses and systematic reviews conducted by entities such as the Campbell Collaboration (Campbell Collaboration, 2009) and the U.S. Task Force on Community Preventive Services (The Community Guide, 2009). There is also a rich, if less-well-organized, research literature on incidental public health law. For example, researchers have studied the unintended consequences of HIV reporting laws on attitudes toward testing, time of testing, and willingness to be tested (Hecht, Chesney, Lehman, et al., 2000; Tesoriero, Battles, Heavner, 2008). Research on the health effects of infrastructural health law has been more limited.

Consistent with ecological models in public health, intervention studies may investigate how laws influence health by changing environments. For example, zoning rules, clean indoor air laws, and laws regulating the condition of rental properties can directly shape residents' exposures to noise, environmental toxins, and stress, as well as their activity patterns, social connections, collective efficacy, and many other factors that appear to influence population health outcomes (Browning & Cagney, 2002; Maantay, 2002; Schilling & Linton, 2005). Occupational health and safety laws affect workers' exposure to hazardous conditions on the job. Product regulations protect consumers from a range of hazards arising from the use of products, from herbal supplements to firearms (Larsen & Berry, 2003; Robson, 2007; Vernick & Teret, 2000).

Interventional research focuses not only on how the law changes physical environments, but also on how it may change social environments in ways that affect health or health behaviors. Law may shape people's health knowledge and attitudes, the way they perceive risks and benefits of different choices, frames through which they view particular choices, and social norms against which their health decisions are set. PHLR can measure any or all of these dependent variables, as well as changes in health behaviors. There are many examples: research on the effects of indoor smoking prohibitions on social expectations about exposure to secondhand smoke in public (Kagan & Skolnick, 1993); the effect of laws requiring disclosure of calorie information on restaurant menus on consumers' awareness of calorie content and attitudes about the role of calorie information in food-purchasing decisions (Bassett, Dumanovsky, Huang, et al., 2008); and the effect of punitive laws concerning substance abuse during pregnancy on the prenatal-care-seeking behavior of pregnant women (Poland, Dombrowski, Ager, & Sokol, 1993), to name a few.

Finally, intervention research can illuminate policy choices under conditions of uncertainty. When problems or policy responses are new, there naturally will be little or no intervention research directly on point. Policy making can still be informed by established theory on mechanisms of legal effects, understandings of how law typically works to influence environments and behaviors, and evidence about analogous policies, although all analogies are, of course, imperfect proxies for the situation at hand. An example is the area of legal restrictions on cell phone use by drivers (Ibrahim, Anderson, Burris, & Wagenaar, 2011). Although public health research recently has provided good evidence of the injury risk associated with this behavior, evidence about the effectiveness of different legal and policy approaches to the problem is not yet available. Until it is, lawmakers seeking to respond to what is clearly a significant health risk might be guided by the lessons learned about the design and enforcement of laws requiring safety belt and helmet use and prohibiting driving under the influence of alcohol. Health impact assessment has also emerged as a useful way to use mixed methods to develop and inform policy decisions with reliable data on possible effects, intended and unintended (Collins & Koplan, 2009; Lee, Ingram, Lock, & McInnes, 2007; Mindell, Sheridan, Joffe, Samson-Barry, & Atkinson, 2004). Monte Carlo simulations, widely in use in the field of decision science but rarely used in PHLR (Studdert, Mello, Gawande, Brennan, & Wang, 2007), offer an intriguing method for accounting for uncertainty about multiple parameters of importance to evaluating the likely effect of law. Economic evaluation that systematically explores the costs and benefits of policy options (or enacted policies) can and generally should influence policy choices. Methods for cost-effectiveness and cost-benefit studies of public health law are described in Chapter 16.

Mechanism Studies

To advance the field, we need to have not only more evidence of law's health effects but a greater understanding of *how* law has the effects it has. There are a number of reasons this is important. Evidence of mechanisms strengthens specific causal claims. Understanding how a particular intervention influences environments and behavior facilitates identification of further interventions, or of alternatives to eliminate superfluous requirements or unintended side effects and strengthen the mechanisms that are working. The better we understand how law works, the better we can deploy it, replicate its successes across jurisdictions, and extend its approach to other kinds of health risks. Informed by theories of health behavior, PHLR can develop and test models to explain the manner in which public health law effects change in health behaviors and ultimately health outcomes.

At a simple level, laws encourage healthy, safe, and socially beneficial behaviors and discourage unhealthy, dangerous, and socially deleterious ones by shaping incentives (rewards) and deterrents (punishments). Though the theory may be simple, the process is not. There are myriad levers and tactics that regulators can use to influence behavior directly or through manipulation of the environment, and each choice in a regulatory system can and should be studied for its effectiveness, both in absolute terms and relative to less burdensome alternatives. The many mechanisms through which law exerts its influence are the focus of Part II of this volume.

With respect to laws imposing outright prohibitions on particular behaviors, many of the key research questions relate to mechanisms of implementation and enforcement: What penalties are applied to violators of legal rules? What processes are used to detect violators? With what degree of certainty and swiftness will sanctions ensue from a violation? Sociolegal research drawing on disciplines such as psychology, criminology, and sociology has a great deal to contribute to mechanism studies in PHLR. The psychological literature has explored contingencies of reinforcement, criminologists have fleshed out the factors influencing deterrence, and sociological research has plumbed the normative effects of standard setting. Tom Tyler's influential work, for example, has shown the importance of experiences of procedural fairness to compliance with law (Tyler, 1990).

A classic example of compliance research in public health law is investigation of primary versus secondary enforcement of safety belt laws. Primary enforcement laws permit police to pull over motorists for not wearing a safety belt, while secondary enforcement laws permit police to issue a ticket for not wearing a belt only when the motorist has been pulled over for another reason. Because secondary enforcement relies primarily on social norms to enforce safety belt use, with the threat of a ticket serving a greatly subordinate role, studies comparing these approaches to enforcement are essentially a test of the relative effectiveness of punishment versus social norms as a means of encouraging compliance (Dinh-Zarr, Sleet, Shults, et al., 2001). Among the most interesting findings of this PHLR is that the relative benefits of primary enforcement laws varied across population subgroups, with the greatest marginal benefit observed for groups that tend to have lower rates of safety belt use, including males, young people, African Americans, and American Indians (Beck, Shults, Mack, & Ryan, 2007).

These and other studies make clear that deterrence is a complex phenomenon. The deterrent effect of law often seems to be assumed, without appreciation of the factors that will influence whether a person's behavior will be influenced by a fear of detection or punishment. Threat of fines may have a different effect than threat of jail (Wagenaar, Maldonado-Molina, Erickson, et al., 2007). Deterrence may be weak or incomplete because people are ill-informed about what the law requires, because they do not believe violation will result in a sanction, because they are insulated from the adverse effects of a sanction (for instance, by insurance coverage), or because the sanction is not strong enough to outweigh the perceived benefits of noncompliance with the law (Mello & Brennan, 2002). Uncertainty about legal standards can also have the opposite effect, fostering overcompliance in an attempt to avoid sanctions (Mello, Powlowski, Nañagas, & Bossert, 2006). Mechanism studies can examine all of these phenomena. Survey methods, interviews, focus groups, and formal decision analysis can be used to deconstruct how people think through the costs and benefits of different actions. Analysis of administrative data on enforcement actions can shed light on the degree to which popular perceptions reflect what actually happens when a law is transgressed.

Another variable of interest in mechanism studies that focus on compliance with legal rules is the perceived legitimacy of the body imposing the legal rule. Weber classically tied obedience to law to the acceptance of the legitimacy of the system. Even people who are aware of the law may not trust the system, or may see strategies other than compliance as more useful to them in achieving their goals (Burris, 1998b). Studies of the perceived legitimacy of public health lawmakers and law enforcers may be particularly useful in understanding differences in compliance across population groups whose historical experience in the United States has led to different levels of trust in government.

Mechanism studies may also focus on understanding how law shapes behavior in ways more subtle than outright prohibitions. How do regulatory tools such as taxes and subsidies, mandated disclosure or receipt of information, default rules, accreditation and certification, and delegations of authority to private institutions shape how individuals and organizations behave? When are these alternatives more effective and desirable than traditional, command-and-control regulation utilizing rigid rules and penalties? For many of these forms of regulation, understanding the cognitive biases and heuristics that affect individual decision making about risk is critical (Kahnemann, Slovic, & Tversky, 1982) and empirical research can examine how these biases operate to influence health outcomes.

PHLR takes a number of forms, each utilizing diverse methods (Table 1.1). By illuminating the paths we have delineated in our causal model, these forms each play important roles in establishing how law is being deployed to promote population health, and how and to what extent it is achieving its intended purpose.

Conclusion

Lawyers have long proclaimed the maxim that "the health of the people is the supreme law," but in practice, making law work for public health is a constant challenge. The contribution of PHLR is to provide the evidentiary foundation for these efforts. Through policy-making studies, PHLR can identify forces that shape public health policy and strategies for effecting policy change. Through mapping studies, it can illuminate what has been done and thus what kind of action it is possible for various government units to take. Through implementation studies, it can provide information about how best to ensure that "law on the books" becomes effective "law on the streets." Through intervention studies, it can determine which legal approaches are most efficacious in improving health environments, behaviors, and outcomes, and identify harmful side effects. Finally, through mechanism studies, it can tell us why laws have the effects they do, and what mechanisms are at our disposal for improving the effectiveness of legal interventions addressing the entire range of public health concerns.

Researchers carrying out this work and collectively advancing this vision face significant challenges. These include increasing methodological rigor, ensuring adequate research funding, identifying data sources, expanding the knowledge base about mediators of health outcomes, and ensuring the effect of PHLR on policy (Ibrahim, Anderson, Burris, & Wagenaar, 2011). Fortunately, a combination of forces has made the potential for overcoming these challenges greater than ever before. The interest of research sponsors, the broader trend toward interdisciplinary research, the increasing number of legal scholars trained in social science disciplines, and signals from Washington that policy will increasingly be driven by evidence and expertise are all cause for optimism (Obama, 2009).

We urge scholars of public health law to explore and recognize the value of empirical methods. We also hope that scholars and policy makers will adopt the philosophy that evidence derived from rigorous research ought to inform, if not drive, health policy decisions. Through the production of knowledge and conscientious efforts to translate research findings for decision makers, PHLR can make the case for laws that improve health.

Summary

Public health law has received considerable attention in recent years and is assuming the role of an essential field within public health. Public health law *research* has received less attention. Public health law research may be defined as the scientific study of the relation of law and legal practices to population health. Its focus encompasses policy making, mapping patterns and distributions of law across jurisdictions and over time, implementation, and effects of all these on physical and social environments, behaviors, and, ultimately, population health. Research on the content and prevalence of public health laws; processes of adopting and implementing laws; and the extent to which and mechanisms through which law affects health outcomes can be pursued using methods drawn from epidemiology, economics, sociology, and other disciplines. Public health law research is a young field, but holds great promise for supporting evidence-based policy making that will improve population health.

Further Reading

Gostin, L. O. (2008). *Public health law: Power, duty, restraint* (2nd ed.). Berkeley: University of California Press.

Jewell, C. A., & Bero, L. A. (2008). Developing good taste in evidence: Facilitators of and hindrances to evidence-informed health policymaking in state government. *The Milbank Quarterly, 86*(2), 177–208.

Moran, M. (2002). Review article: Understanding the regulatory state. *British Journal of Political Science, 32*(2), 391–413.

Moulton, A. D., Mercer, S. L., Popovic, T., et al. (2009). The scientific basis for law as a public health tool. *American Journal of Public Health, 99*(1), 17–24.

Parmet, W. (2009). *Populations, public health, and the law.* Washington, DC: Georgetown University Press.

Note: This chapter is an amended version of the article "Making the Case for Laws That Improve Health: A Framework for Public Health Law Research," published in *The Milbank Quarterly, 88*(2), pp. 169–210. Used with permission.

Chapter 2

Law in Public Health Systems and Services Research

Scott Burris   Glen P. Mays   F. Douglas Scutchfield

Jennifer K. Ibrahim

Learning Objectives

- Differentiate public health law research from public health systems and services research.
- Identify key research questions at the intersection of the two fields.
- Assess quality and coverage of existing infrastructural public health law research.

The role of law in establishing, empowering, and constraining public health agencies has long been a matter of interest to legal scholars and health practitioners (Gostin, 2008; Gostin, Burris, & Lazzarini, 1999; Tobey, 1939). The importance of "legal infrastructure" to public health, and the need to review and possibly update statutes that define the authority of health agencies at the federal, state, and local levels, have now been emphasized in three major Institute of Medicine (IOM) reports since 1988 (Institute of Medicine, 1988, 2002, 2011). Other commentaries have stressed the importance of the public health workforce exhibiting competency in the use of legal authority and the appreciation of its boundaries (Center for Law and the Public's Health, 2001; Gebbie, Rosenstock, & Hernandez, 2003; Moulton, Gottfried, Goodman, Murphy, & Rawson, 2003). *Healthy People 2010's* chapter "Public Health Infrastructure" included as an objective "Increas[ing] the proportion of Federal, Tribal, State, and local jurisdictions that review and evaluate the extent to which their statutes, ordinances, and bylaws ensure the delivery of essential public health services" (Office of Disease Prevention and Health Promotion & U.S. Department of Health and Human Services, 2010). *Healthy People 2020* likewise encouraged the use of public health law research and public health systems and services research to measure and understand improvements in public health system outcomes (Office of Disease Prevention and Health Promotion & U.S. Department of Health and Human Services, 2011).

The importance of law to the effective operation of public health agencies and systems, often and plausibly asserted, has rarely been the subject of academic research. Only a handful of researchers have empirically examined the relationship between law and public health system performance, and the work to date has not been informed by an explicit, shared conceptual framework or research agenda. Filling this void in theory and research will require the integration of public health law research (PHLR) and public health systems and services research (PHSSR).

PHSSR is a "field of study that examines the organization, financing, and delivery of public health services within communities and the impact of those services on public health" (Scutchfield & Patrick, 2007, p. 173; see also Mays, Halverson, & Scutchfield, 2004). Growing from the field of health services research, which focuses on the delivery and financing of medical care, PHSSR is concentrated on parallel concerns within the realm of public health service delivery (Scutchfield, Marks, Perez, & Mays, 2007). The 1998 Institute of Medicine report called for research focused on the solution of "real world problems," including research questions actively derived from public health practice (Institute of Medicine, 1988). Both the 2002 Institute of Medicine report and *Healthy People 2010* noted the need for more research to inform policy making, with a focus on workforce, infrastructure, and financial investments (Institute of Medicine, 2002), as well as better information on the performance and nature of local health departments (Office of Disease Prevention and Health Promotion & U.S. Department of Health and Human Services, 2010). Most recently, the federal Patient Protection and Affordable Care Act of 2010 called attention to the need for PHSSR by authorizing an ongoing, federally funded program of research for "optimizing the delivery of public health services" (ACA Section 4301).

The field of PHSSR focuses on six categories of investigation surrounding public health services: (1) organization and structure of public health agencies, (2) finance, (3) access to services for defined populations, (4) infrastructure and workforce, (5) quality and performance improvement, and (6) evaluation (Scutchfield, Mays, & Lurie, 2009). The causal model for research efforts in each domain takes into account the context in which a local public health department functions; its resources, processes, and services; and the health outcomes achieved. PHSSR recognizes that a health department operates within a larger system of agencies and organizations in communities that contribute to the mission of public health, "assuring conditions in which people can be healthy" (Institute of Medicine, 1988).

Across each of these areas, there is a range of legal considerations, including authority to act or create policies, regulations on routine functions, and even agency composition. The perception of law and its utility among individuals within a health agency and among other members of the public health system may have a powerful effect on effective use of legal powers and tools. While such legal factors have been assumed or implicitly included in previous research, more research is needed to draw out these factors and carefully examine their role in public health systems and the delivery of public health services.

The framework offered in this chapter identifies three broad areas of inquiry at the intersection of PHSSR and PHLR that deserve closer attention:

- The structural role of law in shaping the organization, powers, prerogatives, duties, and limitations of public health agencies, and thereby their functioning and ultimately their impact on public health ("infrastructure")

- How public health system characteristics influence implementation of interventional public health laws ("implementation")

- Individual and system characteristics that influence the ability of public health systems and their community partners to develop and secure enactment of legal initiatives to advance public health ("innovation")

We present a causal diagram illustrating the main domains of interest, which is used to frame a critical discussion of research to date (Figure 2.1). Our analysis demonstrates opportunities for integrating PHLR and PHSSR through common methods drawing upon both health services and empirical legal research traditions, and points the way to a common research agenda. A research agenda at the intersection of these two subfields provides powerful tools to advance public health's efforts to improve public health practice and ultimately the health status of communities.

Integrating PHLR and PHSSR

PHSSR and PHLR both had early support from the CDC (Horton, Birkhead, Bump, et al., 2002; Scutchfield, Marks, Perez, and Mays, 2007) and have been nurtured by the Robert Wood Johnson Foundation (Larkin & McGowan, 2008; Pérez & Larkin, 2009; Scutchfield, Mays, & Lurie, 2009), but the two fields have nevertheless developed independently. Meeting at the intersection of law and public health services, they draw on different research traditions, theories,

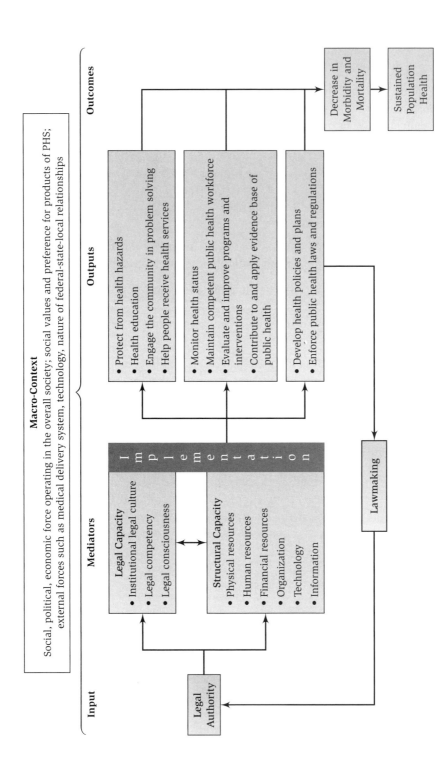

Figure 2.1. Effects of Law and Legal Practices on Public Health System Performance.

and perspectives that have not been sufficiently integrated. To address this challenge, we offer a causal diagram of the relationship among public health law, public health system characteristics, system outputs, and public health outcomes (see Chapter 10 for more on the utility of causal diagrams). We start with the input of law and move to the factors that mediate the performance of public health agencies, including legal culture and legal capacity, authority to act, structural capacity, and implementation of the law. Important outputs include a variety of regulatory and health activities and the development of new health policy tools (Figure 2.1.). The main focus of the causal diagram is on the mechanism by which law and legal authority affect public health agency and system performance. We also recognize that public health agencies operate within a larger context that includes social, political, and economic forces, as well as the system of medical care delivery. The following sections provide detailed explanations of each component of the model.

Law on the Books as a Structural Factor in Public Health System Performance

Is "legal infrastructure," the law that establishes the powers, duties, organization, and jurisdiction of public health agencies, a significant factor in agency performance? The hypothesis that legal infrastructure matters has been repeatedly stated (Gostin, Burris, & Lazzarini, 1999) and put into intervention practice in the form of widely circulated and adopted "model law" provisions (Hartsfield, Moulton, & McKie, 2007). The starting point in Figure 2.1 is, therefore, legal authority. Public health agencies are established by constitutions and laws that set their powers, geographic and topical jurisdiction, procedures, and management structures. Public health departments are organized on state, county, or local levels, or in a variety of combinations; they are established as stand-alone entities or as units within larger health and human services agencies (Beitsch, Brooks, Grigg, & Menachemi, 2006; Beitsch, Grigg, Menachemi, & Brooks, 2006). There may or may not be a board of health, and the powers of boards of health vary from giving advice when asked to formal rulemaking (National Association of Local Boards of Health, 2011). And not all agencies that regulate important public health matters such as education, transportation, and land use planning have "public health"—or even "health"— in their name (Institute of Medicine, 2011).

Although the federal government's role in public health has been steadily increasing for more than a century, the legal infrastructure of state and local health agencies remains almost entirely a matter of state law (Grad, 2005). The heterogeneous legal architecture of public health systems across the states amounts to a long-term experiment in public health management, but one that has not been extensively evaluated. Even in recent textbooks, discussion of law in public health administration is limited to the functions of the agency in the context of the larger governmental bureaucracy (Novick, Morrow, & Mays, 2008), as opposed to a more thorough examination of the internal processes by which the law shapes public health agency performance.

Legal Implementation and Public Health System Performance

The exercise of legal authority—implementation—is mediated by two sets of variables in Figure 2.1: legal capacity and structural capacity. Research over decades in empirical legal studies and implementation has documented the decisive effect of implementation factors on how law on the books is actually expressed in practice (Bardach, 1977). This rich tradition in legal research has not been widely drawn upon in public health law. How actors in public health systems understand and apply the law, and the resources they have to do so, are likely to be powerful mediators of the effect of legal infrastructure on public health system outputs and outcomes.

Perhaps the largest deficit in existing research on the role of law in public health agency performance is its thin conception of legal capacity. There is a small literature that defines "legal competencies" (Center for Law and the Public's Health, 2001; Gebbie, Hodge, Meier, et al., 2008; Lichtveld, Hodge, Gebbie, Thompson, & Loos, 2002). The field has not yet drawn on the theoretically richer sociolegal literature on "legal consciousness" and "legality" of individuals and organizations (Chapter 4.). In this approach, law is not treated simply as a "tool" or "rule" that agents wield or consciously or subconsciously obey, but also as a set of individual beliefs and organizational norms about what the legal system is, how it actually works, and whether and why people should obey its commands. It encompasses what people consciously believe about law but also a range of unconsciously accepted norms and assumptions. Sociolegal theory moves beyond how people "use law," or their explicit legal knowledge, allowing researchers to bring critical empirical attention to bear on how the rule of law is socially constructed, contested, and perpetuated in social fields (Cooper, 1995). At both the individual and the institutional levels, we cannot get a strong grasp on why the law is used to advance public health goals without understanding "when and by whom it is not used" (Silbey, 2005, p. 326). It is as important to study why some health departments avoid law as a tool as it is to identify the determinants of creative and effective regulatory behavior. The sociolegal literature provides powerful theoretical concepts and research methods for getting at how health system agents understand their legal roles and authority to implement laws, their ability to act within a legal framework, and indeed the nature of that legal framework itself (Yngvesson, 1988).

Both objective legal competency—explicit knowledge of the law and one's legal role—and the individual's ideas about law ("legal consciousness") are important determinants of an individual and agency's capacity to use legal authority effectively. Figure 2.1 illustrates that these can be understood both as individual-level attributes and as characteristics of an agency or other organizational unit, and that individual legal consciousness and competencies influence and are influenced by the institution's legal culture. The effect of law on organizations, particularly in terms of compliance, traditionally has been a core concern of empirical legal research, and has produced a distinguished body of theory and evidence (Ayres & Braithwaite, 1995; Braithwaite & Drahos, 2000; Chriqui, O'Connor, & Chaloupka, 2011; Gunningham, 2009b; Power, 1997). Work on law in organizations has shown the value of understanding the construction of law at an organizational level and the processes through which legal decisions are made (Edelman & Suchman, 1997). Organizations are not simply passive recipients of outside legal commands, but are actively engaged in interpreting and reshaping law to make it consistent with organizational imperatives, norms, and beliefs (Edelman, 2005; Teubner, 1987). Strategies of law enforcement and regulation are shaped by politics and even a version of fashion, not just evidence and experience (Power, 1997; Wood, 2004). Understanding the institutional culture and its determinants is essential to a proper assessment of the work of a regulatory agency.

This leads to the second set of mediating variables—the structural capacity of the health department and the public health system in which it operates. In the health services tradition, PHSSR posits that a set of basic structural capacities can be measured and assessed for their effect on the performance of public health systems (Bhandari, Scutchfield, Charnigo, Riddell, & Mays, 2010). These include human, physical, and financial resources; organization and relationships; agency information; and technology. These capacities influence implementation of the system's legally established mission. For example, environmental work such as inspection and citation is dependent on agency budgets, and as the budget drops, so does environmental work at the health department (Arnett, 2011).

Structural capacity interacts with legal capacity and the larger social context. If there are constraints in human or financial resources, there may not be time to think about law or funds available for public health staff to collaborate with legal counsel. If the county executive is running for reelection at the same time the health department is citing influential local business owners for violating health department regulations, there may be more or less subtle pressure on the health department to ignore a major responsibility. If self-regulation and small government are the current fashion, advancing new command-and-control rules enforced by a bureaucracy will be difficult. Health departments *are* bureaucratic regulatory agencies. They operate within a larger administrative system, and may be constrained by competition for rewards or resources, or jurisdictional confusion. Authority may be conferred to other departments or divisions within the bureaucracy (for example, environmental, public safety, or transportation) or the authority to act may be shared.

Public Health System Outputs and Outcomes

Figure 2.1 depicts the outputs of the public health system as ten essential public health services. This typology is now at the center of efforts within PHSSR to develop robust measures of public health agency performance. Their origin is the 1988 IOM report (Institute of Medicine, 1988), which defined public health governmental responsibility as assessment, policy development, and assurance. These were seen as specifically governmental activities, to be carried out by governmental public health agencies in partnership with other organizations that contribute to public health. The IOM report called attention to the unique roles played by governmental public health agencies in mobilizing, coordinating, and monitoring the contributions of other organizations that operate within the larger public health system. Later work elaborated those three governmental responsibilities into the ten essential public health services shown in the figure. The ten essential public health services have become a touchstone for public health activities involving performance and drafting public-health-related documents describing the role of local health departments and their system partners (Erwin, 2008).

Work with the three core responsibilities and the ten essential public health services derived from them has led to new understanding of the mechanisms by which public health infrastructure and inputs influence performance. For example, the services have been used recently to develop an evidence-based typology of local public health systems that allows classification and comparison of systems according to the scope of public health activities performed, the array of organizations involved in performing these activities, and the distribution of effort between the governmental public health agency and other system partners (Mays, Scutchfield, Bhandari, & Smith, 2010). The instruments developed by the National Public Health Performance Standards Program have become vital to the establishment of the Public Health Accreditation Board, which began its initial accreditation efforts in the fall of 2011 (Martin, Conseil, Longstaff, et al., 2010; Mays, Beitsch, Corso, Chang, & Brewer, 2007; Public Health Accreditation Board, 2009).

Public Health Policy Innovation

Health policy is an important *output* as well as an input for public health systems. The practice, experience, and knowledge acquired by actors within the public health system can drive the development of new public health laws, regulations, and enforcement strategies to improve system performance and public health outcomes. Health agencies often have substantial regulatory authority themselves, and can partner with other stakeholders to advance legislative and regulatory initiatives before other policy-making bodies and, in some instances, be involved in litigation. The extent to which individual staff and particular health agencies have an appetite for understanding and using the law, and under what circumstances this occurs, is a gap in the existing literature on policy innovation within health departments.

Existing Research

The PHLR literature has not yet been exhaustively catalogued. The number of studies in incidental and interventional PHLR appears quite large, but we have been able to identify only a handful of studies addressing infrastructural legal questions. A recent review of PHSSR identified seventy-four papers on the organization and structure of public health in the published and gray literatures (Hyde & Shortell, 2012). Most studies looked at the relationship between organization, structure, and performance, but few engaged law in a significant way. While the conceptual connections between PHSSR and PHLR are apparent when one looks for them, research to date has not engaged both disciplines.

The strength of evidence as a guide to practice is customarily assessed with reference to a hierarchy of research design. The criteria of the U.S. Preventative Services Task Force give greatest weight to the randomized controlled trial, followed by quasi-experimental studies, uncontrolled observational studies, qualitative case studies, and expert opinion (Harris, Helfand, &Woolf, 2001). Research at the intersection of PHSSR and PHLR has to date clustered in the lower reaches of this hierarchy. In this respect, the intersection of PHSSR and PHLR is consistent with other areas of empirical health law (Mello & Zeiler, 2008). The limited literature offers instances of ambitious design and rigorous execution, but also weaknesses. Law in general is insufficiently theorized or measured, or a thorough legal analysis is used in a study that does not adequately account for the influence of the public health department or system's organizational characteristics. Strong qualitative findings are not followed up with quantitative research that could yield generalizable results. We will draw on examples from the existing literature addressing infrastructural law in PHSSR to illustrate these weaknesses and suggest topical and methodological directions for integrating the two fields.

Infrastructure Research

The important implications for practice of rigorous infrastructural research at the intersection of PHLR and PHSSR can be seen in studies that have taken on one of the most widely held assumptions in public health law. For quite some time, influential scholars in public health law have pointed to antiquated or technologically superannuated statutes as a barrier to effective public health agency performance (Gostin, Burris, & Lazzarini, 1999). The work in PHSSR to develop measures of public health system performance makes it possible now to investigate that issue empirically, and a few studies have attempted to do so. McCann, for example, examined the core question of how the type and extent of discretion granted by a statute to a public health agency influenced the agency's success in implementing the statute (McCann, 2009). Using a quasi-experimental time-series design, the study defined three forms of discretion in setting standards for newborn screening: to decide which conditions to include in the screening panel; to set the charges assessed on hospitals; and to develop the criteria for including conditions in the panel. The study tested the hypothesis that each of these forms of discretion would be associated with fewer implementation problems. Fiscal discretion and authority to choose what conditions to include were associated with successful implementation, while, interestingly, the discretion to set criteria slowed implementation. The study, as the author puts it, "only scratches the surface of public health law's importance for public health practice" (McCann, 2009). Discretion is well-theorized and has a robust impact, but the contradictory findings suggest that key mediating factors are missing from the theoretical framework.

One widely promoted cure for laws that are out of date or inconsistent with best practices has been the "model law." Model laws are intended to set out clearer requirements in keeping with current technologies, health practices, and legal norms (Erickson, Gostin, Street, & Mills, 2002). Hartsfield and colleagues asked a deceptively simple question: To what extent did the sponsors of model laws provide information on the procedures—and the evidence—used to develop them? Such information was, it turned out, provided for only 7 of 107 model public health laws published between 1907 and 2004 (Hartsfield, Moulton, & McKie, 2007). Model laws can embody evidence-based best practices, but there is apparently no evidence that they do. Simple in design and narrow in scope, the study illustrates valuable insights that can be gleaned from systematic legal research and straightforward content analysis.

Using performance data from the National Public Health Performance Standards (Centers for Disease Control and Prevention, 2011a), Merrill and colleagues examined the congruence among state enabling statutes, the mission and essential services of public health as defined in *Public Health in America* (Public Health Functions Steering Committee Office of Disease Prevention and Health Promotion, 1994), and self-reported delivery of at least some essential services in 207 localities (Merrill, Keeling, Meier, Gebbie, & Jia, 2009). The data in this cross-sectional, observational study were analyzed using binary logistic regression. In most local public health systems, the agency mission and essential services were rated congruent or highly congruent with the state statutory language constituting the agencies' legal infrastructure. The association between congruence and agency performance varied from positive to negative across the ten essential services. As the authors themselves observe, the challenge for future research is to integrate legal variables with the wider range of structural capacity and other factors depicted in Figure 2.1 in a design that will support causal inference.

Most recently, Jacobson and colleagues investigated how federal and state laws influence the preparedness of public health systems as reflected in the knowledge and attitudes of 144 agency staff, their legal counselors, and legislative staffers in nine states (Jacobson, Wasserman, Botoseneanu, Silverstein, & Wu, 2012). Explicit criteria were used to select sites that varied by key characteristics (per capita health expenditure, geographic region, organization of the public health system, and level of emergency preparedness). Semistructured interviews were used to elicit which laws respondents thought were influencing preparedness and how. Although the study did not explicitly deploy sociolegal theories of individual or organizational legal consciousness, the researchers took it as given that there are "gaps between the objective and perceived legal environments" (p. 299), and that much of the explanation of how law influences preparedness would be found in such gaps. The study found that local public health agency practitioners are ill-informed and poorly advised about legal requirements influencing preparedness. Though not statistically generalizable, the study is richly informative of the kinds of legal conundrums health officials worry about, the ways in which they try to resolve them, and the types of effects law has on preparedness. The study exemplifies the potential for qualitative research to address important questions in rigorous ways—and the need for follow-up quantitative research to investigate specific hypotheses emerging from a qualitative study.

The collection of legal data using standardized transparent and reproducible methods required by science is relatively rare. McCann's study included the collection of data on newborn screening statutes in all fifty states over a period of sixteen years. And Meier and colleagues collected basic public health enabling statutes from all the states (Meier, Merrill, & Gebbie, 2009). In neither case, however, was there a detailed description of the legal dataset or how it was created, information on whether inter-coder reliability was assessed, or any indication that the data are available to other researchers to build upon. This is not unusual, and exemplifies an area in which new data-collection standards could benefit the field. In a few topics, notably tobacco control and alcohol policy, excellent scientific datasets are available and information about law is readily accessible to the broad community of researchers and the public (Fishman, Allison, Knowles, et al., 1999; National Institute on Alcohol Abuse and Alcoholism, 2011a). Improving standards for collection of coded legal data would enable each such topic-specific dataset to serve as a brick in building the field: a comprehensive, consistent, continually updated dataset on infrastructural public health law.

Implementation and Enforcement Research

McCann examined the association between discretion and outcomes, but did not study the process of implementation itself, work that perhaps would have helped explain why discretion appears to have varying effects on outputs. Merrill and colleagues found associations between statutory language that matched public health mission and service standards and the delivery of services, but likewise did not examine the processes through which that occurred. Moreover, they used a research design that could not illuminate whether more expansive statutes produce higher-functioning agencies or higher-functioning agencies earn more expansive powers. The study of how legal authority or other legal factors influence the day-to-day practices of health agencies is in its infancy. There are, as far as we know, no studies other than that of Jacobson and colleagues (Jacobson, Wasserman, Botoseneau, Silverstein, & Wu, 2012) that observe and assess the actual day-to-day exercise of general legal authority within health agencies, let alone any that draw upon (and test) the elements posited as important in Figure 2.1.

The impact of particular interventional health laws is the most fully developed topic area of PHLR. The depth of the literature is captured in reviews of such important interventions as safety belt laws (Houston & Richardson, 2005), alcohol taxes (Wagenaar, Tobler, & Komro, 2010), workplace smoking bans (Fichtenberg & Glantz, 2002), and school vaccination requirements (Briss, Rodewald, Hinman, et al., 2000). Some evaluations of interventional health laws include data on implementation, but by no means do all. Few studies consider in depth the effect of health department activities or health system characteristics on implementation. An exception is the rich body of qualitative work that has looked at how power, values, and politics have played out in the enforcement by health and other agencies of smoking restrictions (Ashley, Northrup, & Ferrence, 1998; Howard, Ribisl, Howard-Pitney, Norman, & Rohrbach, 2001; Montini & Bero, 2008).

An excellent example of research on tobacco law implementation is Jacobson and Wasserman's report of case studies in seven states and nineteen local jurisdictions (Jacobson & Wasserman, 1999). They found a sharp divergence in enforcement practice between clean indoor air laws and youth access restrictions. The former were seen by health officials as largely self-enforcing, so most agencies only took action when there was a complaint. Laws that restrict youth access to tobacco, by contrast, were deemed by most agencies to require more active enforcement, though strategies and intensity varied. The authors identified a number of legal and structural capacity issues retarding enforcement, including lack of resources, concerns on the part of counsel that enforcement would not withstand legal challenge, and fragmented enforcement authority. This work illustrates the practical value of research illuminating determinants of effective enforcement. Like McCann's work, though, it offers only tantalizing glimpses of topics that could use much greater systematic attention, such as the nature and quality of the relationship between health officials and their legal advisers, or the gap between counsel's beliefs about litigation success and the actual outcomes (Nixon, Mahmoud, & Glantz, 2004). Like the preparedness work of Jacobson and colleagues, the Jacobson and Wasserman tobacco law implementation case studies invite follow-on confirmatory quantitative research.

Research on Innovation in Policy Making

The role of state and local health agencies in the development of and advocacy for new health laws is another area in which there is a high level of interest and a low level of research. Again, the exception has to be made for anti-smoking policy making, which has been the subject of many useful case studies that identify strategies and mediating factors influencing the success of health agencies in promoting new health laws (Dearlove & Glantz, 2002; Givel, 2005; Ibrahim, Tsoukalas, & Glantz, 2004; Macdonald & Glantz, 1997; Tsoukalas & Glantz, 2003) The HIV epidemic has also produced some strong policy-making research, perhaps most notably the work of political scientist Ronald Bayer (Bayer, 1989).

Putting aside their value as embodiments of best practices, model laws have received attention as a mechanism to "galvanize" lawmaker interest in public health. To test this effect, Meier and colleagues undertook a comparative case study of the process and impact of considering the Turning Point Model Public Health Act in four states (Meier, Hodge, & Gebbie, 2009). The Turning Point model law embodied a comprehensive set of recommendations regarding agency mission and function, infrastructure, collaborations and partnerships, and authorities and powers. The study conceptualized the use of the model law in three stages—use of the act to develop or focus support for reform, drafting of actual state legislation, and enactment—and identified barriers and facilitators at each stage. In two of the states, the model law process did in itself help set the agenda for change; in a third it failed to generate momentum to the second stage, while in the fourth the model law added some impetus to reform efforts that were already under way. The study's careful, qualitative research gives us insight into questions no one has tried to answer before. The next step is to build on the formative findings in more robust, generalizable studies. It will be useful to take a broader view of health policy making and its determinants, for example looking for patterns in the breadth of health issues states choose to regulate and the depth or intensity of their regulations on particular topics.

Policy development outside of legislatures—litigation, administrative rule-making, executive orders, and enforcement strategies—has been almost entirely neglected. The public health work of attorneys general, which has led to such important results as the 1998 Master Settlement Agreement, has not been studied by PHSSR or PHLR researchers (Jacobson & Wasserman, 1999; Rutkow & Teret, 2010). What Kromm and colleagues call "public health advocacy in the courts" encompasses a wide range of "actions by public health professionals that inform and affect how courts approach matters that affect the public's health" (Kromm, Frattaroli, Vernick, & Teret, 2009, p. 889). These include not only filing suits but also providing expertise as witnesses, submitting amicus briefs, educating the judiciary, influencing judicial selection, and monitoring and evaluating court outcomes. The production of administrative law, arguably the most important vehicle for regulation under the control of public health agencies (Kinney, 2002), has likewise not been touched by empirical research in PHLR or PHSSR.

The Path Forward

The 2011 Institute of Medicine report, *For the Public's Health: Revitalizing Law and Policy to Meet New Challenges*, devotes an entire chapter to law and public health infrastructure (Institute of Medicine, 2011). The report recommends once more a review of state and local public health laws to ensure appropriate authority for public health agencies, but it adds some new, important, and quite practical suggestions: ensuring that health officials have adequate access to legal counsel; making evaluation of the health effects and costs associated with legislation, regulations, and policies prior to and following implementation a more frequent practice; and using better research methods to assess the strength of evidence regarding health impacts of public policies (Institute of Medicine, 2011). All of these recommendations speak to the need for an integrated approach between PHLR and PHSSR, and, at their core, point to three primary PHLR-PHSSR research questions.

Three Pressing Questions for Research

What is the relationship between statutory architecture and language and the outputs and outcomes of public health systems? Despite repeated recommendations from the IOM, there are those who doubt that legal infrastructure is a significant factor in agency performance (Richards & Rathbun, 2003), and in the thirty years this has been under discussion, most legislatures have declined to act. Answering the question remains important because if legal infrastructure does matter, understanding how will allow potentially low-cost changes in law that promote greater effectiveness in the delivery of health services. If there is a right way or a best practice in public health infrastructural law, we should do the scientific research required to know what it is. The IOM report (Institute of Medicine, 2011) and many supporters have encouraged states to consider the Turning Point Model Act, but the fact remains that it is based on the wisdom of experience rather than empirical evidence of effectiveness. While innovation and improvement should not await definitive evidence, neither should it proceed in an evidence-free zone. We still do not know whether law works, which law(s) work, or even whether the exercise of law reform is good or bad for public health systems (DeVille, 2009).

The legal relationship of local health departments to each other is an urgent area for integrated PHLR-PHSSR work. Governments across the nation continue to restructure health departments in the face of substantial budget cuts. New organizational structures vary from voluntary shared services among local health departments to regionalization and varying levels of centralization in which multiple local health agencies are joined together under the leadership of the state health department (Libbey & Miyahara, 2011). What is the optimal arrangement to share services? Is it best to be voluntary and flexible, or should strict parameters be mandated by law? Are there certain types of services that should be shared? Are there particular responsibilities—for example fiscal decisions—that should remain under the legal authority of individual local health agencies? How does preemption factor into the considerations? Economics must be balanced with legal requirements for the performance of state and local health departments as outlined in state constitutions and statutes (Baker & Koplan, 2002; Baker, Potter, Jones, et al., 2005; Institute of Medicine, 2002). As state and local agencies experiment with various models of shared governance, real-time evaluations of the performance of health agencies and associated effects on population health will be needed. New structures also call for ongoing monitoring and assessment of the functions of health departments and quality of public health services delivered.

What are the structural and operational determinants of implementation of law by health agencies? Few would disagree with the observation that some health agencies and leaders use legal authority more robustly, and more effectively, than others. But why? Is it an accident of personality, background, geography, or local political culture? Does it reflect the way a public health agency is organized or its resources and capacities? Is there any sign that legal training for health officials, or health training for lawyers, plays a role? Research documenting how legal authority is used and identifying enabling and retarding factors can help increase effective use of legal authority. If we can figure out what the most effective users of legal power know, how they learned it, and how they put it into practice in the context of other governmental agencies and other levels of government, the result may be something to scale up to health agencies nationwide.

The IOM acknowledges the importance of legal capacity and "recommends that every public health agency in the country have adequate access to dedicated governmental legal counsel with public health expertise" (Institute of Medicine, 2011, p. 7). It is a reasonable suggestion, and one that generates plenty of questions. How much of a change would this be—that is, what is the current state of legal representation for health officials? How does the need for and provision of counsel in health agencies fit within the overall design of legal services in local and state governments? The current Association of State and Territorial Health Officials (ASTHO) and National Association of County and City Health Officials (NACCHO) biennial health agency surveys contain two questions addressing the legal counsel arrangement and legal services provided. However, this is merely descriptive and does not explain the logic for the arrangement or the mechanism by which the provision of services occur; future research must address this gap.

Empirical study of regulation and governance, which focuses on effective use of regulatory authority, has largely neglected public health agencies (Braithwaite, Coglianese, & Levi-Faur, 2007). The IOM report mentions two important implementation issues arising from our federal system—preemption and co-enforcement. Preemption is a constraint: federal law can supersede state law, and state law can supersede local. Preemption can bring uniformity, but it can also cut off policy innovation. It is, politically, a weapon of choice for any interest group that wants to set a broadly applicable standard, so is a regular topic of health policy making. Knowing more about how the risk or reality of preemption is managed by public health agencies can help us assess whether its overall effect on enforcement is positive or negative. By contrast, co-enforcement—when state and federal agencies join forces to enforce health and safety regulations—is potentially a source of new practical authority and efficiency; potentially, but so far not shown to be positive by evidence. The need for research on the relationship between federal, state, and local governments reinforces the need for more sophisticated multilevel analyses that account for hierarchical relationships.

Accreditation, which the IOM recommends and which has had an enthusiastic reception in public health practice, is seen as a way of both improving agency performance and increasing agency credibility and influence (Bender & Halverson, 2010). As a moving target, accreditation in recent years presented a number of pressing legal issues relating to how current state law would influence the process. An initial study in this area found an unexpected synergy between the emerging accreditation movement and an interest in regionalization largely driven by increasingly severe budget pressures (Matthews & Markiewicz, 2011). As accreditation settles in, and budgets stabilize, research at the intersection of PHLR and PHSSR will be needed to determine whether accreditation is bearing fruit. With time, we will be able to get a clearer picture of how legal infrastructure influences the choice to be accredited and the success of the process, and how accreditation influences agency performance, including enforcement of law, achievement of basic outputs, and ability to devise and promote new uses of legal authority. The challenge is to ensure that research on accreditation takes on the legal issues in a sophisticated and determined way.

What individual and system characteristics influence the ability of public health systems and their community partners to develop and secure enactment of legal initiatives to advance public health? We have a toe-hold in the climb to understand the role of health agencies in promoting innovation in public health law. Case studies in areas such as tobacco and HIV document the contest between those promoting health regulations and those who oppose them on ideological or economic grounds. There is no magic bullet to be discovered, no secret to winning in the political process. The importance of the research is in increasing the odds for healthy public policy by identifying strategies and habits of mind of agencies and leaders that design and are able to advance laws and regulations that improve the public's health.

The IOM offers a ringing endorsement of a "health in all policies" approach (HIAP). HIAP involves collaboration between government and the private sector to devise and implement coordinated strategies to promote health (Collins & Koplan, 2009; Institute of Medicine, 2011). Operationally, this entails creation of coalitions or councils of the many public and private actors whose activities are important to health. Data on the known or potential effects of policies are seen as essential to moving diverse stakeholders to align their interests and agree on action. Health impact assessment (HIA) is "a combination of procedures, methods, and tools by which a policy, program, or project may be judged as to its potential effects on the health of a population, and the distribution of those effects within the population" (Dannenberg, Bhatia, Cole et al. 2008, p. 241). The objective is to consider and weigh possible health effects in advance of any proposed policy or program. From a research perspective, the question is whether HIA in fact does mobilize and inform stakeholders, get health on the agenda, and produce better policy outcomes for health. Although a new development in the United States, HIA has been used for more than a decade in Europe, and some cautionary findings have emerged (Wright, Parry, & Mathers, 2005).

Improving Research at the Intersection of PHLR and PHSSR

The primary questions discussed in the previous section are the nucleus of a research agenda that will continue to grow as more researchers, practitioners and funders immerse themselves in the field. They imply a number of challenges for the field in producing more, and more rigorous, research.

DATA

Poor availability of legal data has been identified as a general challenge to empirical health law research (Mello & Zeiler, 2008). The lack of legal datasets that capture the features of public health law in a scientifically credible and useable way has been a chronic impediment to sophisticated research on the impact of law in public health systems (Chriqui, O'Connor, & Chaloupka, 2011). Taking up a suggestion made by PHLR researchers (Burris, Wagenaar, Swanson, et al., 2010), the 2011 IOM report called for work to test the feasibility of systematic "policy surveillance" as part of a broader effort to give "evidence-based policy" the same sort of documentary resources as evidence-based medicine (Institute of Medicine, 2011). The IOM committee suggested that the CDC develop a policy surveillance pilot, which would track a set of important laws across states and over time. For its part, the PHLR National Program Office, based at Temple University, has begun the process of building consensus on basic standards and methods for quantitative legal datasets (Chapters 11 and 12). The standard includes a core set of elements such as date of passage, date of enactment, regulatory targets, and the regulatory elements themselves, comprehensively and (for the most part) dichotomously coded. The Program Office also suggests the use of FIPS (Federal Information Processing Standard) codes as unique identifiers for states, facilitating the integration of legal data with data on public health agency performance or population health outcomes. Studies that create such datasets using high-quality reproducible protocols—referred to as "mapping studies" (Burris, Wagenaar, Swanson, et al., 2010)—should be recognized as an important contribution to public health research in themselves, even if the mapping study team does not correlate the legal data with outputs or outcomes (Ibrahim, Anderson, Burris, & Wagenaar, 2011).

The development of PHSSR has faced comparable obstacles. Basic data about health systems have been unavailable. For example, between 1992 and 2008, no data on the current characteristics of state health departments were gathered. In other instances, data are available but not comparable. NACCHO, ASTHO, and the National Association of Local Boards of Health (NALBOH), working with the University of Kentucky's Center for Public Health Systems and Services Research, have established a standardized database for state and local health departments and their governing entities. These data can now be matched with legal data to answer questions posed by PHLR and PHSSR researchers (Scutchfield, Lawhorn, Ingram, et al., 2009).

RESEARCHERS AND PRACTITIONERS

A hallmark of PHSSR has been its organic connection as a research enterprise with public health practice. The ethic of research by practitioners about practice for practitioners remains strong, and is also a value of PHLR. Partnerships with practitioners can drive the appetite for research among practitioners, both as consumers of research findings and participants in research development and implementation. Practitioners can provide valuable insight into the development of research questions and guide the conduct of the research to ensure that findings are relevant and useful. Public health practice-based research networks can facilitate and institutionalize this type of inquiry by bringing multiple public health practice settings together into an ongoing collaboration with academic partners to support the design, implementation, translation, and dissemination of new research (Mays, 2011). The practice setting can provide a real-time "lab" in which to study the development, implementation, and effect of public health laws on public health systems performance, and can even encourage and facilitate experimental field study designs. Adding PHLR to the mix creates a new segment of practice—legal counsel. Unlike health practitioners, lawyers typically are not exposed to empirical research or methods during their professional training, so bringing lawyers into research and practice networks requires openness and willingness to learn on both professional sides. Mello and Zeiler have discussed the many challenges of recruiting and supporting researchers in empirical health law (Mello & Zeiler, 2008).

RESEARCH METHODS

The limited PHLR-PHSSR literature is composed primarily of qualitative studies and uncontrolled observational designs. Most existing PHSSR studies use cross-sectional designs that do not support robust causal inferences (Lenaway, Halverson, Sotnikov, et al., 2006). This is to be expected in a new area of research, in which formative research helps create a foundation for early hypothesis and theory development, as well as the development of measurement tools. More sophisticated methods, including longitudinal analyses and multilevel modeling, can be used to examine change over time and the relationships between different levels of government agencies. Most changes in laws and regulations affecting population health are natural experiments, offering great opportunities for sophisticated quasi-experimental time-series studies that provide a strong basis for assessing the causal impact of law (Chapter 14). Randomized controlled trials of law will always be the exception: the same diversity of lawmaking and executive authority that creates a favorable climate for quasi-experiments makes true experiments difficult to arrange. Researchers are virtually never in a position vis-à-vis legislators or public health officials to randomly assign a set of local health departments to one legal intervention and another group to a control or placebo—though including practitioners in research teams could make it more feasible to roll out implementation of new legal interventions in a controlled manner that would allow experimental designs (Ayres, Listokin, & Abramowicz, 2010).

Care should be taken to ensure that classic epidemiologic methods issues are addressed. Research in PHSSR and PHLR should be sensitive to issues of confounding, bias, and the clear inferential limits of cross-sectional regression analysis. Rigor in scientific method must apply to the research of PHSSR and PHLR if it is to be accepted in the community of science. That said, it is also important to affirm the value of qualitative and observational research, legal mapping studies, and health impact assessments to public health research and practice. Qualitative research provides invaluable insights, rooted in the experience of their peers, to practitioners and policy makers. When extensive longitudinal data are lacking, cross-sectional studies and regression analysis are indispensable to beginning to build an evidence base. HIA and other modes of systematic rapid assessment make up in timeliness what they lack in certainty. The field requires work at every level of the evidentiary hierarchy. Progress means that every study at every level is as well done, as well targeted, and as well timed as possible.

Conclusion

Historically and to the present day, law has largely been treated by empirical researchers as an afterthought to the organization and work of health agencies. Perhaps due to a lack of a clear conceptual framework and supporting research methods, researchers often leave law for discussion sections rather than truly engage and measure effects of law. There can now be no disputing that law is an important force at work in public health systems, and that it requires the same careful study and attention as other drivers of public health agency characteristics, performance, and outcomes. Integration of PHLR and PHSSR is essential because law, for all its importance, is a force that works in interaction with other factors—resources, training, community values—and the effects of law are likely to vary over time, topic, and place. Our vision is not one of a new crop of studies devoted solely to law (although some such formative research is certainly needed) but the emergence of PHLR as an integral part of PHSSR and vice versa.

More and better research is needed—but research remains a means, not the end. Law has enormous potential to improve the delivery of public health services, in terms of both effectiveness and efficiency. In the face of demands for austerity, resistance to a "nanny state," and long-term ideological attacks on the effectiveness of government regulation of any kind, policy makers and public health practitioners must be able to demonstrate that what they are doing works and works cost-effectively. Reorganization of health departments, redrafting of enabling statutes, accreditation, and the development of new legal health interventions have no inherent value: they are justified by results. And so it should be. PHSSR and PHLR must work in partnership with practice to wisely use, credibly justify, and (in so doing) properly increase public funding and political support for further improvements in the health of the population.

Summary

In a 2011 report, the Institute of Medicine (IOM) recommended a review of state and local public health laws to ensure appropriate authority for public health agencies; adequate access to legal counsel for public health agencies; evaluations of health effects and costs associated with legislation, regulations, and policies prior to and following implementation; and enhancement of research methods to assess the strength of evidence regarding health effects of public policies. These recommendations, and their similarity to calls in prior IOM reports, speak to the need for an integrated approach between the emerging fields of public health law research and public health systems and services research. A unified framework for the two fields integrates theory and methods from health services and sociolegal research traditions to pursue three broad areas of inquiry: (1) the structural role of law in shaping the organization, powers, prerogatives, duties and limitations of public health agencies, and thereby their functioning and ultimately their effects on public health ("infrastructure"); (2) how public health system characteristics influence implementation of interventional public health laws ("implementation"); and (3) individual and system characteristics that influence the ability of public health systems and their community partners to develop and secure enactment of legal initiatives to advance public health ("innovation"). Research to date has laid a foundation of evidence, but progress requires better and more accessible data, a new generation of researchers comfortable in both law and health research, and more rigorous methods. The routine integration of law as a salient factor in broader studies of public health system functioning and health outcomes will enhance the usefulness of research in supporting practice and the long-term improvement of system performance.

Further Reading

Hyde, J. K., & Shortell, S. M. (2012). The structure and organization of local and state public health agencies in the U.S.: A systematic review. *American Journal of Preventive Medicine, 42*(5 Suppl. 1), S29–S41.

Institute of Medicine. (2011). *For the public's health: Revitalizing law and policy to meet new challenges*. Washington, DC: The National Academies Press.

Silbey, S. S. (2005). After legal consciousness. *Annual Review of Law and Social Science, 1*(1), 323–368.

Note: This chapter is an amended version of the article "Moving from Intersection to Integration: Public Health Law Research and Public Health Systems and Services Research," published in *The Milbank Quarterly, 90*(2), 375–408. Used with permission.

Part Two

Understanding How Law Influences Environments and Behavior

Many evaluations of public health laws proceed without articulating a theory on how the law is expected to affect health. While such "black box" studies that directly assess the correlation between existence of a particular law and a health outcome often make useful contributions, the quality of a study is substantially enhanced by a clear articulation of *how* a particular law is expected to have an effect on health. Hypothesized mechanisms of legal effect directly influence many processes and decisions of the study. The investigator's theory of how a law affects health (1) shapes selection of specific statutes, regulations, or court cases to study, and indicates which are similar enough to group together and which are so distinct as to represent a different type of law; (2) determines how to code and score relevant dimensions of the law; (3) points to key measures of implementation that are most relevant; (4) suggests specific features of the physical, organizational, and social environment to observe for reactions to the law; (5) indicates high-priority response behaviors for measurement in the population exposed to the law; and (6) affects specific health outcome variables to collect and analyze. Theory on how a law affects population health points to the expected timing, patterns, and diffusion of its effects, directly shaping decisions on the best research design to use. Theory helps the investigators understand the numbers and kinds of intermediate steps that must occur before an effect on health outcomes is expected. It shapes the statistical models analyzed by presenting hypothesized distributions of effects across groups, time, and space. The maxim "there is nothing so practical as a good theory" (Lewin, 1952, p. 169) holds for public health law research as for all areas of scientific inquiry.

Part Two discusses the many mechanisms through which law works to affect the public's health. The diversity and breadth of possible ways law can operate to affect population health are exciting, and illustrate the nascent state of our field and the many opportunities available for important research waiting to be conducted. The chapters that follow suggest hundreds of specific causal paths or links between law and health, links that warrant study across the whole range of contemporary public health problems. In this section we are focused on theory, not in the "legal theory" sense in which the objective is to articulate how a given law might apply to a particular case, but scientific theory, in which the objective is to specify chains of causal links that are supported by a body of scientific research. The theories and perspectives come from numerous distinct disciplines and fields of scholarship, but all are highly relevant for public health law research. At times, multiple theories suggest opposite—or at least different—effects and research is needed to assess which theory fits best for understanding public health effects of law. More often, a law has multiple routes of effect, and understanding the whole range of mechanisms and how they operate in particular contexts is necessary to maximize beneficial public health effects while minimizing deleterious ones. Many theories overlap, with similar mechanisms of action described using quite different terms across disciplines. Other times, the differing terms suggest subtle but important differences in understanding how a law works to affect health. Taken together, they provide a rich menu of theoretical options and practical tools for the public health law researcher.

The section starts with Komro, O'Mara, and Wagenaar presenting perspectives from the field of public health. Public health traditionally focuses on the production of health and illness through the interaction of behavior and environment, each of which can be manipulated to produce healthier outcomes. Major achievements in public health over the past century used law to dramatically reduce the burden of infectious diseases, motor vehicle injuries, dental caries, and chronic disease. Chapter 3 describes ways in which law can affect the fundamental social determinants of health, a pressing issue for public health in the twenty-first century.

The public health perspective emphasizes the outcomes—aggregate health indicators for the population. Traditionally, public health focuses somewhat less on the mechanisms by which law affects particular individuals. Stryker describes how scholars in the law and society tradition approach the question of how law affects health. Chapter 4 offers a view of law as more than just specific rules regulating particular behaviors; law also works by shaping culture and shared meanings in a society, with important consequences for population health. Thus, perhaps pollution laws reduce exposure to toxic chemicals, but also over time create the notion of a human right to clean air and water not subject to the vagaries and uncertainties of the market.

Jennings and Mieczkowski review key concepts from the field of criminology in Chapter 5, describing how laws deter unhealthy or unsafe behaviors and how law's role in labeling particular individuals or groups as dangerous can affect their behavior. Tyler and Mentovich, presenting procedural justice theory in Chapter 6, draw on research emerging from social psychology to suggest that deterrence is not always the best way to explain obedience to law. They describe how the public's perception of a law as legitimate, and the perceived fairness of procedures attendant to its implementation, have powerful effects on people's willingness to obey.

Chaloupka describes in Chapter 7 how economic theory applies to public health law research, beginning with the assumption of a rational individual maximizing his or her own well-being and analyzing the need for and use of law in relation to the concept of market failure. Flay and Schure follow in Chapter 8, building from a base in social psychology to present an ambitious theory that integrates concepts from many social science disciplines. The theory of triadic influence facilitates a coherent understanding of many ways laws operate to affect population health. Part Two concludes with Burris and Wagenaar drawing together the ideas from all these perspectives and illustrating their application to a few specific public health issues.

Careful attention to testing particular theory-based mechanisms of legal effect advances the field of PHLR as well as science more broadly. When we demonstrate through carefully designed scientific research that a particular law affected a particular population health outcome, but also discover the causal pathways by which that effect was achieved, we create more general knowledge that can be applied to ameliorating the entire range of public health problems. We are also then effectively using the real-world laboratory of public health law across local, state, and national levels to contribute improved theory back to the basic science disciplines from which we draw.

Chapter 3

Perspectives from Public Health

Kelli A. Komro   Ryan J. O'Mara   Alexander C. Wagenaar

Learning Objectives

- Identify the central processes through which law can influence population health outcomes from a public health perspective.
- Illustrate the influence of law on economic, social, and physical environments, and, in turn, effects on population-level risks and protections.
- Formulate study hypotheses on specific causal pathways by which law affects population health outcomes.
- Access measures to study effects of laws on the environment, exposures, health behaviors, and health outcomes.

The advent of public health can be traced back to the late eighteenth century, when the first organized attempts were made to confront disease collectively. With the rise of industrialism and globalization, people shifted to urban centers and seaports, producing dense populations living and working in unsanitary conditions ideal for spreading infectious diseases. As incidences of typhoid, smallpox, influenza, cholera, tuberculosis, and other diseases reached unacceptable levels, the first boards of health were formed in urban centers to respond to the epidemics (McNeill, 1977). The formation of boards of health illustrated the start of infrastructural public health law, and their actions in quarantining ill persons illustrate early use of police powers on behalf of public health. Right from the start, law was central to public health action.

Public health pioneer John Snow implemented corrective environmental actions long before science determined that microorganisms were the causes of widespread infectious diseases. In 1854, Snow traced a cholera outbreak in London to well water drawn from the Broad Street pump. By simply removing the pump handle, he prevented perhaps thousands of additional cases (Brody, Rip, Vinten-Johansen, Paneth, & Rachman, 2000). Snow's action illustrates the practical orientation of the field—preventive action need not wait until all the detailed mechanisms and mediators are understood. More important, Snow's action illustrates the simplicity and effectiveness of changing the physical environment to improve the public's health, in contrast to attempts to change the behavior of thousands or millions of individuals, in the cholera case by boiling water thoroughly every time before drinking.

During the twentieth century, major public health achievements were realized through law. Vaccination laws resulted in the control of many preventable diseases, including smallpox and polio. Smallpox and polio were eliminated, and morbidity associated with seven other vaccine-preventable diseases reduced by nearly 100 percent (Centers for Disease Control and Prevention, 1999b). Annual death rates per vehicle miles traveled declined 90 percent as a result of mandated improvements in vehicle and road design and laws shaping driver behavior, such as safety belt use and drinking and driving (Centers for Disease Control and Prevention, 1999c).

As public health, safety, and medical breakthroughs of the early to mid-twentieth century controlled infectious disease epidemics, increased safety, and expanded life expectancy (Centers for Disease Control and Prevention, 1999e), public health shifted attention to chronic disease prevention (Omran, 1971). Epidemiological studies of chronic disease showed that most cases in the population do not occur among those at high risk but rather among those at moderate risk, because there are more people with moderate risk levels than there are with very high risk levels (Epstein, 1996; Rose, 1985). Recognition of the widespread distribution of risk might have led to a return to addressing the environmental and social conditions that elevated risks in so much of the population, but in the second half of the twentieth century, chronic disease prevention efforts focused primarily on individual-level strategies designed to alter specific risk factors that are proximal causes of disease, such as education on risk factors, screening, and use of antihypertensive and lipid-lowering drugs (Centers for Disease Control and Prevention, 1999a). In the late twentieth century, population-level strategies using law to prevent chronic diseases emerged, with particularly notable achievements in tobacco control (Centers for Disease Control and Prevention, 1999d, 2011b).

A limitation of the focus on proximal risk factors is the de-emphasis of "fundamental" or antecedent determinants of population health (such as environmental conditions and social class) that influence multiple proximal risks and maintain an association with disease even when specific proximal risks change (Link & Phelan, 1995). Although an intervention may temporarily reduce proximal risk factors for those individuals exposed to a particular intervention (for example, health education, screening), new people continue to enter the at-risk population at the same rate if the intervention fails to intervene on forces in the community that cause the problems in the first place (Syme, 2004). The field of social epidemiology (Berkman & Kawachi, 2000) and the growing recognition of "social determinants of health" (Marmot, 2005) and "structural interventions" (Blackenship, Friedman, Dworkin, & Mantell, 2006) signify that public health increasingly is returning to its classic emphasis on environmental and social conditions. Because law is such an important influence on such environmental and social conditions, a return to classic public health action is also elevating empirical research on law's public health effects as an increasingly recognizable field of study.

How Laws Affect Population Health

Figure 3.1 illustrates the central processes through which law can influence population health outcomes from a public health perspective. The causal diagram highlights the central public health focus on altering the economic, social, and physical environments in ways that reduce toxic exposures and increase protective exposures, and ways that facilitate healthy behaviors and impede unhealthy behaviors. These many dimensions of the environment drive exposures and behaviors that, moderated by individual-level factors, ultimately affect aggregate levels of population health.

Law shapes environments through its effects on institutions, organizations, and other implementation structures and processes. Obviously, law can also have direct effects on individual behavior, as illustrated in the many other chapters in this volume. This chapter highlights the centrality of enhancing environments as a key role for law in improving population health. For simplicity, the many possible interactions across dimensions of the environments, and the cybernetic nature of this causal system, are not depicted. Our goal is much more modest than a complete depiction of how law affects health. Because history shows most public health gains have been achieved by altering social and physical environments, we highlight the central role of law in shaping those environments. Following a description of the conceptual framework, we present three detailed examples.

Law

Law affects the full range of institutions, organizations, and structures in society, and the resulting characteristics and actions of those organizations and structures

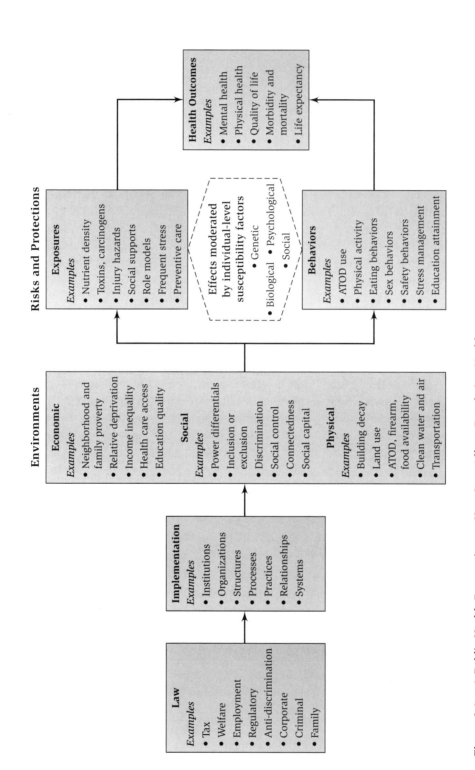

Figure 3.1. A Public Health Perspective on How Law Affects Population Health.

affect the economic, social, and physical environments that the population experiences. Law shapes families, schools, churches, community organizations, businesses, and corporations. By affecting actions within such organizations and institutions, law influences the distribution of wealth, employment, health care, education, and other resources across a population. Economic factors such as family income, relative income, degree of inequality, employment status, occupation, and education level have been independently linked with health outcomes (Adler & Newman, 2002). Tax law and welfare regulations have direct effects on family income and resources, and on the distribution of wealth within a society. One example is the Earned Income Tax Credit (EITC), first enacted in 1975, with federal and state expansions since then. The goal of the EITC is to incentivize work and raise the effective wages of low-income workers (Hotz, 2003). Several studies have indicated that the EITC has positive effects on maternal and child health outcomes (Arno, Sohler, Viola, & Schecter, 2009; Evans & Garthwaite, 2010; Strully, Rehkopf, & Xuan, 2010). An example of a policy influencing the distribution of wealth is Social Security. As a result of the Social Security Act (and its amendments), monthly cash benefits are provided to the majority of retired workers in the United States, and constitute the major source of income for most of the elderly. Social Security dramatically lowered the rate of poverty and reduced health disparities among the elderly (Adler & Newman, 2002). Another example of law influencing the distribution of resources is food assistance programs (food stamps, school lunch requirements), which have been found to have a protective effect for low-income children's health (Jones, Jahns, Laraia, & Haughton, 2003).

Laws influence job creation, minimum wage, and collective bargaining rights. Enterprise Zone laws create special (typically blighted) geographic areas where normal tax and regulatory laws are lifted, in an attempt to increase employment and business in distressed areas (Greenbaum & Landers, 2009). Minimum wage and other labor laws reduce inequality at the lower end of the wage distribution (Autor, Manning, & Smith, 2010). Collective bargaining and trade union laws structure workplace relations in ways that influence wages, income inequality, and worker participation, all of which appear to affect health (Hirsch, 2008; Kahn, 2000). Occupational health and safety regulations directly affect workplace dangerous exposures, and other workplace regulations can encourage (or conversely discourage) healthy practices such as breastfeeding.

Federal securities laws and state corporate governance standards influence corporate conduct and affect relations between corporate executives, investors, and the public. Law attempts to curb undesirable effects of markets by reducing health, safety, and environmental risks; limiting market power; and preventing unfair discrimination. Laws that influence collective bargaining and the rights of, or limitations on, unions have an effect on power dynamics between employers and employees. Anti-discrimination and diversity policies promote the rights and freedoms of disadvantaged groups (Kalev, Dobbin, & Kelly, 2006; Moreau, 2010). Criminal law sets standards of conduct necessary to protect individuals and the community and defines formal social control structures and practices to minimize violence and injury.

Family law in the United States includes a complex mixture of state and federal laws (Estin, 2010), defining what constitutes a family, family responsibilities, and protections for children. Bogenschneider and Corbett (Bogenschneider & Corbett, 2010) argue for a much-expanded view of family policy, and advocate for a whole field of inquiry examining social policy effects on family functioning. They define four main functions of families: family creation, economic support, childrearing, and caregiving, all of which contribute to the health and well-being of its members.

The family is only one example of a social structure affected by law. Laws define and shape a wide range of social and institutional structures and functions in society. Such laws affect population health by directly influencing broad social conditions within a society, including power dynamics, social stratification, inclusion or exclusion of specific subpopulations, and connectedness and social capital in the population, that in turn affect health outcomes (Sampson, Morenoff, & Gannon-Rowley, 2002).

Laws and regulations provide guidelines and rules that directly alter physical conditions, thereby influencing exposures to risks or protections. Laws prohibit or regulate dangerous products. For example, many states and local governments prohibit or limit consumer fireworks due to the risk of injury and death. Laws are often successfully used to reduce the amount of hazard in products or the environment, such as regulations on the design and manufacture of products (for example, car air bags, safety locks on firearms, alcohol concentration, number of pills per prescription).

Laws and regulations protect food supplies and provide safe housing. For example, the U.S. Food Safety Modernization Act of 2011 will build a new system of food safety oversight for the prevention of foodborne illnesses. Local and state governments define building codes and housing quality standards to protect the safety and health of residents.

Many laws directly change the physical environment, such as road design, alcohol outlet density regulation, building codes, and pollution control standards. Rules imbedded in law are also used to separate hazards from people, such as smoke-free rules to limit exposure to environmental tobacco smoke (Brownson, Eriksen, Davis, & Warner, 1997; Global Smokefree Partnership, 2009), minimum legal drinking age to reduce availability of alcohol to underage youth (Wagenaar, Finnegan, Wolfson, et al., 1993), and pool fence requirements to protect children from drowning (Deal, Gomby, Zippiroli, & Behrman, 2000). Urban design and land use rules determine walkability and safety of neighborhoods and are shaped by public health professionals to create safe and walkable communities.

These examples illustrate the wide range of laws and regulations that affect the environments in which the population lives. We turn now to a brief mention of implementation considerations, followed by a detailed look at environments, the most important intervening concept between law and population health when viewed from a public health perspective. Our most notable public health successes have used law to shape those environments, rather than using law to shape individual health behavior directly.

Implementation

As with all public health preventive interventions, how effective a law is in improving health depends on how well the law is implemented. Implementation fidelity is a key component to the effectiveness of any program, practice, or policy, and implementation science is an entire field of study in itself (Fixsen, Naoom, Blase, Friedman, & Wallace, 2005; Rabin, Brownson, Haire-Joshu, Kreuter, & Weaver, 2008), to which Brownson and colleagues (2012) provide a comprehensive introduction. Laws shape environments through effects on institutions, organizations, personal and professional practices, relationships, and systems. Fidelity of implementation can be assessed through measures of exposure, awareness, receptivity, participation, enforcement, and compliance. Effects of any statute or regulation are necessarily mediated by many dimensions of the way it is implemented.

Environments

We distinguish three broad types of environments relevant to health: economic, social, and physical. We have previously summarized the links between these three domains of environmental conditions and child health and developmental outcomes (Komro, Flay, Biglan, and the Promise Neighborhoods Research Consortium, 2011). Here, we expand upon our previous work on how environmental conditions affect health outcomes more broadly across the lifespan.

ECONOMIC ENVIRONMENT

Low income and lack of resources put individuals and families at increased risk of exposure to a multitude of health-compromising factors. Socioeconomic status is linked to a wide range of health outcomes and all-cause mortality (Adler & Rehkopf, 2008). Higher incomes promote exposure to health protections, such as better nutrition, housing, education, and recreation (Adler & Newman, 2002). Lower-status jobs expose workers to both physical and psychosocial risks (Adler &

Newman, 2002). Families face multiple challenges when they live in neighborhoods with a high poverty rate (Sampson, Morenoff, & Gannon-Rowley, 2002). Residents of high-poverty neighborhoods are more likely to be exposed to health risk factors, less likely to be exposed to health protection factors, and more likely to have poor health outcomes (Krieger, Chen, Waterman, Rehkopf, & Subramanian, 2005; Sampson, Morenoff, & Gannon-Rowley, 2002).

In addition to absolute poverty, relative deprivation and income inequality affect exposures to risks and health outcomes. Wilkinson and Pickett (2009) provide an overview of the relationship between economic inequality and various measures of health and well-being. Countries and U.S. states with greater inequality in wealth have higher levels of health and social problems. They have lower life expectancy and higher rates of teenage births, obesity, mental illness, and homicides. In an analysis of the fifty U.S. states, income inequality was associated with all indicators of child well-being (Wilkinson & Pickett, 2009).

Low-income families are much less likely to have health insurance or access to dental and medical care, which results in many consequences, including being unlikely to have a regular source of health care; unhealthy parents, which adds to financial distress; less prenatal care, resulting in unhealthy infants and increased infant mortality; less medical and dental care for children; and poorer health outcomes among children (National Research Council & Institute of Medicine, 2002).

Household income is also linked with the quality of schools that children attend and, through earnings of offspring, contributes to the growth of income inequality in the United States. (Chetty & Friedman, 2011). Numerous studies have found a link between educational attainment and health outcomes (Egerter, Braveman, Sadegh-Nobari, Grossman-Khan, & Dekker, 2009). Educational attainment affects health outcomes through health knowledge, literacy, and behaviors; better employment opportunities and higher income; and social and psychological factors (Egerter, Braveman, Sadegh-Nobari, Grossman-Khan, & Dekker, 2009).

Social Environment

Social cohesion and social capital are defined as the extent of connectedness and solidarity within groups, enhancing the ability to reinforce social norms and provide help and support (McNeill, Kreuter, & Subramanian, 2006). Communities with greater social cohesion and social capital have lower overall population mortality (Lochner, Kawachi, Brennan & Buka, 2003). Social support has been defined as a related, yet separate dimension of the social environment (associated with but distinct from social cohesion or social capital) (McNeill, Kreuter, & Subramanian, 2006). Social support enhances access to resources, material goods, and coping responses (McNeill, Kreuter, & Subramanian, 2006). There is strong empirical support for the association between greater social integration and lower mortality risk (Seeman & Crimmins, 2001).

Social exclusion and discrimination break social cohesion. Discrimination creates psychological trauma, limits opportunities for advancement, and increases exposures to risks (McNeill, Kreuter, & Subramanian, 2006). Perceived discrimination is linked to multiple deleterious health outcomes (Williams & Mohammed, 2009). Discriminatory policies and practices limit the power, status, and wealth of particular subgroups, contributing to patterns of social isolation and concentrated poverty (Wilson, 2009). As a result, residents in high-poverty neighborhoods tend to experience lower levels of physical and mental health, educational attainment, and employment than residents of other neighborhoods (Lamberty, Pachter, & Crnic, 2000; Pachter & Coll, 2009).

PHYSICAL ENVIRONMENT

Many aspects of the physical environment affect exposures to risks and health outcomes. Neighborhoods with greater physical disorder and decay (that is, abandoned buildings, trash, and crumbling structures) have higher levels of social and health problems, including crime, higher levels of fear, lack of social cohesion, and more physical illness (Sampson, Morenoff, & Gannon-Rowley, 2002). Evidence suggests that improving neighborhood physical conditions can increase social cohesion and mental health outcomes (Williams, Costa, Odunlami, & Mohammed, 2008). Changing community- and street-scale urban design, and land use laws such as zoning, can achieve significant increases in physical activity and social interaction (Heath, Brownson, Kruger, et al., 2006).

Availability of health-compromising products poses a significant risk for health outcomes. Tobacco availability and promotion are associated with all stages of smoking among children and adolescents, from experimentation through addiction (U.S. Department of Health and Human Services, 2004). Ease of access and low cost of alcohol influence patterns of alcohol use and alcohol-related problems (Popova, Giesbrecht, Bekmuradov, & Patra, 2009; Wagenaar & Perry, 1994). Firearm availability, affected by numerous laws and regulations, similarly affects health. A ten-year time-series analysis of data from the fifty states indicated a significant association between firearm availability and the rates of unintentional firearm deaths, suicides, and homicides among five-to-fourteen-year-olds (Miller, Azrael, & Hemenway, 2002).

Residents of low-income and minority neighborhoods have limited access to supermarkets and healthy foods, and greater access to fast-food restaurants and energy-dense foods (Powell, Chaloupka, & Bao, 2007). Increasing fruit and vegetable availability in low-access neighborhoods appears to improve dietary choices (Glanz & Yarock, 2004). Research suggests that neighborhood residents with better access to supermarkets and limited access to convenience stores tend to have healthier diets and lower levels of obesity (Larson, Story, & Nelson, 2009). Residents of majority-minority and high-poverty neighborhoods face a greater risk of exposure to a range of physical toxins and carcinogens (Crowder & Downey, 2010). Living near toxic exposures is related to an increased risk for adverse health outcomes (Braun, Kahn, Froelich, Auinger, & Lamphear, 2006; Brender, Maantay, & Chakraborty, 2011).

Risks, Protections, and Health Outcomes

Economic, social, and physical environmental conditions affect exposures to health risk and protection factors, as well as affect health behaviors. Income and resources affect multiple risks and protections including affordability of nutritious food; safe housing and neighborhood quality; stress; preventive health care, screening and treatment; and educational attainment. Social conditions affect exposure to social support, positive or negative role models, norms, and stress. The physical environment affects exposure to high-fat and high-sugar (that is, low-nutrient-density) food, physical toxins, and injury hazards. Environments not only have direct effects shaping health-relevant behaviors, but also have indirect effects operating through exposures to risks and protections, and those effects are moderated by other individual-level susceptibility factors (for example, genetic, biological, psychological, social). Finally, some physical and social toxic exposures have particularly large and long-lasting deleterious effects if the exposure occurs at particularly vulnerable times in the lifespan, such as during pregnancy or early child development.

The leading causes of morbidity and mortality are heavily influenced by exposures to risks and protections and health behaviors. Major types of exposures include physical and biological contaminants such as chemicals, gases, metals, radiation of various types, smoke, and infectious bacteria, protozoa, and viruses (related to cancers, other chronic disease, and infectious disease); access to specific foods and demands or opportunities for exercise (related to obesity and its consequences); access to alcohol, tobacco, and other drugs for human consumption (related to many acute and chronic health problems); amounts and concentrations of kinetic, thermal, and other types of energy (concentrated energy is the fundamental cause of injuries of all types); and social supports and role models. Major categories of health behaviors include alcohol, tobacco, and other drug use; physical activity; eating behaviors; sexual behaviors such as partner selection and use of condoms and contraceptives; and safety behaviors such as driving under the influence of alcohol or drugs and safety belt use.

Laws affect environments in many ways, and the resulting changes in environmental conditions and ultimate population health outcomes are complex and involve a large number of causal paths. Understanding these complex mechanisms requires drawing on knowledge and theory across many disciplines, including biological sciences, medical and clinical sciences, environmental sciences, epidemiology, psychology, sociology, anthropology, economics engineering, urban planning, architecture, education, and social work. Nevertheless, all social and physical environmental influences on health outcomes operate broadly via two causal pathways—affecting exposures to risks and protections and affecting health-related behaviors.

Studying Causal Mechanisms

We now use smoke-free laws, anti-discrimination laws, and the Earned Income Tax Credit to illustrate ways laws might affect environments, the distribution of risky and protective exposures, and health-related behaviors. In each case we draw on the overall model in Figure 3.1 to hypothesize specific causal chains that could be empirically evaluated to better understand how law influences population health.

Smoke-Free Laws

Smoke-free laws provide a straightforward example of law promoting better public health outcomes by engineering the physical and social environment. Smoke-free policies restrict smoking in venues such as workplaces, public transportation, and restaurants. There is a growing movement in the United States and other countries to extend smoke-free restrictions to outdoor public spaces such as college campuses and hospital grounds (Global Smokefree Partnership, 2009), thus creating expansive areas of involuntary tobacco abstinence.

Smoke-free laws operate primarily by influencing social and physical environments. Laws that restrict smoking influence the physical environment via the simple expedient of making it harder to find places where smoking is allowed. They also promote and support a social norm against exposing others to smoke in public spaces. The force of social norms not to smoke, and to obey the rules, appears to contribute to widespread compliance even without enforcement (Kagan & Skolnick, 1993). After implementing campus-wide smoke-free requirements, for example, hospital administrators reported more support, less difficulty, and lower costs than anticipated, as well as few negative effects and numerous positive effects on employee performance and retention (Sheffer, Stitzer, & Wheeler, 2009).

These laws are designed to reduce environmental tobacco smoke in public areas where smokers congregate (Klepeis, Ott, & Switzer, 2007). Even brief exposure to smoke can have immediate physiological effects, such as constricting blood vessels and causing platelets to clump together to form clots, which can trigger a heart attack or stroke in particularly susceptible individuals (U.S. Department of Health and Human Services, 2006). These clinical findings are corroborated by a growing body of population-based studies documenting that hospital admission rates for cardiovascular events decline significantly in municipalities after public smoking bans are implemented (Pell, Haw, Cobbe, et al., 2008), and these declines appear to be most pronounced among younger individuals and nonsmokers (Meyers, Neuberger, & He, 2009). Reduced access to places where smoking is allowed may also lead to less smoking, which may lead to better health outcomes for smokers as well.

The general idea is simple, but research is needed to elucidate more precisely the means through which these effects are won by legal intervention. Implementation is a key mediating factor. Barriers to implementing smoke-free policies include lack of administrative and staff support to guide planners through the policy implementation process at their institution; lack of employee, student, or patient support and involvement; and lack of resources and tools to instruct planners how to initiate a smoke-free movement (for example, a step-by-step guide, media templates, and model local ordinances) (Harbison & Whitman, 2008; Whitman & Harbison, 2010). Increasing compliance with an outdoor smoking ban may require multiple enforcement strategies such as moving cigarette receptacles away from building entranceways, adding signage about the smoking ban, and specifying the smoke-free zone with prominent ground markings (Harris, Stearns, Kovach, & Harrar, 2009).

The major goal of smoke-free policies is to reduce exposure to second-hand smoke and its deleterious consequences. Therefore, a logical hypothesized causal pathway for the effect of smoke-free laws on population health is

Smoke-free policies → implementation fidelity → reduced tobacco smoking → reduced exposure to smoke in public places → decreased cardiovascular risk factors or events

In addition to reducing tobacco smoke in public spaces, outdoor smoke-free policies may have other beneficial effects on the physical environment, such as reduced unintentional fires, the vast majority of which are caused by cigarettes being abandoned or carelessly disposed (Hall, 2010). Aside from the fire hazard, cigarette butt waste—the single most common form of litter, constituting up to 40 percent by weight of all litter (Chapman, 2006)—has become a growing environmental concern (Healton, Cummings, O'Connor, & Novotny, 2011). Cigarette filters are made of non-biodegradable cellulose acetate designed to capture the toxic chemicals found in cigarettes (Novotny, Lum, Smith, Wang, & Barnes, 2009), and disposed cigarette filters may leach these toxins into the environment, including groundwater supplies, causing harmful effects (Moerman & Potts, 2011; Slaughter, Gersberg, Watanabe, et al., 2011). Outdoor smoking bans might reduce exposure to such environmental hazards. We are not aware of any studies to date that have examined the health effects of outdoor smoke-free policies mediated through water-borne exposures to toxins. A hypothesized causal pathway is

> Outdoor smoke-free policy → implementation fidelity → decreased cigarette butt waste → decreased exposure to toxins in water → reduced health risk

Beyond modifying the physical environment, smoke-free policies may also affect positively the social and economic environments. For example, smoking bans at workplaces may increase employee attendance and productivity (Parrott, Godfrey, & Raw, 2000); bans at hospitals may improve patient outcomes and hospital profits (Whitman & Harbison, 2010); bans at restaurants or bars may have positive effects on sales and employment (Scollo, Lal, Hyland, & Glantz, 2003); bans on beaches may increase tourism revenue (Ariza & Leatherman, 2012); and bans in any municipality may reduce cleanup and maintenance costs associated with litter abatement (Schneider, Peterson, Kiss, Ebeid, & Doyle, 2011). These economic effects could be examined on outcomes beyond smoke exposure, such as

> Outdoor smoke-free policies → implementation fidelity → increased community resources → increased health protection factors and decreased health risk factors → enhanced population health

Most important, smoking bans directly reduce prevalence and amount of tobacco use (Fichtenberg & Glantz, 2002) and indirectly affect public attitudes about smoking, making the practice less socially acceptable (Albers, Siegel, Cheng, Biener, & Rigotti, 2004; Heloma & Jaakkola, 2003). In turn, lower tobacco use reduces health care costs and productivity losses attributed to smoking (Centers for Disease Control and Prevention, 2008).

Anti-Discrimination Laws

Discrimination—the differential treatment of groups by individuals and social institutions (Bonilla-Silva, 1997)—represents one of the most studied social determinants of health and health inequalities. Perceived racial discrimination has received substantial empirical attention as a psychological stressor that could have important consequences for health (Williams & Mohammed, 2009). The stress literature indicates that discrimination affects health by causing negative emotional states such as depression and anxiety, which create biological and behavioral stress responses that undermine health (Cohen, Kessler, & Underwood-Gordon, 1995). Consistent with this theorized stress mechanism, recent systematic reviews find robust associations between perceived racial discrimination and a broad array of adverse health consequences (Paradies, 2006; Pascoe & Richman, 2009; Williams & Mohammed, 2009; Williams, Neighbors, & Jackson, 2003). The most persistent findings from these reviews are strong associations between perceived discrimination and negative mental health outcomes including depression and anxiety, psychological distress, and general well-being (for example, self-esteem, life satisfaction, quality of life). Weaker but consistent associations exist for physical health outcomes including hypertension, cardiovascular disease, low birth weight and prematurity, numerous diseases, physical conditions, and general indicators of illness. Furthermore, evidence from longitudinal studies suggests that discrimination precedes poor health status (Gee & Walsemann, 2009).

Intuitively, anti-discrimination laws are expected to reduce social and institutional exposure to discrimination, and therefore lessen the resulting health consequences of this psychological stressor. However, despite the consistency of findings that link perceived discrimination with poor health, few published studies examine the effects of anti-discrimination laws on perceptions of discrimination and related health outcomes. And there are challenges in assessing implementation fidelity and compliance with anti-discrimination laws. Many lessons about implementing anti-discrimination policies can be gleaned from experiences with the Americans with Disabilities Act of 1990 (ADA), a wide-ranging civil rights law that prohibits, under certain circumstances, discrimination based on a physical or mental impairment. Obstacles to ADA implementation include accommodations that entail substantial cost (for example, wheelchair accessibility in a public transit system), lingering questions about who is covered, challenges and prejudices regarding mental disability, and insufficient capacity to monitor implementation and compliance (Percy, 2001). Assessing implementation fidelity of such a wide-ranging anti-discrimination law requires an examination of many processes along the implementation pipeline such as ensuring that ADA language covers the full set of organizational and individual practices that can lead to discrimination based on handicap, confirming that administrative regulations are in place and enforced, measuring adherence to implementation guidelines, monitoring compliance by governing units and business enterprises, registering complaints, and tracking settlements that have been negotiated or imposed (Percy, 2001).

Several studies have examined the effects of anti-discrimination laws on health outcomes. In an analysis of women's health policies, Wisdom and colleagues (2008) found that state-level anti-discrimination laws were associated with population health status indicators for women. For example, state laws prohibiting insurance discrimination against domestic violence victims were associated with lower rates of hypertension and diabetes, while sexual orientation discrimination laws were associated with lower rates of smoking

(Wisdom, Michael, Ramsey, & Berline, 2008). The study authors conclude that state efforts to safeguard female residents from discrimination may not only protect civil rights but also protect public health by reducing stress for women. Similarly, King, Dawson, Kravitz, & Gulick, (2012) found that diversity training policies at workplaces ameliorate minorities' experiences of discrimination as well as improve their job satisfaction, both of which could potentially reduce stress and improve health. Workplace anti-discrimination policies may also affect income and resources by mitigating financial costs of litigation (Goldman, Gutek, Stein, & Lewis, 2006), job turnover (Nunez-Smith, Pilgrim, Wynia, et al., 2009), and social isolation of women and minority workers (Kalev, Dobbin, & Kelly, 2006). Therefore, a testable mediation model is

> Anti-discrimination policies → implementation fidelity → reduced discrimination → reduced stress → improved health outcomes

In addition to reducing perceptions of discrimination and associated psychological stressors, anti-discrimination law may also alter economic and physical conditions, reducing subtle non-perceived institutional forms of discrimination that foster differential access to societal goods, services, and opportunities. For example, anti-discrimination law can target racial residential segregation—the physical separation of races by imposed residence in certain areas (Williams & Collins, 2001). Racial segregation, which remains exceedingly high for African Americans in the United States, is a well-established contributor to racial differences in socioeconomic status by limiting access to education and employment opportunities (Acevedo-Garcia, Osypuk, McArdle, & Williams, 2008; Williams & Collins, 2001). A recent housing experiment to address racial segregation showed that single-parent, minority women who took advantage of rent-subsidy vouchers (to help relocate their families to more affluent neighborhoods) were less likely to become obese or develop diabetes than were women who remained in poor neighborhoods (Ludwig, Sanbonmatsu, Gennetian, et al., 2011). A hypothesized mediation model is

> Anti-discrimination policies → implementation fidelity → enhanced living and working conditions → reduced exposure to risks, increased exposure to protections → improved health outcomes

Anti-discrimination laws go far beyond racial forms of discrimination, including unfair treatment attributed to gender, sexual orientation, religion, disability, or other group identification. For example, the growing movement to enact anti-stigma and anti-discrimination legislation for people with mental disabilities may provide critical avenues for eliminating social barriers and promoting adequate and equitable access to mental health treatment (Cobigo & Stuart, 2010). But, we know that simply passing such laws is not enough (Burris,

Swanson, Moss, Ullman, & Ranney, 2006). Careful study of implementation structures and processes, and the subtle and complex prejudices of actors in the implementation systems, are also warranted.

Earned Income Tax Credit

The federal Earned Income Tax Credit is the largest U.S. cash-transfer program for lower-income families. The EITC has been successful at promoting entry into the labor force of single parents, especially mothers, and increasing income among poor working families (Eissa & Hoynes, 2006; Neumark & Wascher, 2001), though the extent of its impact is debated (Alstott, 2010). Inasmuch as it has been credited with lifting more children out of poverty than any other government program (Eissa & Hoynes, 2006), it offers an example of how law in the form of the federal tax code can be used in a public health model to influence health outcomes.

The EITC works primarily through altering the economic environment. The EITC is designed and implemented to promote work and lift families out of poverty. As such, most of the literature is focused on evaluating the effectiveness on labor force involvement and poverty indicators. Evidence linking income support policies to health outcomes is scarce (Arno, Sohler, Viola, & Schecter, 2009), highlighting the need for research that explores this possible relationship and its mechanisms. A primary focus of the EITC is income support to families with young children, hypothesized to provide material resources at a critical period of child development. Those increased resources are expected to improve many dimensions of the immediate environment experienced by such families (for example, more nutritious food, improved child care, lower stress) with long-term positive outcomes expected as a result (Arno, Sohler, Viola, & Schecter, 2009). One hypothesized causal chain to examine the effects of the EITC on health outcomes is

> EITC → implementation fidelity → decreased family poverty → increased material resources → improved child development and child health → adult and lifelong health and quality of life

Alternatively, Arno and colleagues (2009) examined the effect of EITC on health insurance coverage for children, as a hypothesized mediator of an effect on child health outcomes. They found that single mothers with low or moderate incomes who were ineligible for the EITC program were 1.4 times more likely to lack health insurance for all of their children than single mothers who were eligible to receive the credit. They also examined EITC direct effects on infant mortality and found a statistically significant inverse association between EITC penetration and infant mortality. A causal interpretation of these results would be enhanced if they were to combine the two studies, directly examining the mediating influence of health insurance coverage on prenatal care and infant mortality, depicted as

> EITC penetration → implementation fidelity → increased health insurance coverage → increased prenatal care → decreased infant mortality

Strully, Rehkopf, and Xuan (2010) published an exemplary study examining the health effects of the EITC on birth weight mediated through maternal smoking during pregnancy. Low birth weight was chosen as an important outcome variable since it is predictive of various negative outcomes across the life course (for example, infant mortality, poor child health, and lifelong low educational attainment and earnings). Results of their analyses supported the mediational hypothesis. First, they found that those participants who received EITC experienced an increase in maternal employment and income, which was then associated with an increase in birth weight. They then performed a mediation analysis and found that the association between EITC and increased birth weight was partially explained by a reduction in maternal smoking during pregnancy. The mediation model tested was

> EITC → implementation fidelity → increased maternal employment or income → reduced maternal smoking during pregnancy → increased birth weight

Evans and Garthwaite (2010) examined direct health effects of the EITC on mothers' health outcomes. Using national datasets (that is, Behavioral Risk Factors Surveillance System and the National Health Examination and Nutrition Survey), they compared low-educated mothers with two or more children, who are eligible for the maximum EITC benefits, to mothers with only one child. They found evidence of positive health effects among those mothers eligible for maximum benefits, including fewer days with poor mental health, greater percentage reporting excellent or very good health, and lower levels of bio-markers that indicate inflammation, which is associated with stress and is a risk for cardiovascular disease. However, they did not examine mediational hypotheses. On the basis of our conceptual framework and the work by Evans and Garthwaite, we present two potential causal pathways, one examining effects on access to health care and one on social conditions:

> EITC → implementation fidelity → increased social inclusion, connectedness → decreased stress → maternal health

and

> EITC → implementation fidelity → increased access to health care → preventive services → maternal health

Potential health effects of the EITC may also operate via economic effects on high-poverty neighborhoods. It has been estimated that federal and state EITC refunds put $9.3 million per square mile into New York City communities (Arno, Sohler, Viola, & Schecter, 2009). And Spencer (2007) examined the effect of the EITC on the economies of poor neighborhoods in Los Angeles. Results indicate a positive effect on poor neighborhoods, with increased EITC income associated with retail job gains. More distal effects on health indicators in the neighborhoods were not examined. A hypothesized causal chain for effects of the EITC on health outcomes within high-poverty neighborhoods is

EITC → implementation fidelity → decreased neighborhood poverty → job and business generation → increased neighborhood protective exposures → improved neighborhood health

The earned income tax credit, anti-discrimination laws, and smoke-free laws each have many possible health effects deserving further study, and we have depicted only a few possible causal paths. These are just three examples from hundreds of laws that deserve careful theorizing and empirical testing of the many possible dimensions of economic, social, and physical environments affected by a law, and how those environmental changes are reflected in aggregate levels of population health and well-being.

Measures to Study the Effects of Laws

To evaluate the broad range of legal interventions that could affect population health, public health law researchers must determine relevant measures including primary health outcomes, proximal behaviors and exposures, and more distal indicators of environmental change. The relevant measures depend on hypothesized causal mechanisms of legal effect. Consider the smoke-free policy example illustrated earlier. One hypothesized causal pathway for the effect of a smoke-free law on population health is that the smoking ban reduces tobacco smoking in a public area, which reduces non-smokers' exposure to secondhand smoke, which in turn reduces the physiological effects that can trigger asthmatic or cardiovascular events in susceptible non-smokers who share the public space. Each of these links in the causal chain can be measured. For example, a comprehensive list of U.S. municipalities with local 100 percent smoke-free laws (by type of locale, that is, restaurants, bar, or non-hospitality workplaces) can be found at the Americans for Nonsmokers' Rights (ANR) website (http://www.no-smoke.org/). Similarly, the CDC's State Tobacco Activities Tracking and Evaluation (STATE) System allows comparison of state smoke-free legislation ranging from public school campuses to private vehicles. Further along the causal pathway, tobacco smoking prevalence in states and municipalities can be assessed longitudinally (before and after implementation of the law) using a variety of CDC-sponsored tobacco surveillance systems for both youth and adults, such as the Behavioral Risk Factor Surveillance System (BRFSS), National Health and Nutrition Examination Survey (NHANES), National Health Interview Survey (NHIS), National Youth Tobacco Survey (NYTS), and Youth Risk Behavior Surveillance System (YRBSS). Furthermore, some of these surveys have items that assess exposure to secondhand smoke. Last, numbers of asthmatic and cardiovascular events can be measured using claims data supplied by the Centers for Medicare & Medicaid Services (CMS) or using hospital and non-hospital patient medical record data supplied by the CDC-sponsored National Hospital Ambulatory Medical Care Survey (NHAMCS), National Ambulatory Medical Care Survey (NAMCS), and National Hospital Discharge Survey (NHDS). Measuring multiple links in the hypothesized causal pathway (as opposed to examining only the legal intervention and the ultimate health outcomes) maximizes understanding of the mechanisms of legal effect. If the observed pattern of effects matches the theoretically expected pattern, confidence is strengthened in causally attributing the observed effect to the law.

Before considering expensive and time-consuming primary data collection to address a research question, researchers should explore the gamut of secondary data sources. The availability of data (including its periodicity, time span, and geographic levels) limits research design options. Some data sources provide extensive longitudinal data, which can allow incorporation of multiple research design elements for strengthening causal inference such as the ability to use many repeated measures or comparison jurisdictions, groups, or outcomes (see Chapter 14). A wealth of high-quality data sources exists measuring a range of health-related indicators over varying time periods and geographic levels of analysis. For example, the U.S. Census Bureau provides Small Area Income and Poverty Estimates (SAIPE)—combining data from administrative records, inter-census population estimates, and the decennial census with direct estimates from the American Community Survey—to provide consistent and reliable single-year estimates (since 1995) of income and poverty statistics for U.S. states, counties, and school districts. The U.S. Consumer Product Safety Commission (CPSC) oversees the National Electronic Injury Surveillance System (NEISS), which (since 1978) monitors hospital emergency department records for consumer product-related injuries including demographic data, cause or mechanism of injury, locale where injury occurred, and product involved.

A useful list of data sources for public health law research can be found at the Health Indicator Warehouse (HIW) website (http://www.healthindicators. gov/Resources/DataSources). The HIW—a collaboration of agencies and offices within the Department of Health and Human Services, and maintained by the CDC's National Center for Health Statistics—was created to provide a single source for national, state, and community health indicators. Table 3.1— adapted from the HIW's comprehensive list of data sources—describes fifty-five

(*Text continues on page 85*)

Table 3.1. Data Sources for Measuring Population Health and Related Outcomes.

Data Source	Supplier	Years or Periodicity	Mode	Measures	Population	Website
American Community Survey (ACS)	U.S. Census Bureau (Census)	2005–present; annual	Mail survey; telephone and personal follow-up	Demographic characteristics, gnomonic and labor force characteristics (for example, income, occupation), housing characteristics (for example, type of housing unit, number of rooms), and health insurance coverage	U.S. population, including the population living in group quarters	http://www.census.gov/acs/www
American Housing Survey (AHS)	Department of Housing and Urban Development (HUD); U.S. Census Bureau (Census)	1973–present; biennial	In-person and telephone interviews	Characteristics of housing unit (for example, age, condition, size, type of fuel); neighborhood characteristics; household composition; demographic and economic characteristics of household members; previous unit of recent movers	Housing units in the United States	http://www.census.gov/housing/ahs/
Area Resource File (ARF)	Health Resources and Services Administration, Bureau of Health Professions (HRSA, BHPr)	1970–present; annual	Compilation of data sources	Geographic codes and classifications; health professions supply and demographics; health facility numbers and types; hospital utilization; population characteristics and economic data; land use and housing density; and health professions training resources	One record for each county and independent city in the United States; one record for each county equivalent in the U.S. territories	http://www.arf.hrsa.gov/

Behavioral Risk Factor Surveillance System (BRFSS)	Centers for Disease Control and Prevention, Public Health Surveillance Program Office (CDC, PHSPO)	1984–present; annual; all states participating since 2001	Telephone interview	Tobacco use, health care coverage, HIV/AIDS knowledge and prevention, physical activity, and fruit and vegetable consumption	U.S. civilian noninstitutionalized population aged eighteen and older residing in households	http://www .cdc.gov/brfss
Common Core of Data (CCD)	Department of Education, National Center for Education Statistics (ED, NCES)	1986–present; annual	Administrative records and surveys	General descriptive information on schools and school districts (name, location, type); data on students and staff (including demographic characteristics); and fiscal data (revenues and current expenditures)	All public elementary and secondary schools in the United States	http://nces .ed.gov/ccd/
Current Population Survey (CPS)	Department of Labor, Bureau of Labor Statistics (DOL, BLS); U.S. Census Bureau (Census)	1945–present; monthly and annual	Household survey; one adult in the household responds for all household members	Employment, unemployment, earnings, hours of work, and other indicators, available by a variety of demographic characteristics; data also collected on occupation, industry, and class of worker	U.S. civilian noninstitutionalized population aged sixteen and older	http://www .census.gov/ cps
Drug Abuse Warning Network (DAWN)	Substance Abuse and Mental Health Services Administration (SAMHSA)	1994–present; annual	Emergency department medical records and death investigation case files	Drug-related visits to hospital emergency departments and drug-related deaths investigated by medical examiners and coroners	U.S. population and selected metropolitan areas	http://www .samhsa.gov/ data/DAWN .aspx

(continued)

Table 3.1. (*continued*)

Data Source	Supplier	Years or Periodicity	Mode	Measures	Population	Website
Fatality Analysis Reporting System (FARS)	Department of Transportation, National Highway Traffic Safety Administration (DOT, NHTSA)	1975–present; annual	Official state records	Data regarding fatal injuries suffered in motor vehicle traffic crashes including time and location of crash, numbers of people and vehicles involved, vehicle type(s), impact points, driver's license status of all drivers, demographics of all persons involved, their role in crash (driver, passenger), injury severity, safety belt use, driver blood alcohol content	U.S. population	http://www .nhtsa.gov/ FARS
General Estimates System (GES)	Department of Transportation, National Highway Traffic Safety Administration (DOT, NHTSA)	1988–present; annual	Official state records	Time and location of crash, numbers of people and vehicles involved, vehicle type(s), impact points, age and gender of all persons involved, their role in crash (driver, passenger), injury severity, seatbelt restraint use, and alcohol or drug involvement	U.S. population	http://www .nhtsa.gov/ NASS
General Social Survey (GSS)	National Opinion Research Center (NORC)	1972–present; annual	Computer-assisted personal interviewing (CAPI) conducted in households	Core demographic and attitudinal questions to track changes in social indicators, plus topics of special interest such as the Quality of Worklife Module, which covers topics such as hours of work, workload, worker autonomy, layoffs and job security, job satisfaction and stress, and worker well-being	Representative sample of U.S. households	http://www .gss.norc.org/

Dataset	Agency/Source	Years; Frequency	Source Records	Content	Coverage	URL
HIV/AIDS Surveillance System	Centers for Disease Control and Prevention, National Center for HIV/AIDS, Viral Hepatitis, STD, and TB Prevention (CDC, NCHHSTP)	1981–present; annual	State and territorial health departments report HIV/AIDS cases to CDC using uniform surveillance case definitions and case report form	Demographic characteristics, living status, mode of exposure to HIV, case definition category, and other clinical information	All fifty states, the District of Columbia, U.S. dependencies and possessions, and independent nations in free association with the United States	http://www.cdc.gov/hiv/topics/surveillance/
Linked Birth/Infant Death Dataset	Centers for Disease Control and Prevention, National Center for Health Statistics (CDC, NCHS)	1983–present; period and birth cohort linked files available since 1995	Birth and death certificate records	All variables on the birth file, including racial and ethnic information, birth weight, and maternal smoking; all variables on the mortality file, including cause of death and age at death	To be included in the linked file, both birth and death must have occurred in the fifty U.S. states or the District of Columbia	http://www.cdc.gov/nchs/linked.htm
Local Area Unemployment Statistics (LAUS)	Department of Labor, Bureau of Labor Statistics (DOL, BLS)	1990–present; monthly	Compilation of data from Current Population Survey (CPS), Current Employment Statistics (CES) program, and state unemployment insurance (UI) systems	Employment, unemployment, and labor force data for Census regions and divisions, states, counties, metropolitan areas, and many cities, by place of residence	U.S. population	http://www.bls.gov/lau/
Medicare Administrative Data	Centers for Medicare & Medicaid Services (CMS)	1991–present; annual	Medicare claims records	Claims data include type of service, procedures, diagnoses, dates of service, charge amounts, and payment amounts; enrollment data include date of birth, sex, race or ethnicity, and reason for entitlement	All persons enrolled in the Medicare program; claims data include data for Medicare beneficiaries who filed claims	http://www.resdac.org/medicare/index.asp

(continued)

Table 3.1. (*continued*)

Data Source	Supplier	Years or Periodicity	Mode	Measures	Population	Website
Monitoring the Future Study (MTF)	National Institutes of Health, National Institute on Drug Abuse (NIH, NIDA)	1975–present for twelfth graders; 1991–present for eighth and tenth graders	Self-administered survey completed in the classroom	Lifetime, annual, and thirty-day prevalence of use of specific illegal drugs, inhalants, tobacco, and alcohol; perceived risks; and opinions about availability of substances	Seniors, tenth graders, and eighth graders in U.S. public and private high schools	http://www .monitoring thefuture.org/
National Ambulatory Medical Care Survey (NAMCS)	Centers for Disease Control and Prevention, National Center for Health Statistics (CDC, NCHS)	1973–1981, 1989–present	Field personnel meet with physicians and instruct them in survey data-collection methods; physicians complete forms for a sample of office visits during an assigned reporting period	Type of providers seen; reason for visit; diagnoses; drugs ordered, provided, or continued; and selected procedures and tests ordered or provided; patient demographics, method of payment, and selected characteristics of physician practices	Patient encounters in offices of non-federally employed, office-based, patient care physicians in the United States	http://www .cdc.gov/ nchs/ahcd. htm
National Hospital Ambulatory Medical Care Survey (NHAMCS)	Centers for Disease Control and Prevention, National Center for Health Statistics (CDC, NCHS)	1992–present; annual	Hospital staff complete a Patient Record Form for a sample of patient visits during an assigned reporting period	Types of providers seen, reason for visit, diagnoses, drugs ordered, provided, or continued, and selected procedures and tests performed during the visit; patient demographics, method of payment, and selected characteristics of the hospital	Visits to emergency departments and outpatient departments of nonfederal, short-stay, or general hospitals in the United States	http://www .cdc.gov/ nchs/ahcd .htm

Name	Organization	Dates/Frequency	Method	Description	Population	URL
National Assessment of Educational Progress (NAEP), also known as The Nation's Report Card	Department of Education, National Center for Education Statistics (ED, NCES)	National: 1969–present; State level: 1990–present; annual	Assessments completed in the classroom	Student proficiency in academic subjects including mathematics, reading, science, writing the art, civics, economics, geography, and U.S. history	U.S. students in grades 4, 8, 12	http://nces.ed.gov/nationsreportcard/about/
National College Health Assessment (NCHA)	American College Health Association (ACHA)	2000–present; biannual	Paper and web-based surveys	Alcohol, tobacco, and other drug use; sexual health; weight, nutrition, and exercise; mental health; personal safety and violence	Students in self-selected U.S. colleges and universities	http://www.achancha.org/data_highlights.html
National Crime Victimization Survey (NCVS)	Department of Justice, Bureau of Justice Statistics (DOJ, BJS)	1973–present; annual	In-person and telephone interviews	Demographics; reports of incidents of criminal victimization by rape, sexual assault, robbery, assault, theft, household burglary, and motor vehicle theft	U.S. resident population aged twelve and older	http://bjs.ojp.usdoj.gov/index.cfm?ty=dcdetail&iid=245
National Death Index (NDI)	Centers for Disease Control and Prevention, National Center for Health Statistics (CDC, NCHS)	1979–present; annual	Death records	All information pertinent to death records	U.S. population	http://www.cdc.gov/nchs/ndi.htm
National Electronic Injury Surveillance System (NEISS)	Consumer Product Safety Commission (CPSC)	1978–present; annual	Hospital emergency department records	Consumer product-related injuries including demographic data, cause or mechanism of injury, locale where injury occurred, and product involved	U.S. civilian noninstitutionalized population	http://www.cpsc.gov/cpscpub/pubs/3002.html

(continued)

Table 3.1. (*continued*)

Data Source	Supplier	Years or Periodicity	Mode	Measures	Population	Website
National Electronic Injury Surveillance System-Work Supplement (NEISS-WORK)	Centers for Disease Control and Prevention, National Institute for Occupational Safety and Health (CDC, NIOSH)	1998–present; annual	Hospital emergency department records	Work-related nonfatal injuries and illness including demographic data, diagnosis, body part affected, ED disposition, information about the event or exposure, and the source of the illness or injury	U.S. civilian noninstitutionalized workers	http:// www2a.cdc .gov/risqs/ wrtechinfo .asp
National Health and Nutrition Examination Survey (NHANES)	Centers for Disease Control and Prevention, National Center for Health Statistics (CDC, NCHS)	1999–present; continuously, but at least two data years required for analyses	In-person interviews in households or in mobile examination center; Standardized physical examinations and medical tests in mobile examination centers	Chronic disease prevalence (including undiagnosed conditions) and risk factors such as obesity and smoking, serum cholesterol levels, hypertension, diet and nutritional status, immunization status, infectious disease prevalence, health insurance, and measures of environmental exposure; hearing, vision, mental health, anemia, diabetes, cardiovascular disease, osteoporosis, oral health, mental health, dietary and pharmaceuticals supplement use, and physical fitness	U.S. civilian noninstitutionalized population	http://www. cdc.gov/nchs/ nhanes.htm
National Health Interview Survey (NHIS)	Centers for Disease Control and Prevention, National Center	1957–present; annual	Computer-assisted personal interviewing (CAPI) conducted in households	Demographics, illnesses, injuries, impairments, chronic conditions, utilization of health resources, health insurance, and other health topics	U.S. civilian noninstitutionalized population	http://www .cdc.gov/ nchs/nhis .htm

Survey	Organization	Years/Frequency	Data collection method	Content	Population	URL
	for Health Statistics (CDC, NCHS)			(such as chronic health conditions and limitations in activity, health behaviors, health care access, health care provider contacts, immunizations, and AIDS knowledge and attitudes)		
National Hospital Discharge Survey (NHDS)	Centers for Disease Control and Prevention, National Center for Health Statistics (CDC, NCHS)	1965–present; annual	Manual selection of inpatient medical records by field personnel, or automated data collection through electronic files from abstracting sources, states, or hospitals	Patient information including demographics, length of stay, diagnoses, and procedures; hospital characteristics collected include region, ownership, and bed size	Nonfederal U.S. hospitals with an average length of stay of less than thirty days for all inpatients, general hospitals, and children hospitals	http://www.cdc.gov/nchs/nhds.htm
National Immunization Survey (NIS)	Centers for Disease Control and Prevention, National Center for Health Statistics (CDC, NCHS); National Center for Immunization and Respiratory Diseases (CDC, NCIRD)	1994–present; annual; teenagers participating since 2006	Telephone interviews of households with age-eligible children, followed by a mail survey of children's vaccination providers	Vaccination status and date of vaccination for selected vaccines, demographic characteristics, and geographic area of residence	Children aged nineteen–thirty-five months and teenagers aged thirteen–seventeen years in the U.S. civilian noninstitutionalized population	http://www.cdc.gov/nchs/nis.htm

(continued)

Table 3.1. (*continued*)

Data Source	Supplier	Years or Periodicity	Mode	Measures	Population	Website
National Notifiable Diseases Surveillance System (NNDSS)	Centers for Disease Control and Prevention, Public Health Surveillance Program Office (CDC, PHSPO)	1912–present; weekly	State epidemiologists report cases of notifiable diseases to CDC, which tabulates data into weekly and annual summaries	Incidence of reportable diseases using uniform case definitions, such as infectious diseases, cancer, elevated blood lead levels	All fifty states, five U.S. territories, New York City, and the District of Columbia	http://www .cdc.gov/ osels/ph_ surveillance/ nndss/ nndsshis.htm
National Poison Data System (NPDS)	American Association of Poison Control Centers (AAPCC)	1985–present; annual	Case reports from poison control centers	Confirmed human exposures, animal exposures, information calls, and cases that were later confirmed to be non-exposures	sixty-one U.S. poison control centers	http://www .aapcc.org/ dnn/NPDS PoisonData .aspx
National Profile of Local Health Departments (NPLHD)	National Association of County and City Health Officials (NACCHO)	1989, 1992–93, 1996–97, 2005, 2008; periodically	Web-based survey, with paper option	Core components include activities, community assessment and planning, emergency preparedness, funding, governance, jurisdictional information, and workforce	All health departments in the U.S. meeting the definition of a local health department	http://www .naccho.org/ topics/ infrastruc ture/profile/ index.cfm
National Program of Cancer Registries (NPCR)	Centers for Disease Control and Prevention, National Center for Chronic Disease Prevention and Health Promotion (CDC)	1994–present; annual	State cancer registries collect data on cases of cancer reported by medical facilities within the state	Occurrence of cancer; the type, extent, and location of the cancer; and the type of initial treatment	The central registries participating in the NPCR cover 96 percent of the U.S. population	http://www .cdc.gov/ cancer/npcr/

Data System	Source	Years/Frequency	Data Collection Method	Content	Population	URL
National Survey of Family Growth (NSFG)	Centers for Disease Control and Prevention, National Center for Health Statistics (CDC, NCHS)	1976–2002, 2006–present; continuously, but at least two data years required for analyses	Computer-assisted personal interviews (CAPI) conducted by female interviewers; also, an audio computer-assisted self-interviewing (ACASI) section is used for more sensitive topics	Sexual activity, marriage, divorce and remarriage, unmarried cohabitation, forced sexual intercourse, contraception and sterilization, infertility, breastfeeding, pregnancy loss, low birth weight, and use of medical care for family planning and fertility	Men and women aged fifteen–forty-four years in the U.S. household population	http://www.cdc.gov/nchs/nsfg.htm
National Vital Statistics System-Fetal Death	Centers for Disease Control and Prevention, National Center for Health Statistics (CDC, NCHS)	1922–present; annual	Nearly complete census of fetal deaths of twenty weeks of gestation or more and/or 350 grams birth weight, with additional reporting of fetal deaths of earlier gestations	Maternal age, marital status, race, Hispanic origin, state of residence; gestational age at delivery, birth weight, plurality, sex, medical risk factors, method of delivery, obstetric procedures	All reported fetal deaths occurring in the fifty states, District of Columbia, New York City, Puerto Rico, and Guam to U.S. residents and nonresidents	http://www.cdc.gov/nchs/fetal_death.htm
National Vital Statistics System-Mortality (NVSS-M)	Centers for Disease Control and Prevention, National Center for Health Statistics (CDC, NCHS)	1910–present; annual; all states participating since 1933	Death certificates are completed by physicians, coroners, medical examiners, and funeral directors, then filed with state vital statistics offices	Demographics about the decedent and medical information on cause of death	U.S. population; death data refer to events occurring within the United States; data for geographic areas are by place of residence	http://www.cdc.gov/nchs/deaths.htm

(continued)

Table 3.1. (*continued*)

Data Source	Supplier	Years or Periodicity	Mode	Measures	Population	Website
National Vital Statistics System-Natality (NVSS-N)	Centers for Disease Control and Prevention, National Center for Health Statistics (CDC, NCHS)	1915–present; annual; all states participating since 1933	Hospitals and attendants at delivery are responsible for completing birth certificates; demographic information is provided by the mother; medical information is based on hospital and other records	Place of birth, prenatal care, demographics and health status of the baby; demographics of mother and father; pregnancy history of mother; medical and health data about the delivery, pregnancy, and mother	All registered births occurring in the United States	http://www.cdc.gov/nchs/births.htm
National Youth Tobacco Survey (NYTS)	Centers for Disease Control and Prevention, National Center for Chronic Disease Prevention and Health Promotion, Office on Smoking and Health (CDC, NCCDPHP, OSH)	2000–present; biennial	Self-administered survey completed in the classroom	Use of cigarettes, cigars, smokeless tobacco, and other tobacco products within the past thirty days; smoking cessation, tobacco-related knowledge and attitudes, access to tobacco, media and advertising, and secondhand smoke exposure	U.S. students in grades 6 through 12	http://www.cdc.gov/tobacco/data_statistics/surveys/nyts/index.htm

Population and Housing Unit Estimates	U.S. Census Bureau (Census)	1900–present; annual	Census enumeration and modeled adjustments	Counts of the number of people and housing units at the national, state, county, and sub-county level, including race data for thirty-one race groups	All U.S. residents	http://www.census.gov/popest/
Pregnancy Risk Assessment Monitoring System (PRAMS)	Centers for Disease Control and Prevention, National Center for Chronic Disease Prevention and Health Promotion (CDC, NCCDPHP)	1988–present; annual	Combines data from birth certificates with mail survey data obtained from a sample of women who had a recent birth	Demographics, barriers to and content of prenatal care, obstetric history, maternal use of alcohol and cigarettes, maternal stress, and early infant development and health status	Mothers and infants in participating states	http://www.cdc.gov/prams/
Projects for Assistance in Transition from Homelessness (PATH)	Substance Abuse and Mental Health Services Administration, Center for Mental Health Services (SAMHSA, CMHS)	2001–present; annual	State reports submitted annually to SAMHSA	Demographics of enrollees, principal diagnosis, length of time homeless; percentage of enrollees receiving services by type (for example, community mental health, substance abuse); staffing, and funding	Homeless persons with serious mental illness in the U.S. and its territories	http://pathprogram.samhsa.gov/
Racial and Ethnic Approaches to Community Health (REACH)	Centers for Disease Control and Prevention (CDC)	2009–present; annual	Phone, mail, and in-person interviews	Health, chronic diseases, diet, exercise, preventive services, and adult immunizations	Adults aged eighteen years or older residing in twenty-eight REACH communities across the United States	http://www.cdc.gov/reach/

(continued)

Table 3.1. (*continued*)

Data Source	Supplier	Years or Periodicity	Mode	Measures	Population	Website
Risk Factor Survey						
Safe Drinking Water Information System (SDWIS)	Environmental Protection Agency, Office of Water (EPA, OW)	1998–present; annual	Compilation of data submitted by states, EPA regions, and public water systems in conformance with reporting requirements established by the Safe Drinking Water Act (SDWA) and related regulations	Included for each water system: basic information (name, location, type of system, number of people served); violation information (compliance with monitoring and treatment schedules, and so on); enforcement information (actions taken to return system to compliance); sampling information (for unregulated and regulated contaminants)	156,000 U.S. public water systems	http://water. epa.gov/ scitech/ datait/ databases/ drink/ sdwisfed/ index.cfm
School Health Policies and Practices Study (SHPPS)	Centers for Disease Control and Prevention, National Center for Chronic Disease Prevention and Health Promotion (CDC, NCCDPHP)	1994, 2000, 2006; every six years	Computer-assisted telephone interviews and mail surveys completed by personnel in state education departments, school districts, and schools	Health education, physical education and activity, health services, mental health and social services, nutrition services, healthy and safe school environment, faculty and staff health promotion, and family and community involvement	Public and private elementary, middle, and high schools in the United States	http://www .cdc.gov/ Healthy Youth/ shpps/index .htm
School Survey on Crime and Safety (SSOCS)	Department of Education, National Center for Education Statistics (ED, NCES)	2000–present, biennial since 2004	Self-administered survey completed by school principals in the spring of even-numbered school years	School practices and programs, parent and community involvement at school, school security, staff training, limitations on crime prevention, frequency of crime and violence at school, incidents reported to police or law enforcement, hate crimes and gang-related crimes,	Public primary, middle, and high schools in the United States	http://nces .ed.gov/ surveys/ ssocs/

Name	Agency	Time period	Description	Details	Coverage	URL
				disciplinary problems and actions, and other school characteristics related to school crime		
Small Area Health Insurance Estimates (SAHIE)	U.S. Census Bureau (Census)	2005–present; annual	Models health insurance coverage by combining survey data with population estimates and administrative records	County-level estimates of persons with no health insurance by age, sex, poverty level, race, and ethnicity	All U.S. states and counties	http://www.census.gov/did/www/sahie/
Small Area Income and Poverty Estimates (SAIPE)	U.S. Census Bureau (Census)	State and county estimates are available since 1993; school district estimates are available since 1995	Model-based single-year estimates combine data from administrative records, inter-censal population estimates, and the decennial census with estimates from American Community Survey	Estimates of selected income and poverty statistics for school districts, counties, and states	All U.S. states and counties	http://www.census.gov/did/www/saipe/index.html
State Tobacco Activities Tracking and Evaluation (STATE) System	Centers for Disease Control and Prevention, National Center for Chronic Disease Prevention and Health Promotion (CDC, NCCDPHP)	1996–present; annual	State-level data on tobacco use are compiled from a variety of surveys and other sources	Cigarette and other tobacco use, population estimates, tobacco manufacturing and sales, health consequences and cost, and state tobacco-control legislation	All U.S. states	http://apps.nccd.cdc.gov/statesystem/Default/Default.aspx

(continued)

Table 3.1. *(continued)*

Data Source	Supplier	Years or Periodicity	Mode	Measures	Population	Website
STD Surveillance System (STDSS)	Centers for Disease Control and Prevention, National Center for HIV/AIDS, Viral Hepatitis, STD, and TB Prevention (CDC, NCHHSTP)	1941–present; annual	Case reports of STDs reported to CDC by surveillance systems operated by state and local STD control programs and state and local health departments	Case reports of STDs, including demographics	All reported cases of STDs in the fifty states, District of Columbia, and U.S. dependencies, possessions, and independent nations in free association with the United States	http://www.cdc.gov/std/
Surveillance, Epidemiology, and End Results Program (SEER)	National Institutes of Health, National Cancer Institute (NIH, NCI)	1973–present; annual	Cancer registries collect and report new cases of cancer (and follow-up information on previously reported cases) to National Cancer Institute	Cancer patient demographics, primary tumor site, morphology, stage at diagnosis, first course of treatment, and follow-up for vital status	Seventeen population-based cancer registries currently reporting SEER data cover approximately 26 percent of the U.S. population	http://www.seer.cancer.gov/
Survey of Occupational Injuries and Illnesses (SOII)	Department of Labor, Bureau of Labor Statistics (DOL, BLS)	1971–present; annual	Mandatory reports of occupational fatalities, injuries, and illnesses by a sample of employers	Number of new nonfatal injuries and illnesses by industry; demographic data are collected on workers injured, the nature of the disabling condition, and the event and source producing that condition for cases that involve one or more days away from work	Persons employed in private industry establishments in the United States; survey excludes the self-employed, farms with fewer than eleven employees, private households, and federal, state, and local government agencies	http://www.bls.gov/iif/

Toxics Release Inventory (TRI)	Environmental Protection Agency (EPA)	1987–present; annual	Compilation of data reported by certain industries and federal facilities	Toxic chemical releases and waste management activities, including facility name and location, chemical identification, on-site release quantities, off-site transfer quantities for release and disposal, summary pollution prevention quantities	Chemical releases of nearly 650 chemicals and chemical categories from industries including manufacturing, metal and coal mining, electric utilities, and commercial hazardous waste treatment	http://www.epa.gov/tri/
Treatment Episode Data Set (TEDS)	Substance Abuse and Mental Health Services Administration (SAMHSA)	1995–present; annual	Data routinely collected by state administrative systems and submitted to SAMHSA in a standard format	Demographic and substance abuse characteristics of admissions to (and discharges from) substance abuse treatment, including characteristics of client, type of service, number of prior treatment episodes, substance problem, principal source of referral	Admissions reported by over ten thousand facilities to all fifty states, the District of Columbia, and Puerto Rico	http://oas.samhsa.gov/dasis.htm#teds2
Uniform Crime Reporting Program (UCR)	Department of Justice, Federal Bureau of Investigation (DOJ, FBI)	1995–present; annual	Law enforcement agencies voluntarily report data on crime using a handbook that provides uniform crime definitions and explains how to classify and score offenses	Eight classifications of crime, known as the crime index, are tracked to gauge fluctuations in the overall volume and rate of crime; these include violent crimes of murder and non-negligent manslaughter, forcible rape, robbery, and aggravated assault, and property crimes of burglary, larceny-theft, motor vehicle theft, and arson	Seventeen thousand city, county, and state law enforcement agencies active in the UCR represent 93 percent of the total U.S. population	http://www.fbi.gov/about-us/cjis/ucr/ucr

(continued)

Table 3.1. *(continued)*

Data Source	Supplier	Years or Periodicity	Mode	Measures	Population	Website
Youth Risk Behavior Surveillance System (YRBSS)	Centers for Disease Control and Prevention, National Center for Chronic Disease Prevention and Health Promotion (CDC, NCCDPHP)	1990–present; biennially since 1991	Self-administered survey completed in the classroom	Tobacco use, dietary behaviors, physical activity, alcohol and other drug use, risky sexual behaviors, and behaviors that contribute to unintentional injury and violence	High school students in public and private schools in the United States	http://www .cdc.gov/yrbs
ZIP Business Patterns (ZBP)	U.S. Census Bureau (Census)	1994–present; annual	Data extracted from Business Register (BR)	Business counts by industries, plus summaries by ZIP code (without industry breakdown) for employment, payroll, and counts by employment size	ZBP databases cover businesses in about forty thousand five-digit ZIP codes nationwide	http://www .census.gov/ econ/cbp/ index.html

high-quality data sources including supplier, years available and periodicity, mode of data collection, selected measures, population covered, and a website where one can obtain additional information.

Conclusion

The field of public health is fundamentally interdisciplinary, integrating knowledge and theory from many sciences and disciplines to develop effective ways to create the conditions that maximize the health and well-being of the entire population. Law is a critically important force in shaping the social, economic, and physical environments in which people live, and historically, most major public health accomplishments were achieved with the help of good law. Because law shapes so many dimensions of society, and because so many dimensions of the economic, social, and physical environment affect one's odds of optimal health, opportunities for research on how law affects health abound. But research also needs to move beyond common "black box" studies that simply assess whether a given law is related to a given health outcome, as important as they are initially on new or understudied topics. Understanding the many ways law affects population health would be enhanced by increased focus on more-complex mediation studies testing specific theory-based, and potentially widely generalizable, mechanisms of effect.

Summary

Public health approaches dating back to the late eighteenth century were primarily focused on environmental conditions that increase risk of morbidity and mortality. As public health and medical breakthroughs of the early twentieth century controlled infectious diseases and expanded life expectancy, public health shifted its attention from infectious to chronic disease. For several decades public health primarily focused on individual-level risk factors and intervention approaches. More recently there has been a movement to reemphasize the importance of fundamental determinants of health and disease—the environments that allow people to be optimally healthy.

The public health perspective highlights many mechanisms through which laws affect economic, social, and physical conditions that, in turn, affect population distributions of risky or protective exposures and risky or protective behaviors. Exposures and behaviors, in turn, affect population health outcomes. Smoke-free laws, anti-discrimination laws, and the Earned Income Tax Credit (EITC) illustrate causal pathways from law to population health outcomes. A wide variety of data are available for exploring mechanisms of legal effects on population distributions of exposures, the health-related behaviors of individuals and organizations, and health outcomes.

Further Reading

Braveman, P., Egerter, S., & Barclay, C. (2011). How social factors shape health: Income, wealth and health. *Robert Wood Johnson Foundation Issue Brief: Exploring the Social Determinants of Health*. Retrieved September 1, 2012, from http://www.rwjf.org/files/research/4%20Income%20and%20wealth%20health%20Issue%20brief%20.pdf

Centers for Disease Control and Prevention. (1999e). Ten great public health achievements—United States, 1900–1999. *Morbidity and Mortality Weekly Report, 48*(12), 241–243. Retrieved September 1, 2012, from www.cdc.gov/about/history/tengpha.htm

MacKinnon, D. P. (2008). *Introduction to statistical mediation analysis*. New York: Taylor & Francis Group.

Rose, G. (1985). Sick individuals and sick populations. *International Journal of Epidemiology, 14*(1), 32–38.

Williams, D. R., Costa, M. V., Odunlami, A. O., & Mohammed, S. A. (2008). Moving upstream: How interventions that address the social determinants of health can improve health and reduce disparities. *Journal of Public Health Management and Practice, 14*(6 Suppl.), S8–S17.

Chapter 4

Law and Society Approaches

Robin Stryker

Learning Objectives

- Identify and discuss key concepts in the law and society approach.
- Explain the way law influences public health through meaning-making, organizational politics, and "fundamental causes." Give concrete examples.
- Identify two ways in which the law and society approach dramatically expands the research agenda for law and public health research.

"Law and society" is the name given to scholarship using a wide variety of social science perspectives and methods to study law and legal institutions (Friedman, 2005). Many such approaches, including law and economics, law and psychology, and criminology, are tied loosely together through the inter-disciplinary Law and Society Association (LSA). Sociologists of law founded the LSA in 1964, and sociological preoccupations with law and inequality, the politics of law, and the workings of legal culture and institutions and their effects remain central to the law and society tradition (Edelman & Stryker, 2005; Friedman, 2005; Scheingold, 2004; Silbey, 2002; Stryker, 2007). This chapter shows how theory and methods yielding insight into these core issues likewise improve our understanding of how law can diminish or improve public health. The chapter first explores key concepts and mechanisms of legal effect emphasized by law and society researchers, highlighting methodological strategies appropriate for leveraging these concepts in public health research. Second, it develops the potentially far-reaching implications of the law and society approach for policy interventions dealing with "fundamental causes" of variation in health outcomes (Burris, Kawachi, & Sarat, 2002; Link & Phelan, 1995; Lutfey & Freese, 2005).

Concepts, Methods, and Mechanisms

Law and society researchers recognize that, as assumed by economists and criminologists emphasizing deterrence, law affects social action by shaping the instrumental costs and benefits of alternative behaviors. The unique contribution of the law and society approach, however, is to suggest mechanisms of legal effect emphasizing *meaning-making*. Key law and society concepts including legal consciousness, law as legality, organizational legalization, organizational politics and the difference between law "on the books" and "law in action" all implicate meaning-making (Edelman & Stryker, 2005; Stryker, 2007). Meaning-making may involve either an overt politics of contested meanings or the exercise of covert power, and it is an avenue for establishing both power and resistance (Edelman & Stryker, 2005; Ewick & Silbey, 1998).

Legal Consciousness and Legality

From its beginnings, law and society research distinguished between law's meanings and practices as understood, experienced, and enacted by lawyers, judges, and other actors within legal institutions (legal culture) and those meanings and practices as understood and experienced by ordinary citizens (popular legal culture) (Friedman, 1989). Research on legal consciousness derives from interest in the latter. Scholars such as Tom Tyler (1990) investigated through survey research how attitudes about procedural and distributive justice, and support for and sense of internalized obligation to obey legal authorities, shaped obedience to law (see Chapter 6). But scholars of legal consciousness, including Austin Sarat (1990), Sally Merry (1990), and Patricia Ewick and Susan Silbey (1998) went in a somewhat different direction. They used the term *legal consciousness* to highlight how ordinary people, in interaction with each other as well as with formal legal authorities, constructed, experienced, and enacted legal meanings. Using qualitative data gathering and analytic techniques including observation, in-depth interviewing, and detailed narrative and interpretive accounts, they showed that citizen understandings of law were complex and often contradictory.

For example, Sarat (1990) conducted field research in a local welfare office and found that "the welfare poor understood that law and legal services are deeply implicated in the welfare system and are highly politicized" (p. 374). At the same time that the welfare poor experienced fear and uncertainty in the face of the welfare bureaucracy, many of them also expressed hope that (at least partly because of law) their needs would be met. Welfare bureaucrats might be seen as embodying mindless technical rule-following or as agents of need-based, substantive justice.

On the basis of in-depth, face-to-face interviews with more than a hundred persons in four New Jersey counties, Ewick and Silbey (1998) found three types of everyday legal consciousness that together worked to produce what these researchers labeled "law as legality." Where *"before the law"* legal consciousness was marked by awe at law as a "serious and hallowed space . . . removed from ordinary affairs by its objectivity," *"with the law"* legal consciousness saw the legal arena as a game and law as a resource to be mobilized strategically (pp. 47–48). *"Against the law"* legal consciousness was marked by a "sense of being caught within the law or being up against the law" and trying to "forge moments of respite from the power of law" (p. 48). The same individuals attributed multiple—and often contradictory—meanings to law in their every-day lives. The various meanings and their interrelationships formed a cultural repertoire available to be drawn on variably within and across persons and situations. The very concept of *legality* blurred the boundary between meanings attributed to law by formal legal actors and those by actors outside the formal legal system, and between formal law and the "law like" meanings that worked in and through other institutions, including the economy, education, religion, health and medicine, and the family. Ewick and Silbey argued that the very plurality and contradictory character of legal consciousness helped explain the power of law and the durability of legal institutions.

Building on Ewick and Silbey's explication of legality, Kathleen Hull (2003) found that many same-sex couples denied a formal legal right to marry held commitment ceremonies combining religious ritual and broader cultural enactments of the wedding ceremony as an alternative source of legality. The point of the commitment ceremony was to assert that they were "normal," just like heterosexuals, and to transform their social status and identities from that of single individuals to that of members of a married couple. In this case, even though the formal law did *not* recognize or endorse the identity and status transformation, enactment of the commitment ritual and the meanings attached to it by the community of participants ensured that "social roles and statuses . . . relationships . . . obligations, prerogatives, and responsibilities . . . [and] identities and behaviors" nonetheless bore an "imprint of law" (Ewick & Silbey, 1998, p. 20).

Given that commitment rituals enhance social support for the primary relationship recognized and symbolized therein and that social support typically is positively related to health (for example, Lakey, 2010; Uchino, 2009), such rituals may well have unintended positive consequences for the physical and mental well-being of people who celebrate them. Indeed, we might go further and hypothesize that if formal law itself were to recognize and validate same-sex marriage, the health of gay men and lesbians would improve, whether or not they chose to get married (Burris, 1998a). Perceptions and experiences of marginalization and discrimination are associated with greater stress and feelings of insecurity (Schnittker & McLeod, 2005). By "caus[ing] wear and tear on the cardiovascular, endocrine, immunologic and metabolic systems," experiencing chronic stress increases the long-term risk of maladies including hypertension, obesity, diabetes, depression, asthma, and infections (Burris, Kawachi, & Sarat, 2002, p. 513). By reducing perceptions and experiences of marginalization, then, the removal of federal legislation defining marriage as between a man and a woman, the further diffusion of state laws validating same-sex marriage, and a Supreme Court decision affirming the right of gays and lesbians to marry just like anyone else may be expected to improve aggregate health outcomes among gays and lesbians.

Figure 4.1 provides a causal diagram capturing this particular hypothesized process, and any similar process through which formal law or enactment of legality makes meaning that affects social status or identity, which in turn affects mental and physical health. For the sake of simplicity, this diagram does not include the more proximate risk and protective factors, including social support and chronic stress, that may mediate between status and identity transformation and individual and group-level health outcomes.

To the extent that either formal law or broader concepts of legality do transform social status or identity, or create new social categories or other types of cultural meanings, law and society scholars refer to law's "constitutive" power or effects—that is, law's power to make, and make sense of, the social world (Edelman & Stryker, 2005; Scheingold, 2004). Research on disability by David Engel and Frank Munger (2003) illustrates the promise of concepts such as legality, legal consciousness, and the constitutive power of law for research on law and public health. Where much research on the efficacy of the Americans with Disabilities Act of 1990 investigated quantitatively the statute's impact on employment outcomes of the disabled, Engel and Munger focused instead on the impact of the ADA as a vehicle for individual identity transformation. Using a narrative, life history approach, they did in-depth interviews with sixty people with diverse learning and physical disabilities. They found that the rights granted by the ADA "had a powerful effect on many of the

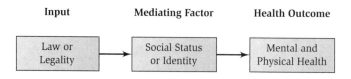

Figure 4.1. How Formal Law and Legality Influence Health.

interviewees by fostering their self-image as capable and potentially successful employees" (Stein, 2004, p. 1156, discussing Engel & Munger, 2003). However, for the ADA to enhance self-image and well-being, the disabled had to understand the rights it bestowed and that their previous exclusion from employment had been a rights violation.

Engel and Munger were not researching law and health outcomes per se. But their study, like Hull's similar study of law and same-sex couples, encourages broader investigation of potential public health consequences of law-promoted status and identity change. At the same time, it shows that the meanings individuals draw from any particular health-related law in everyday life will be contingent upon their prior life roles, experiences, and understandings. So, for example, the ADA and other disabilities-related law can be expected to shape images of disabilities and of the disabled somewhat differently for the disabled themselves, their family members, employers, and health care providers (see Engel & Munger, 1996; Stein, 2004).

Organizational Legalization

Using different methods, including surveys of organizations and various statistical modeling techniques, law and society research on law and organizations also emphasizes meaning-making as a key mechanism of legal effect. The concept of organizational legalization drew from seminal work on industrial justice by Philip Selznick (Selznick, Nonet, & Vollmer, 1969) and focused initially on the due process grievance procedures that American firms adopted in response to post–World War II legislation and judicial rulings governing the workplace and social welfare (Dobbin & Sutton, 1998; Sutton, Dobbin, Meyer, & Scott, 1994). Organizational legalization signals that organizations *not* part of the formal legal system—for example, schools, workplaces, doctors' offices, hospitals and clinics, insurance companies, health maintenance organizations, pharmacies, day care centers, churches, and synagogues and mosques—may operate in a formal-rational way. That is, they enact and implement internally sets of "law-like" organizational rules, structures, and procedures that define and effect the rights and responsibilities of actors within the organization to each other and to the organization itself (Edelman & Stryker, 2005). Examining processes and effects of organizational legalization in response to state regulatory laws including labor, pension, employment, occupational safety, environmental, tax, insurance, information technology, health privacy and security, and family leave law has become a cottage industry (for example, Dobbin, 2009; Dobbin & Sutton, 1998; Edelman, Krieger, Eliason, Albiston, & Mellema, 2011; Kalev, Dobbin, & Kelly, 2006; Suchman, 2010).

Some of this research is qualitative, including field research and in-depth interviews attempting to assess directly the attribution and transformation of legal meaning by organizational actors, including affirmative action officers, human resource personnel, and medical professionals (Edelman, Erlanger, & Lande, 1993; Suchman, 2010). One research project observed privacy and security policy planning meetings and training sessions, toured numerous hospital clinics and wards with the hospital privacy officer, and interviewed hospital decision makers and selected front-line doctors and nurses to glean how the 1996 Health Insurance Portability and Accountability Act (HIPAA)'s security and privacy provisions were understood and were reshaping hospital practices (Suchman, 2010). This field study of a single 500-bed teaching hospital was accompanied by a survey of 320 hospitals using a multilevel stratified random sampling design that captured variations in governing state and federal law. Suchman (2010) assumed that HIPAA would affect both costs and quality of health care, and that these in turn would affect health. However, it would be impossible to say what direction these health effects would take or how large they would be without first understanding how organizational actors, meanings, and practices shaped on-the-ground implementation of HIPAA.

Figure 4.2 diagrams the causal logic of this argument, in which upstream change in regulatory law affects organization-level meaning attribution. This in turn affects organization-level policies and practices, which affect interaction among medical professionals and between medical professionals and patients. These interactions affect the quality of health care provided and ultimately the health of individual patients. Suchman's field research and in-depth interviews provide empirical evidence on the first causal link only. In the full multilevel process theorized, law's effect on organizational policies and practices is mediated by (that is, works through) organization-level meaning attribution. Interaction patterns within the organization then mediate between organization-level policies and practices and health care quality.

While Suchman examined meaning-making empirically, much research on organizational legalization examines some relationship between formal legal change and organizational outcomes, while *hypothesizing* but not directly *testing* a mediating meaning-attribution process suggested by other literature. So, for example, Edelman (1992) collected survey data on organizations and then used event history analysis to model the diffusion of affirmative action policies and offices through organizational fields, as a consequence of

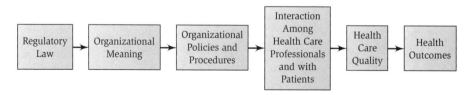

Figure 4.2. How Upstream Change in Regulatory Law Ultimately Affects Health.

enactment of Title VII (the employment title) of the Civil Rights Act of 1964 and of Executive Order 11246 requiring government contractors to undertake affirmative action. By 2010, Suchman had used his field research at one hospital to help him design appropriate organization-level survey questions for quantitative research that would assess systematically how a more representative sample of hospitals responded to HIPAA. To the extent that compliance with HIPAA is construed to impede efficient communication among the often decentralized collection of doctors with different specializations, treatment clinics, and diagnostic laboratories, one can imagine that the continuity and quality of care could be affected unintentionally and adversely, increasing patient risks of mortality or sustained morbidity.

With respect to Title VII, Edelman (1992) argued that managers and human resource professionals would assimilate new federal legislation and executive orders into their prior understanding of what constituted good business practice. From the managerial perspective, a "legalized" workplace, emphasizing formalized rules and due process grievance procedures, would ensure smooth operation of the business and employee productivity. Thus managers and human resource professionals constructed strategies of compliance that involved adding affirmative action rules and offices to other aspects of formalization within their organizations.

Much other research on organization-level meaning attribution also emphasizes this type of process, typically dubbed "managerialization" (Edelman, 1992). However, other research shows that it is not just personnel managers and human resource professionals, but also other kinds of professionals, including scientific-technical staff, who use positions in organizations as well as in their professional networks and associations to promote interpretations of regulatory law that are consistent with their professional norms, values, and identities, and also with their professional interests in expanding their authority, influence, and status (Dobbin, 2009; Kelly, Moen, & Tranby, 2011; Stryker, Docka-Filipek, & Wald, 2011). One would expect health care professionals in diverse organizational settings to be no different. And while Edelman (1992) presumed that elite meaning-making reflected covert power, others have shown how meaning-making also results from interest-based strategic action and from overt organizational and professional conflicts over the meaning of law within organizations and organizational fields, including health care (Dobbin, 2009; Kellogg, 2011; Pedriana & Stryker, 2004; Scott, Ruef, Mendel, & Caronna, 2000; Stryker, 2000).

From Organizational Legalization to Organizational Politics

To be of maximal utility for research linking law and public health, research on the legalization of organizational fields *external* to the formal legal system must be brought together with understanding of how *internal* organizational politics may affect meaning attribution within single organizations. Similarly, one must consider how variation *between* organizations in internal organizational politics and consequent meaning attribution may reverberate back to influence organizational structures, policies, and practices across the broader organizational field (Kellogg, 2011; Scott, Ruef, Mendel, & Caronna, 2000; Stryker, 1994; Stryker, 2000).

Different professions train their members according to their own sets of professional norms and practices. Examining how the introduction of scientific-technical expertise into the legal system influenced formal legal decisions and the legitimacy of law, Stryker (1994, 2000) showed that legal and scientific meanings, norms, and practices often competed to provide alternative solutions to legal issues. Parties engaged in adversarial litigation could mobilize each set of meanings, norms, and practices as resources to influence judges to rule in their favor. She termed this situation one of "competing institutional logics of law and science." More recently, she has shown how political processes of mobilization, counter-mobilization, and conflict among the competing institutional logics of law and science helped shape judicial doctrine interpreting Title VII of the 1964 Civil Rights Act (Stryker, Docka-Filipek, & Wald, 2011).

Carol Heimer (1999) showed that a similar kind of competing institutional logics analysis is fruitfully applied to health law research. She used comparative ethnographic research to study medical decision making in the neonatal intensive care units (NICUs) of two teaching hospitals in Illinois in the late 1980s and early 1990s. She showed that formal law "gain[ed] influence by working through internal organizational processes," and that decision making in NICUs was influenced by three separate sets of meanings, norms, and practices—those pertaining to the often competing institutions of law, medicine, and family (p. 17).

As Heimer's study shows, the quantity of law that could potentially affect medical treatment and infant health outcomes in the NICU is fairly mind-boggling. The civil law of torts operates through insurance companies, accreditation bodies, rules about standards of care, quality assurance monitoring, incident reports, hospital risk managers, hospital legal counsel, and medical malpractice litigation. Regulatory law governing medical practice operates through "consent procedures in hospitals and coordination with state officials when consent is not given by families, rules about DNR (do not resuscitate) orders, inspections, record keeping, [and] review committees [with] much overlap with mechanisms and agents of civil law" (Heimer 1999, p. 47). Baby Doe regulations, outlawing discrimination against infants who are handicapped, and child abuse regulations that prohibit being neglectful of infants who are handicapped, exemplify the category of "fiscal law—regulations about expenditure of state and federal monies" and influence infant health outcomes in the NICU through such means as withdrawal of funds, ethics committees, infant care review committees, and hotlines (Heimer 1999, p. 47). Meanwhile, such criminal laws as those against murder and manslaughter, child abuse, and child neglect also impinge on the NICU to help protect infant patients from harm; one way they do so, for example, is through custody hearings for abusive parents.

However, Heimer found wide variability of legal penetration into the day-to-day practice of medicine in NICUs. What legitimated NICUs in the eyes of government regulators and funders was often not the same as what legitimated them to the parents of infants and professional bodies such as the American Academy of Pediatrics. Government regulatory agents were on site in NICUs very infrequently, whereas medical professionals were on site all the time. Parents mobilizing law to affect their child's treatment were, in the famous language of Marc Galanter (1974), typically "one shot players" against the "repeat player" medical professionals who had been in similar decision-making situations many times before.

Unsurprisingly, Heimer found that, although "[f]amilies, the state and hospital staff members all claim[ed] the right to make decisions about infants in NICUs, and each trie[d] to influence both individual decisions and decision-making procedures . . . laws end[ed] up mainly being used for the purposes of the repeat players in hospital settings—physicians rather than parents or agents of the state" (1999, pp. 61–62). Those laws that hospital staff found less useful had much less effect. The ways that law could penetrate the NICU varied depending on the type of law and the skills possessed by those interested in using it in the medical setting, but the impact of law diminished "where legal and other institutions work[ed] at cross purposes, as when families or physicians resisted judicial intrusion" (Heimer 1999, p. 59).

Themes of law, power, and resistance as they pertain to public health likewise are emphasized in Katherine Kellogg's field research on the impact of regulatory change restricting work hours by hospital residents (2011). From the outside, regulating residents' working hours seems like a no-brainer. Indeed patients' rights and residents' rights groups pushed for limiting resident work hours because residents were "overworked, sleep deprived and unduly stressed. The result [was] damage to their well-being, to medical education, to patient care, and to the entire profession" (Kellogg, 2011, p. 2, quoting commentary in the *New England Journal of Medicine*). New York passed the Bell Regulation, limiting work hours for residents to 80 per week, with no reduction in pay, rather than the 100 to 120 hours per week typically worked. Though the Bell Regulation failed to go national, the American Council for Graduate Medical Education (ACGME) did enact a similar nation-wide regulation on hours worked.

Despite the new regulation's worthy goal of improving health outcomes for patients and residents, Kellogg found such substantial resistance to reform by defenders of the status quo within the surgical units of three teaching hospitals that two of the hospitals successfully resisted changing residents' work hours. She reported that "changing the daily work practices targeted by this regulation proved difficult because it required challenging long-standing beliefs, roles, and authority relations" (Kellogg, 2011, p. 8). Those residents with the highest status in the surgical world maintained high commitment to the "Iron Man" forged through weekends spent on continuous call from Friday morning until Monday night. They pushed to maintain the traditional practices buttressing their status and identity in the surgical world, and many truly believed the traditional practices were best for medical training and for patients. Reformers inside surgical units in hospitals tended to come from among those who were just starting out as interns and had not yet grasped the rules of the surgical world; female residents, who were excluded from adopting the Iron Man label; residents who did not intend to make a career path of general surgery; and male residents who were especially patient-centered or who wanted to take on more responsibilities outside the hospital.

Administrators in all three hospitals planned similar compliance programs, and for a few months, change processes were similar across all three hospitals. However, over the two-and-a-half-year duration of the study, "members acted quite differently in each hospital and outcomes diverged radically" (Kellogg, 2011, p. 8). In two of the three hospitals, reformers were able to build coalitions across work conditions to promote the reduction in resident work hours, but in one of the hospitals, reformers did not achieve this key step to successful change. In only one of the two hospitals that mobilized an initial broad-based internal constituency for change could that constituency be sustained through repeated attempts to divide and undermine it by defenders of the status quo.

In short, explaining which of the three hospitals embraced the change mandated by the work hours regulation, and explaining how and why implementing the change failed in two of the hospitals, required Kellogg to examine how external legal pressures reverberated into an internal politics of contested meaning in the everyday life of the hospitals. Kellogg (2011) devotes much of her book to charting the relevant actors, resources, strategies, and tactics involved in promoting or resisting work hours change in the three hospitals, and to showing what factors accounted for differences in hospital change processes and outcomes. Kellogg's own interest is in change in health care delivery, rather than in the causal link between health care delivery and health outcomes for residents and patients. However, her research exemplifies mechanisms of legal effect that operate through an everyday politics of contested meanings. These mechanisms are likely to influence on-the-ground policies and practices in many different organizational settings for health care delivery.

Figure 4.3 diagrams the more general process through which enactment of new health-related formal law sets off an internal organizational politics of

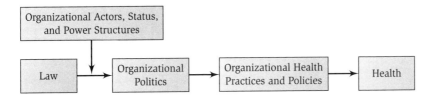

Figure 4.3. Process by Which New Health-Related Law Influences Health Through Organizational Politics.

contested meaning in health care organizations. As Kellogg's research shows, such internal organizational politics are not likely to be resolved uniformly. Indeed the paths and resolutions of internal organizational politics are likely to vary systematically depending upon exogenous variability in types and distributions of actors inside organizations and their resources, including the organization-level status and power structure prior to the advent of the new law. Different organization-level political resolutions in turn are likely to have different effects on organization-level health practices, and these in turn will affect the health of persons treated in each health care organization.

As in Figure 4.2, the horizontal arrows in Figure 4.3 signal that law has its effects on health *through* organization-level practices (that is, these practices mediate law's impact on health). However, unlike in Figure 4.2, law has its effects on organization-level health practices through internal organizational politics, and law's impact on organizational politics is itself *moderated* by variability in extant within-organization actors, status, and power structures that preexisted the law. In other words, just as each additional year of education may produce *different* returns in income depending upon sex or race, law may produce a *different* set of within-organization political processes and outcomes depending on the between-organization variability in actors, status, and power structures inside organizations.

To retain focus on the causal meaning of moderate versus mediate, Figure 4.3 does not depict an added complexity often characterizing legal effects through meaning attribution: that a politics of contested meanings may take place simultaneously in single organizations and at the level of the organizational field. The two are interrelated. Field-level activity influences individual organizations. But interaction internal to key individual organizations, including those that are "first movers" in constructing compliance with law, feeds back to influence the entire field (Stryker, 1994, 2000). Aggregate health outcomes for some population of individuals receiving health care across a population of health care organizations (say all surgical hospitals, for example) will depend heavily on which of a set of multiple organization-level policies and practices resulting from organizational meanings attributed through organizational politics come to dominate the organizational field.

Law on the Books and Law in Action

Whether highlighting the concept of legal consciousness, legality, organizational legalization, or organizational politics, we have seen that one way law operates in action is through meaning-making outside the formal legal system. As does Kellogg's (2011) study, many studies of law in action illuminate sizeable gaps between statutes, directives, regulations, executive orders and judicial opinions, and how compliance with them is constructed (or not) by regulated organizations. But law in action research also focuses on gaps that emerge within the formal legal system itself. Legislative law must be implemented and enforced through meaning-making by other formal legal actors including administrative agencies, courts, police, prosecutors, and prisons. Such further meaning-making will be consequential for the public health impact of all health-related legislation.

Shep Melnick's (1983) qualitative analysis of air pollution control standard-setting and enforcement in U.S. appellate and trial courts illustrates the import of formal legal meaning-making for public health. He showed that the adversarial, narrow, and reactive processes through which U.S. pollution control takes place paradoxically led courts to extend the scope of Environmental Protection Agency (EPA) programs but diminish EPA resources to achieve pollution control. Appellate judges upheld stringent general anti-pollution standards set by the EPA, but the standards still had to be enforced in any particular situation through lawsuits heard in the first instance in federal district court. In such individual enforcement actions, trial judges typically engaged in equity-balancing, considering both the standards' potential health benefits and their potential economic costs to local businesses being sued. Over time, the U.S. judiciary collectively made it clear that while general anti-pollution standard-setting itself allowed little role for such equity balancing, equity balancing could play a role in judicial decisions about how those general standards should apply in any particular case. Judicial interpretation of anti-pollution law, then, has been complex, and public health gains potentially achieved through strict standard setting may have been partially undermined through a case-by-case, equity-balancing enforcement of those standards.

Similarly, writing about water pollution control, Peter Yeager (1990) combined interpretive analysis of evolving legal doctrine with quantitative modeling of pollution charges, violations, and sanctions to show how the culture and politics of enforcement limited federal water pollution control law from substantially improving public health. Because enforcers attributed moral ambivalence rather than unqualified harm to the conduct they regulated, they adopted a more technical, less aggressive orientation to compliance rather than a possible more punitive approach. Yeager argues that in so doing, enforcers may have lessened the positive public health impact of federal clean water legislation.

Yeager also found that large corporations that were the largest polluters had the most financial and technical resources to combat the EPA in administrative enforcement. Larger companies had more access to administrative hearings than did smaller companies, and these hearings often changed pollution control requirements in favor of regulated companies. Bigger polluters thus ended up with fewer legal violations than smaller polluters. The EPA sometimes avoided going after the largest polluters because the agency knew it could win more easily in court against resource-poor smaller companies. In Yeager's estimation, the overt politics of contested meaning that played itself out through administrative and judicial enforcement, and also the more covert power of administrative enforcers to decide on targets for enforcement, ended up reproducing the very public health problems that motivated federal anti-pollution legislation in the first place.

Figure 4.4 combines the insights afforded by the different strands of research on law in action—the one focusing on formal legal actors and the other focusing on actors in organizations outside formal law—to depict a causal process linking law to public health through multiple and mutually influencing pathways of meaning construction.

As shown in Figure 4.4, health-related legislation is likely to set off parallel meaning construction among organizations both in the formal legal arena and outside of it. Relevant organizations outside formal law include health care providers, employing organizations, insurers, schools, churches, and families. Indeed, substantial law and society research shows that meaning-making by organizations outside the formal legal system is influenced not only by legislation but also by variation over time in interpretation and enforcement by administrative agencies and courts (Dobbin, 2009; Pedriana & Abraham, 2006; Pedriana & Stryker, 2004). At the same time, if meaning-making with respect to health-related legislation resembles meaning-making with respect to Title VII,

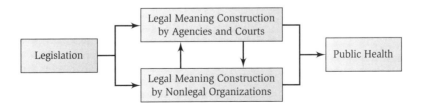

Figure 4.4. How Law Is Linked to Health Through Multiple Pathways of Meaning-Making.

agencies and courts interpreting and enforcing the legislation likewise will be influenced by how the organizations they are regulating construct compliance (see Edelman, Krieger, Eliason, Albiston, & Mellema, 2011, on judicial deference to the policies, structures, and practices put in place by business organizations constructing compliance with Title VII).

Consistent with this added complexity, Figure 4.4 illustrates that the impact of legislation on public health works through the combination of formal legal meaning-making and the making of broader, culturally infused legal meanings by regulated organizations. The two-way vertical causal arrows in Figure 4.4 are meant to signal that the "combined" meaning attribution process that intervenes and mediates between law and public health involves a two-way street between formal legal actors and regulated actors external to the legal system.

Law, Inequality, and Health

Within the literature on the social determinants of health, one important line of research focuses on describing and explaining health disparities based on socioeconomic status (SES) (Lutfey & Freese, 2005). Findings of health gradients by income, education, and occupational prestige are commonplace, as is the knowledge that inadequate economic resources tend to translate into less and less good health care; poorer health-related education and information networks; poorer diet and lifestyle; and greater exposure to environmental toxins, crime, and violence (Burris, Kawachi, & Sarat, 2002; Graham, 2004; House, Kessler, & Herzog, 1990; Link & Phelan, 1995; Schnittker & McLeod, 2005).

In 1995, Bruce Link and Jo Phelan proposed that socioeconomic status be considered a "fundamental cause" of variability in individual health outcomes. By this they did *not* mean that the virtually ubiquitous positive association between SES and health (higher SES is associated with better health) invariably worked through the same mediating causal pathway. They meant instead, as Lutfey and Freese wrote, that

> some *meta-mechanism(s)* is [or are] responsible for how specific and varied mechanisms are continuously generated over historical time in such a way that the direction of the enduring association is observed. . . . If an explanatory variable is a fundamental cause of an outcome, then the association cannot be successfully reduced to [any one] set of more proximate, intervening causes because the association *persists* even while the relative influence of various proximate mechanisms *changes* [Lutfey & Freese, 2005, pp. 1327–1328, emphasis in original].

Karen Lutfey and Jeremy Freese investigated and built on the notion of SES as a fundamental cause of health with respect to one narrowly defined health domain: treatment of diabetes. The starting points of their research were the oft-replicated findings showing that incidence of and complications and mortality from diabetes are inversely associated with SES in the United States and other developed countries. The researchers hypothesized that in-depth qualitative, comparative research could illuminate multiple potential mediating mechanisms through which these statistical associations could work. Therefore they conducted a comparative ethnography of diabetes treatment in two endocrinology clinics, one of which treated a mostly white, middle- and upper-class population, the other of which served a mostly minority, working-class, and under-insured population. They did indeed identify a multiplicity of interconnected mediating mechanisms that would tend to reproduce poorer health outcomes among lower-SES, relative to higher-SES, diabetics. Some of these mechanisms operated at the clinic level, at which Lutfey and Freese found systematic differences in continuity of care, in-clinic educational resources, and the division of labor among doctors. These differences worked to advantage patients treated at the clinic disproportionately serving those of high SES. Other mechanisms included "differences in external constraints on potential [treatment] regimens [and] those manifesting as [between patient] differences in patient motivation . . . and [apparent] patient cognitive capabilities" (Lutfey & Freese, 2005, p. 1338).

Each of these factors in turn could matter for health outcomes for multiple reasons. For example, the high continuity of care characterizing the clinic disproportionately serving a high-SES population allowed the doctors in that clinic to have better information about the patient prior to the medical interview and to get better information during the medical interview process. Because these doctors knew that they would be able to follow up personally on individual cases, they felt free to recommend more aggressive treatment regimens that provided greater control over patients' glucose levels and so had a better chance of improving patients' longer-term health outcomes than did less aggressive treatments. Meanwhile, in the low-continuity-of-care clinic disproportionately serving a low-SES population, doctors had trouble acquiring basic information about patients, learning about patient habits, and identifying connections between patient habits and diabetes management. Treatment under a low-continuity-of-care regime was predicated on the assumption that all subsequent doctors who saw the patient would have the same problems. This favored a more conservative treatment regimen that provided weaker control over glucose levels, and in turn increased the risk of long-term complications (Lutfey & Freese, 2005).

The point here is not to provide a detailed accounting of all the pathways mediating between SES and health outcomes as identified in the research of

Lutfey and Freese. Rather, it is to highlight just how many alternative mechanisms might contribute to the association between SES and health, and to point out that, as any one such mechanism is eliminated, another might emerge in its place, reproducing the positive association between SES and health.

This does *not* mean that addressing fundamental causes of health disparities is futile. Instead it suggests that when possible, one might want to tackle the fundamental cause itself, rather than tackling only the mediating mechanisms. If variability in the fundamental cause—in this case SES—is reduced, health disparities likewise will be reduced and probably through multiple specific pathways. One also could consider putting in place potential intervening or mediating factors that would operate as countervailing or compensatory mechanisms, reducing the more typical effect of the fundamental cause (see Lutfey & Freese, 2005).

Law provides a vehicle for both kinds of interventions. With respect to tackling directly the fundamental cause itself, if, for example, tax law were used to narrow individual-level variability in income and wealth, there would be less such variability available to act as a fundamental cause of health disparities. Instead, however, in the United States tax law has been moving in the opposite direction. Since 1981, federal tax law has increased, rather than decreased, economic inequality, and tax law may likewise have contributed to reproducing substantial wealth inequality between blacks and whites (Burris, Kawachi, & Sarat, 2002).

Meanwhile, where law establishes universal health insurance, this would operate in countervailing or compensatory fashion to undermine at least one of the pathways through which individual-level disparities in SES translate into individual-level health disparities. Thus, *other things equal*, the historical lack of universal health insurance in the United States (Quadagno, 2005) should make for greater health disparities associated with SES in the United States than in countries providing universal health insurance.

In *The Spirit Level*, Richard Wilkinson and Kate Pickett (2009) encourage thinking about law and fundamental causes of health—indeed about law and the social determinants of health more generally—at the aggregate level as well as in terms of individual-level health disparities. The *Spirit Level* is reminiscent of Emile Durkheim's *Suicide* ([1897] 1951) in mining different types and levels of data to converge repeatedly on the same argument. For Wilkinson and Pickett, as for Durkheim, the type and character of our social environments have profound social-psychological implications, shaping each individual's mental and physical health. Like law and society researchers, Wilkinson and Picket also highlight the roles of status, identity, and meaning-making as mediating mechanisms, in this case between economic inequality and health, rather than between law and health.

Wilkinson and Pickett argue that aggregate levels of economic inequality are associated with aggregate levels of public health through inequality's effects on social inclusion or exclusion, social status, and friendship. Increased inequality removes opportunities and inclinations for protective social interactions involving reciprocity, mutuality, sharing, social obligation, trust, recognition, and understanding of the other and others' needs. Conversely, increased inequality exacerbates status-driven comparison processes; competition and hostility; and an incapacity to perceive obligations, to trust, take the role of the other, to involve oneself in the community, and to perceive things in terms of the community good. Increased inequality aggravates individual insecurities, the emotions of pride and shame, low self-esteem, and low sense of efficacy or high sense of grandiosity and self-aggrandizement. In short, Wilkinson and Pickett hypothesize that aggregate economic inequality relates to aggregate public health through meaning attribution embedded in situational opportunities and constraints and the nature of social interaction. These processes include socialization, behavioral experiences and attributions, individual and collective identity processes, status processes, and comparison processes.

Though the argument and evidence in *The Spirit Level* focus explicitly on economic inequality, the basic argument, by logical implication, also should apply to other social determinants of health, including race. This is so because the theorized pathways of *mediation* through meaning attribution, whether through self and identity processes, status and comparison processes, or other meaning attribution processes, flow from the "social fact" of aggregate inequality levels, whether social or economic. There is, in fact, substantial research to show that health disparities are based on race, as well as on socioeconomic status (Burris, Kawachi, & Sarat, 2002; Schnittker & McLeod, 2005; Williams & Collins, 1995). Much, though not all, such research shows that race differences in health persist after controlling for socioeconomic status (Schnittker & McLeod, 2005).

The Spirit Level has been criticized for methodological shortcomings and has been something of a lightning rod for contending ideologies (Snowdon, 2010). Whatever one's judgment about such controversies, however, the book's underlying social scientific argument is powerful. It also is consistent with the law and society tradition's focus on meaning-making as a central mechanism by which law affects individual and aggregate health outcomes. And it is consistent with a law and society approach to the question of how law, inequality, and public health interrelate.

Above all, and paralleling the implications of SES as a fundamental cause of individual-level health disparities, Wilkinson and Pickett's theoretical argument suggests that *any* law that exacerbates or mitigates economic or social inequality is likely to enhance or conversely shrink dispersion in individual health outcomes

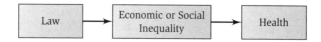

Figure 4.5. Law Affects Health Through Inequality.

within the population, while also affecting mean aggregate health. Figure 4.5 illustrates this causal argument.

Laws that explicitly are health related and laws that apparently have nothing to do with health (for example, tax law) will have consequences for health, through their consequences for inequality. Law will have such consequences whether or not these are intended and whether or not these are recognized by lawmakers or the general public, as long as the law in question affects economic or social inequality. For simplicity, Figure 4.5 omits the many and varied mediating pathways by which SES inequality as a fundamental cause of health is known to affect health-relevant environments and behaviors and health outcomes. Guided by Figure 4.5, it only makes sense that public health effects be factored into debates over both the tax and spending sides of fiscal policy, as well as over environmental law, occupational safety and health law, disabilities law, health privacy and security law, and any law pertaining to health care, health insurance, and other health benefits.

Conclusion

The law and society tradition lays fertile ground for research on law and public health, and especially for research focused on mechanisms of legal effect emphasizing meaning-making. This chapter has shown that law affects health through meaning-making at the levels of both the individual and the organization. Likewise, it has shown that meaning-making promoted by law can operate covertly or through an overt politics of contesting meanings. It also has shown that law promotes meaning-making within the formal legal system and outside of it. The two meaning-making processes mediating between law and public health (that is, the one within the formal legal system and the other outside of it) are interrelated systematically. Each influences the other in a recursive causal fashion. Each of the various concepts emphasized within the law and society tradition, including legal consciousness, organizational legalization, and organizational politics, are associated with particular types of meaning-making at the individual level, the organizational level, or both. All of these core law and society concepts are derived from the traditional law and society concern with how law works "in action." As shown in Figures 4.1 to 4.5, all meaning-making processes elaborated in this chapter generate theoretical hypotheses and guide associated empirical research that links legal inputs to health outcomes.

This chapter also shows that a diversity of qualitative and quantitative methods is useful for research on law and public health framed within the law and society tradition. This is all to the good because it allows all the research design and analytic methods traditionally used in the social and behavioral sciences of health to make appropriate contributions to theory building and theory testing in the field of law and public health. Ideally, research teams are formed in which qualitative and quantitative researchers work in tandem to elucidate the various paths of meaning-making mediating between law and public health. As this chapter has shown, numerous law and society scholars whose work has been foundational use qualitative methods for grounded theorizing about legal meaning-making. But other law and society scholars have used various statistical modeling techniques to test hypotheses consistent with particular pathways of meaning-making. And, as illustrated by research on the social psychology of identity formation and its consequences, including consequences for health, it *is* possible to develop and test identity and other meaning-making processes quantitatively (for example, Stryker & Serpe, 1982; Thoits, 1986). Consistent with the proposed causal processes outlined in this chapter, various types of multilevel and dynamic modeling also can be useful.

In addition to its core emphasis on meaning-making, the law and society tradition stands out among diverse approaches to law and public health by broadening the concept of law so that it includes both formal law and law as legality. The latter concept especially calls for an appreciation of the ways beyond the most obvious that law can be "imprinted" on everyday life, whether at the level of individuals or of organizations, through cultural meanings and practices far beyond the formal legal system itself. That law truly may be "all over"—as in Austin Sarat's famous phrase (1990)—in the production of public health is a boon to research linking law and health. It is so in two far-reaching ways. First, armed with the law and society tradition's insight that the law-like rulemaking by organizations outside the formal legal system is, in fact, a form of law as legality, research on law and public health can expand its focus to the health implications of virtually all organization-level rulemaking, whether such rulemaking occurs in direct response to change in that organization's formal legal environment or not.

A recent example of this type of fruitful organization-based research is that of Phyllis Moen and Erin Kelly (Kelly, Moen, & Tranby, 2011; Moen, Kelly, Huang, & Tranby, 2011). The researchers took advantage of a natural experiment undertaken at the Twin Cities metropolitan headquarters of Best Buy, a Fortune 500 retail company, to study the impact of an organization-level policy initiative intended to create a new norm of flexibility about where and when employees worked (Kelly, Moen, & Tranby, 2011). Treating those participating early in the initiative as the intervention or treatment group, and those who continued prior work practices for a longer time period as the comparison group, the researchers collected pre- and post-intervention survey data and combined their survey research with qualitative observational study and interviews. Selection problems inherent in the design were lessened because employees themselves did *not* select in or out of participating in the policy initiative earlier versus later. Instead, unit supervisors committed to the initiative earlier versus later depending on factors that should have been unrelated to employee health outcomes (Kelly, Moen, & Tranby, 2011; Moen, Kelly, Huang, & Tranby, 2011).

While Moen and Kelly did not frame their research within the law and society tradition, their findings nonetheless are consistent with that tradition's emphasis on meaning-making as a central pathway by which law affects health. Employees participating in the policy initiative experienced reduced work-family conflict and enhanced sense of control over their schedules (Kelly, Moen, & Tranby, 2011, p. 265). Hypothesizing that variation in work-family conflict and schedule control reflected broader notions of variations in job strain and stress, the researchers also found that employees participating in the policy initiative slept more, exercised more, saw a doctor more when they were ill, and refrained more from coming to work when ill than did employees who did not participate in the initiative. The policy effects were mediated in part by the meaning-making inherent in perceiving negative spillovers between work and home and in perceiving schedule control (Moen, Kelly, Huang, & Tranby, 2011).

The second way that the law and society tradition dramatically expands research on law and public health stems from the insight that any law affecting economic and social inequality is also likely to affect public health. Here, the mechanism of legal effect is through inequality as a mediating "fundamental cause" of health disparities. Inequality itself then influences health through a multiplicity of resource and meaning-making mechanisms such as those signaled by Link and Phelan (1995, 2005), Lutfey and Freese (2005), and Wilkinson and Picket (2009). In short, law and public health researchers are encouraged to consider how many laws apparently unrelated to health may nonetheless have substantial public health effects. Indeed, those who are concerned about public health might want to promote considerations of health impact, akin to analogous considerations of environmental impact, across a wide swath of public policy making.

Summary

"Law and society" is the term for scholarship using a variety of social science methods to study law and legal institutions. The unique contribution of this approach is its focus on meaning-making as a mechanism of legal effect.

A foundational assumption is the need to focus on law in action rather than solely on law on the books. The latter ("law on the books") refers to the institutionalized doctrine of legal codes and judicial opinions; the former ("law in action") shows how law operates in practice. Key law and society concepts, including legal consciousness, law as legality, organizational legalization, and organizational politics, elaborate how law operates in action through meaning-making. Meaning-making may involve an overt politics of contested meanings or the exercise of covert power, and is an avenue both for establishing power and for resisting authority. Meaning-making happens both within the formal legal system, for example, through administrative and court enforcement, and outside formal law, for example, through construction of compliance by regulated organizations. Each of these meaning-making processes influences the other.

The concept of legal consciousness highlights how ordinary people construct legal meanings. The same individuals attribute multiple—and often contradictory—meanings to law in their everyday lives. The various meanings and their interrelationships form a cultural repertoire available to be drawn on variably in different situations. To the extent that either formal law or broader concepts of legality transform social status or identity, or create new social categories or other types of cultural meanings, law and society scholars refer to law's "constitutive" effects—that is, law's power to make, and make sense of, the social world.

Law and society research on law and organizations also emphasizes meaning-making. Organizations that are not part of the formal legal system may enact and implement internally sets of law-like organizational rules, structures, and procedures that define and effect the rights and responsibilities of actors within the organization. From the managerial perspective, a "legalized" workplace, emphasizing formalized rules and due process grievance procedures, ensures smooth operation of the business.

To be of maximal utility for research linking law and public health, research on the legalization of organizational fields external to the formal legal system must be brought together with understanding how *internal* organizational politics may affect meaning attribution within single organizations. Similarly, one must consider how variation between organizations in internal organizational politics and consequent meaning attribution may reverberate back to influence organizational structures, policies, and practices across the broader organizational field.

Law and society research can further inquiry into how law operates as or upon social determinants of health. The "fundamental cause" framework of social epidemiology is consistent with the law and society tradition's focus on meaning-making as a central mechanism by which law affects individual and aggregate health outcomes. And it is consistent with a law and society approach to the question of how law, inequality, and public health interrelate. Any law that affects economic or social inequality also is likely to affect mean aggregate public health as well as dispersion in health outcomes within the population.

Further Reading

Burris, S., Kawachi, I., & Sarat, A. (2002). Integrating law and social epidemiology. *Journal of Law, Medicine & Ethics, 30*, 510–521.

Kellogg, K. C. (2011). *Challenging operations: Medical reform and resistance in surgery.* Chicago: University of Chicago Press.

Sarat, A. (1990). ". . . The law is all over": Power, resistance and the legal consciousness of the welfare poor. *Yale Journal of Law & the Humanities, 2*, 343–379.

Chapter 5

Criminological Theories

Wesley G. Jennings   Tom Mieczkowski

Learning Objectives

- Identify how deterrence and labeling theory inform public health law research.

- Illustrate conceptual mechanisms through which deterrence and labeling affect public health outcomes.

- Assess how deterrence and labeling theory can be applied to criminal and non-criminal events from a public health perspective.

Criminology is the scientific study of the nature, extent, causes, and control of criminal behavior. Criminal law and public health overlap in a number of important ways. Crime causes both physical and psychological harm to victims. Violent crimes—murder, rape, assault—cause millions of deaths and injuries every year (Burris, 2006). Criminal laws and their enforcement can cause unintended harm, as exemplified by the negative impact of drug control measures on HIV risks for injection drug users (Burris, Blankenship, Donoghoe, et al., 2004; Davis, Burris, Kraut-Becher, Lynch, & Metzger, 2005). Criminal law is an important regulatory tool used to discourage unsafe behavior, such as driving while intoxicated.

Criminology as a field of research also has important connections to public health science. Epidemiology and criminology overlap both in methods and substantive scope in the effort to investigate the nature, causes, extent, and control of harmful behavior. Some criminologists have gone so far as to propose a framework of "epidemiological criminology" to link the fields

(Akers & Lanier, 2009). For students and practitioners of PHLR, criminology offers theoretical models and research tools for understanding how all regulatory rules—criminal, administrative, and civil—influence behavior. This chapter focuses on two key theories—deterrence and labeling—that can be used in public health law research to improve rigor and explanatory power. The chapter begins with a detailed description of these two key theoretical approaches. This is followed by a presentation of causal diagrams based on deterrence and labeling perspectives, as well as a diagram that integrates both. The discussion includes examples of ways to empirically examine these concepts. We close by pointing to broader applications.

Theory in Criminology

Theory in criminology builds on key propositions emerging over the past few centuries—ideas that also informed other social science disciplines. And theoretical developments in closely related fields such as sociology and psychology shaped the development of criminological theory.

Theoretical Roots of Deterrence

The possibility of an empirical criminology was created by the emergence of two intellectual forces—naturalism and rationalism—both of which are associated with the historic period of the seventeenth century commonly referred to as "The Enlightenment." Both of these strands are essential in understanding the foundation of the explicit and implicit theoretical dynamics of deterrence within contemporary criminology.

Prior to The Enlightenment any set of ideas that might be called a "proto-criminology" would exclusively be identified with mystical views of the nature of causation in the physical world and supernatural causation of human behavior. In to the case of overt, specific, and recognizable deviant and criminal behaviors, the sources of these were regarded as Satanic—either primarily mediated through spirit forces, such as possession by devils or demons, or secondarily induced by an actor or set of actors. These actors were mediators of supernatural forces and brought these forces into the persona by some form of act—for example, through sorcery, witchcraft, or the like.

Furthermore, there existed for more than a millennium an official Christian doctrine regarding innate and universal human characteristics that were criminogenic. Mystical Christian views imbued humankind with an "inclination towards evil" in an anticipation of the Hobbesian view, which suggested that evil, criminal, or deviant behavior itself ought not to be viewed as aberrant but was rather the natural expression of human nature as formed by the Deity. Thus conformity to societal norms expressing "good" behavior was something that needed to be compelled—largely by a combination of self-discipline and internalization of norms, coupled with threats of supernatural punishment—in effect, a deterrence theory.

The Enlightenment began replacing these views in a gradual fashion, selectively negating many of the underlying assumptions of medieval supernaturalism. Perhaps with the exception of Beccaria (1764), it did so moving on a slow pace of displacement rather than revolutionary transformation. Among the foundations of this change were the arguments that causation of events was the result of a logical order to the world—once the underlying logical mechanism was known to the perceiver, the dynamics of events generally were not random and were comprehensible within a naturalistic paradigm. From this circumstance two critical ideas became established in comprehending the meaning of crime. First, human conduct obeyed a logic of cause and effect. Second, this sequence of causation was embodied within a natural as opposed to supernatural view of the world. The correct and consistent perception of this logic is the basis of rationality and consequently predictability in nature. Implicitly (but not explicitly) supernatural factors are dismissed, or saved as some ultimate or ontological principle.

When the rationality of this view was extended to human behavior, two behavioral elements were established as explanations of human criminality. The first was that responsibility rested within the criminal actor—that such people were not acting under the influence of a force alien to them (such as possession by a spirit) and that there was logic to the choices they made. This logic was identified by Bentham (1789) as a "hedonistic calculus," an element built into the very nature of human beings. The choice to act out criminally was a product of the rational summing of the coexisting elements of pleasure and pain, the anticipated rewards of the criminality combined with the potential risk of apprehension.

Influenced by this conceptualization of "human nature," criminological ideas (still reflected in current deterrence theory) used this logic of motivation as the basis of human action in a completely naturalistic paradigm. Indeed, the history of all criminology can be seen as a movement from supernatural and mystical explanations toward naturalistic and secular conceptions of human conduct. This was neither sudden nor abrupt—indeed, it is still linked in the form of conceptions of the morality of law in contrast to purely behavioral law. However, causation outside of a naturalistic paradigm is no longer a part of the actual legal sphere.

LEGAL DETERRENCE

Two fundamental ideas are linked together in the concept that undergirds legal deterrence. These are the hedonism of Hobbes and the utilitarianism of Bentham.

These two ideas created and allowed for a purely naturalistic setting in which the behavior of humans can be reduced to two governing principles—one active, and one passive, one micro-oriented, one macro-oriented. The Benthamite principle of utilitarianism focuses on the logic of the individual actor and uses this as the foundation of criminal behavior. Any subsequently observed large-scale social effects emerged from these individual properties. Characterizations of the large order consistent with this view are best expressed by Hobbes, who saw the emergence of civil society as itself an extension of the principle of rationality—a rational agreement in the form of a contract designed to shape and especially to deter violent and destructive human conduct.

UTILITY

Benthamite utility is a mechanism that explains individual conduct as a rational choice that is the net outcome of an assessment of pain and pleasure. Its role in modern criminology is incorporated in behavioral psychological mechanics as applied to criminal conduct and the imagination and prospective thinking of the criminal actor. Manipulating this utility (via a punishment-or-pleasure schedule or structure) is the underlying basis of deterrence. It is complicated by a variety of nuances around Bentham's ground-state mechanism of a hedonistic calculus. Among these are a series of elaborations that include differentials in perception of what is pleasurable and what is painful, how the temporal ordering of experiences of pleasure and pain influence behavior (such as lag), and the complexity of phenomena that contain simultaneous elements of both pleasure and pain.

CONFLICT

The Hobbesian belief in the fundamentally anarchic and self-serving orientation of the human psyche can be coupled with the Benthamite hedonistic calculus. It is the fusion of these two views that completes the intellectual foundation of deterrence. Utility shapes the individual behavioral dynamic and Hobbesian control shapes the social policy component.

The Hobbesian view of the "natural state" of human life is grim. Hobbes's most noted observation comes from his work *Leviathan* and its most famed paraphrase, the "war of all against all," which would be the defining characteristic of social life without constraints. The motive of survival and the pursuit therefore of self-interest and self-advancement determine the dynamic of human conduct. In criminology, this most often is colloquially expressed by the statement that it is not criminal behavior which begs an explanation, but rather non-criminal behavior that is enigmatic. Indeed, Hobbesian views are comfortable with this quip. Conformity to the law is extracted through the threat of punishment. Absent that, one would fully expect an anarchic "war of all against all" as the natural product of human nature. The law serves as a protective buffer or insulator against the natural enmity that one human most likely will feel toward others. It is only through a filter of self-utility that relationships exist in the state of nature. Other forms of human conduct are compelled by the law and rely on Bentham's calculus to extract conformity. The law shifts the assessment of pleasure and pain from a variety of interactions sufficiently into the "pain" category and thus extracts obedience and conformity in ways that would be absent in natural settings.

In law, the utilization of deterrence as a social management strategy is based on the ideal of a functional consequence arising out of the act of punishment. It is therefore distinguished from retribution—which sees the pain of punishment as an end in and of itself—and incapacitation in that deterrence is anticipatory and forward looking while incapacitation is reactive. Deterrence arises out of the pain of punishment inflicted by law, and is generally considered to have two objectives, the so-called specific deterrent effect and the general deterrent effect. These two objectives differ in their targeting and typically are assessed using different units of analysis. Specific deterrence focuses on the individual actor, while general deterrence focuses on the aggregate. An evaluation of the deterrent effect of a particular punishment (or the threat of a punishment) on an individual would measure the reduction in offending by that person. A general deterrent effect would be observed as a drop in the crime rate over the aggregate of individuals who are under the domain of that particular law.

Since deterrence is "forward looking" and seeks to prevent criminal behavior, it intrinsically involves the notion of risk. A person can only be deterred from a crime by a complex consideration of the relative risks and rewards of a particular crime. Thus deterrence is always imperfect, since it involves prediction of an outcome that cannot be known with certainty. In addition, it is clearly the perception of risk that is critical in forming intent to commit a crime or desist from criminal behavior. If one assumes that the perceptive mechanisms are functioning appropriately (that there are shared social perceptions of risks and rewards), then the evaluation of risk is based on a calculation involving several elements or variables. These are variations on the context variables identified by Bentham as the basis for the assessment of pleasure or pain. Within criminology the most important of these are certainty (the degree to which the person believes the authorities will detect and respond to the act) and celerity or propinquity (that the time between the act and the response will be short, therefore little time will be had to enjoy the reward of the behavior or avoid punishment). The severity of punishments were to be meted out in relation to the pleasures or social harms associated with the crime—the measure of punishment being defined by the amount of pain necessary to negate the pleasure gain from the criminal act. The principle of equity is also at play in that the punishment is determined by the nature of the act and not the nature of the actor. The social status of the person does not play a role in determining the nature of the punishment, but solely the nature of the crime itself.

These fundamental properties of deterrence are largely identified with the classical school in criminology (Bentham and Beccaria), and in Beccaria's work "On Crimes and Punishments" were summarized as the cornerstone of an equitable and effective criminal justice system. Tied to a belief in the fundamental rationality of humankind, this model would in almost all cases expect that a rational offender will be deterred from criminality because it would always engender a higher cost than gain. This deterrent effect would operate directly on the individual (specific) as well by example on the society as a whole (general). Only the irrational, viewed effectively as "insane," would be exempt from this governor of behavior. Careful calibration of crimes and pleasures would deter all others.

Theoretical Roots of Labeling

Labeling, as the term is used in criminology, is a theoretical paradigm that is a complex amalgamation of philosophical, sociological, and psychological dimensions primarily concerned with the organization and influences of perception on action (Lemert, 1951, 1967). It considers how meaning is attached to perception, and how a series of perceptions and their associated meaning is organized into a coherent set of abstract forms and expectations that then constitute or influence the basis of human social and psychological activity. Labeling is primarily concerned with the negative consequences that come from classifying—via language—human actors as "criminals," "deviants," or similar pejoratives and how these labels then shape the person's future behavior. It incorporates elements of symbolic interactionism—how social exchange itself forms realities and identities in the spirit of Mead's (1934) *Mind, Self, & Society*—and power theory.

Power theory is incorporated into labeling because the creation and meaningful application of specific labels have varying consequences to the extent that institutions of power are the creators of the labels. In effect, not all labelers can create equivalent consequences for the labeled. The reification of a criminal identity, for example, has greater consequences to the extent an institution of power, such as the criminal justice system, is the creator of a label, as compared to a neighbor or casual acquaintance. Thus labeling's criminological ideas come from phenomenology, and much of its language is found particularly in interactionist perspectives within sociology. It also has applications in various conflict and power theories.

Labeling as it applies to criminology is best thought of as a perspective that is infused into a variety of criminological theories. In its most radical form it can be seen as essentially a postmodernist perspective that largely rejects what has often been called the "received view" that an empirical and objective reality can be ascertained and described without regard to the orientation of the perceiver. Postmodern and associated labeling theories generally do recognize that some components of the physical world are imposed or "objective" (and cannot be modified by perception). However, the meaning attached to these empirical experiences is not contained within the experiences themselves, but rather in the interpretation of those experiences. While objective conditions may be recognized as existing, notably in the physical world, the meaning of these objective conditions arises from their perception, context, and other interpretative dynamics. Since a great deal of human life occurs within social and psychological contexts, the phenomenological aspects of labeling cannot be dismissed as sophistry, which some critics have done.

It is also important to mention that labeling is distinct from, yet similar to, the rational choice perspective. Essentially, labeling theory adds a layer of complexity to the rational choice perspective by focusing on how individuals respond to and internalize identities that are applied to them by others. This response often can be counterproductive, or, in other words, law and social control have the potential to backfire due to labeling effects, which is unique from what Hobbesian thinkers would theorize. More specifically, labeling in criminology typically combines both power perspectives and phenomenological perspectives, and can be seen as in some sense a tautological dynamic system. In some ways both of these perspectives can be integrated, but at times the different emphasis (alternately on power or on phenomenon) can create very distinct and opposed ideas of the nature of crime.

Power Perspective

The power perspective, as it involves criminological labeling, adds the dimension of consequence. If one accepts that perceptions themselves lack intrinsic meanings (and meaning comes from the integration of these perspectives into a coherent "narrative" of the world), the power perspective notes that not all constructed narratives carry the same consequences. Some come to have more power than others and are thus deterministic of what constitutes reality. Power theory added to labeling focuses on how any activity is organized and then infused with meaning that has a consequence for all members of a society.

Thus it can be said that no act is intrinsically criminal. Criminal acts come to be labeled as such because of the context in which they occur, and the meaning is associated with the activity and its context. Those who control this process of contextualization are the determiners of what is criminal. Meaning is constructed and then imbued into activity, but not all meanings have the same weight, consequences, or validity. For example, homicide—an objective act— may be criminal (in a robbery attempt) or may be honored (in warfare). This is a relativist theory of moral or criminal conduct that is malleable and for which the concept of absolute evil is greatly reduced if not entirely absent.

PHENOMENOLOGICAL APPROACH

Philosophically, labeling arises out of phenomenology. Phenomenology as a philosophy is concerned with the nature of consciousness, how the experience of the conscious is organized, and how meaning is derived from or arises from the experiences of perception and sensation. Phenomenology is itself not an entirely unified philosophical perspective. The basic ideas on phenomenology as applied to social experience are associated with a nominalist view of the social world. This influence, the shaping of reality of perception and organizing acts of perception into a coherent system, leads to constructionist ideas of social reality.

The phenomenological approach to labeling that is also relatively well established is in social constructionist ideas of crime on the aggregate level. The aggregate level of social construction focuses on the reification of social institutions and the concepts of order and meaning that are gleaned through socialization. For criminological purposes, for example, the concept of a "criminal justice system" is a reified social institution—in effect, a separate reality. It is passed on generationally; it consists of physical structures and an aggregation of individuals, it is spoken of as an objectified entity, and so on.

This dynamic can be extended to both individuals and aggregations; in criminology this has been vigorously applied to subcultural groups. This is especially of interest in criminology, since much of criminality is analyzed in reference to the power of organized criminality and the developmental influences that crime-prone organizations have on developing criminal definitions within the individual. Indeed, one of the most practical implications of labeling theory is the degree to which identity can coalesce around criminal group life. Ultimately, the labeling perspective in criminology can be summarized as a theoretical framework for explaining crime and criminal law and the notion of the label "criminals" itself as a direct result of social construction. Furthermore, those individuals who create these labels can be in positions of power, and those that are labeled can respond to this negative labeling process by developing and internationalizing deviant identities.

Theory for Public Health Law Research

Recognizing that there is a considerable amount of geographical variability and complexity in how laws and legal practices affect populations, it is not possible to develop a "one size fits all" schematic design. Nevertheless, it is possible to categorize and depict two causal diagrams (one diagram from a deterrence theory framework and one diagram from a labeling theory framework) when there is some degree of communality in the process of how laws and legal practices affect population-based public health outcomes. These two theoretically distinct yet complementary causal diagrams are shown in Figures 5.1 and 5.2, in which the independent variables on the left-hand side of the causal diagrams can generally be considered as laws, actions of legal agents, or both, and the dependent variables on the right side can be any of a number of population-based public health outcomes. However, relationships between laws and legal practices and population-based public health outcomes are not necessarily this direct or parsimonious. Rather, a series of key mediators plays a role in how this relationship occurs. Following a description of these two causal diagrams, a theoretically integrated causal diagram meshing deterrence and labeling theories is also presented.

Deterrence Theory Causal Diagram

The first path of the deterrence-based causal diagram (path A in Figure 5.1) assumes that individuals make rational choices about behavior. The rational criminal actor is assumed to be guided by a utilitarian assessment of pain and pleasure, which forms the basis of legal deterrence (path B). Paths C and C' represent the two distinct forms of deterrence-based laws and legal practices: general deterrence or specific deterrence. Paths D and D' depict the operation of these two distinct forms of deterrence: general-deterrence-based laws and legal practices target an aggregate-level unit of analysis (speed limit signs aimed at all drivers), whereas specific deterrence-based laws and legal practices target specific individuals as the unit of analysis (electronic monitoring devices ordered for individual offenders).

Paths E and E' and F and F' represent the key mediators in the causal chain between deterrence-based laws and legal practices and population-based public health outcomes. Specifically, paths E and E' signify that both direct and indirect forms of exposure to deterrence-relevant processes can ultimately have an effect on behavior, and it is possible that these two modes of deterrence (aggregate-level and individual-level) can operate simultaneously (Stafford & Warr, 1993) and be considered as a feedback loop. That is, direct personal experience of being pulled over by the police or arrested affects that person. In addition, the direct experience of particular individuals affects others when they witness the experiences of others, or hear about enforcement or punishment actions through other secondary or tertiary communication channels such as the media. Finally, just as deterrence effects on individuals can shape social diffusion to the population, the degree of general deterrence can shape how individuals respond to threats of punishments.

Although paths E and E' are categorized as important mediators in the relationship between deterrence-based laws and legal practices and population-based public health outcomes, their roles are affected by the variability in the

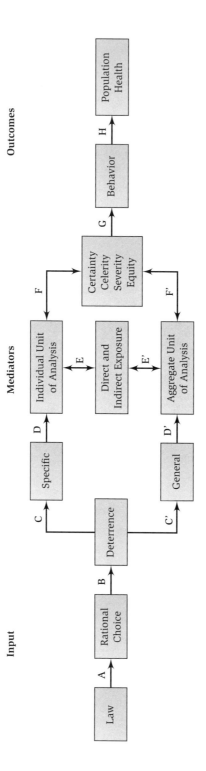

Figure 5.1. Deterrence Theory.

core deterrence-based theoretical components of certainty, celerity, severity, and equity. Behavior is affected along path G by the degree to which people believe that (1) legal authorities will detect and respond to the crime (certainty); (2) time between the crime and the non-pleasurable punishing response will be short (celerity); (3) punishment for harm associated with the crime outweighs the pleasure involved in the commission of the crime (severity); and (4) punishment is determined by the nature of the act, not the nature of the actor (equity). Note that the notion of equity may also be conceived as a moral principle guiding the operations of punishment rather than deterrence.

The relative strengths of effect of certainty, celerity, severity, and equity on behavior is not fully known. Neither is exactly how the four components interact to synergistically increase or diminish effects. The death penalty lacks celerity but is viewed as having the ultimate degree of severity and is presumed to influence an individual's decision to commit homicide and to deter homicides in the aggregate among members of the general population. Nevertheless, the subject of the death penalty remains controversial among researchers and policy makers, particularly concerning its relative ineffectiveness as a mechanism for realizing deterrence without preventing a deleterious side effect, brutalization. In summary, deterrence-based laws and legal practices ultimately affect population-based public health outcomes, such as violence (path H), through a series of mediating mechanisms operating at the individual and aggregate levels of analysis.

Labeling Theory Causal Diagram

The first path of the labeling-based causal diagram (path A in Figure 5.2) indicates that laws and legal practices prescribe labels for criminal actors. For example, the word *delinquent* or *criminal* is a label that distinguishes the actor from *non-delinquents* or *non-criminals*. Path B and B' represent two complementary, but distinct, labeling paradigms through which laws and legal practices can operate. In the power paradigm, the effect of the label is influenced by the consequence associated with the activity on which the label is applied. Labels emerging from laws and legal practices often differentially target groups with the least amount of power in society. For example, vagrancy is labeled a crime because the actors are predominantly poor and transient individuals with little to no power in comparison to those who are actively involved in the lawmaking. In contrast, path B', from the phenomenological paradigm, focuses on the reification of social institutions. Social institutions are created as a result of laws and legal practices that apply labels to different forms of behavior. For instance, special gang police units form because the label "gang" has been applied to individuals who are involved in a variety of "socially unacceptable"

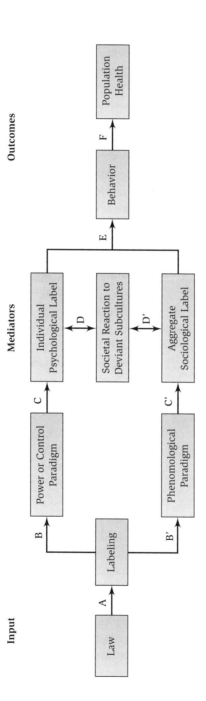

Figure 5.2. Labeling Theory.

behaviors such as graffiti and violence and do so in a group context with an organizational structure.

Labeling can affect an individual's self-concept or identity (path C). This process has been succinctly characterized by American sociologist W. I. Thomas as a "situation defined as real is real in its consequences" (Thomas & Thomas 1928, p. 572). The label applied from the external source becomes incorporated into one's self-identity. Thus the label becomes a self-fulfilling process. For example, an individual has been labeled a deviant because he frequently gambles; therefore, he internalizes this label and continues to gamble because he has been labeled a deviant. Labeling also operates in the aggregate (path C'). For instance, a juvenile spending a great deal of time hanging out with her peers in an unsupervised capacity has been socially constructed as deviant in the sense that unstructured socializing is assumed to be a direct correlate for criminal behavior. Therefore, this behavior that has been socially constructed as deviant behavior has an effect on group behavior in the aggregate.

Although effects of labeling have been described separately for the individual and aggregate levels, it is important to acknowledge a possible feedback loop between social reaction to deviant subcultures (path D') and individual psychological labels (path D). For example, socially constructed labels can also possess power—sometimes great power. The expression of this is described in criminology as "societal reaction"—the label attached to persons, events, or institutions evokes specific responses from a general audience of observers. These observers then proceed to organize their beliefs and behaviors toward the labeled object in accordance with accepted and reified social constructs. Situations and persons, for example, may be perceived as threatening or comforting depending on a series of visible signs that are present to an observer. This is the process of labeling as a reactive state. Taken together, these mediating sociological and psychological mechanisms attenuate the relationship between the labeling that directly results from laws and legal practices (on the left side of Figure 5.2) and health-relevant behavior and, ultimately, population health.

Integrating Deterrence and Labeling Theory

While deterrence- and labeling-based theories of legal effects can be considered separately, and are at times diametrically opposed to one another, there is room for conceptual integration. First, in a theoretically integrated model, the left-hand side of the causal diagram remains unchanged from the deterrence model. Specifically, path A (Figure 5.3) represents the link between laws and legal practices and deterrence (path B) via rational choice assumptions. The next phase of the causal diagram presenting the key mediators disaggregates deterrence into its individual-level form aimed at achieving specific deterrence (path C) and its aggregate-level form, in which the intention is general deterrence (path C').

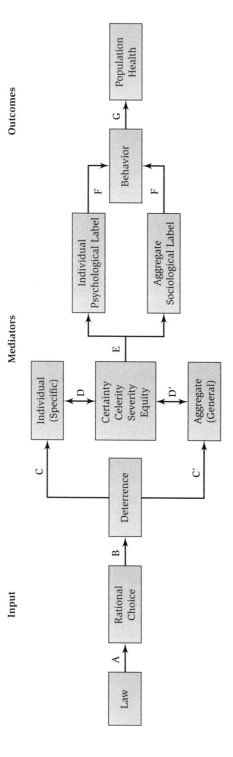

Figure 5.3. An Integrated Model from Criminology.

Acknowledging the possible varying levels of influence and application of the recursive components of deterrence theory exhibited in paths D and D' (certainty, celerity, severity, and equity), the next key mediating mechanism is drawn from the labeling perspective. Similar to the deterrence perspective, these mechanisms can operate at the individual psychological level or the aggregate sociological level (path E). Therefore, this integrated causal diagram is conditioned on the primacy of deterrence in laws and legal practices, yet this causal chain also permits the meditational effects of both deterrence and labeling concepts in ultimately affecting behavior (path F) and population public health outcomes (path G).

These effects are not necessarily operating in a purely linear fashion. The synergistic relationship between deterrence and labeling could be conceptually considered in relation to what regulatory researchers call the enforcement pyramid (Ayres & Braithwaite, 1995). At the base are well-intentioned actors who are attempting to obey the law because they accept that as the right thing to do. Above them is a smaller group of "rational actors" who will obey because they calculate that the benefits of disobedience are lower than the costs of lawbreaking. At the top of the pyramid are a small group of bad actors who, for reasons of their own, are determined not to obey the law. These distinct types of actors require different regulatory strategies, and the key to regulatory efficiency is to apply the correct strategy or mix of strategies.

Actors disposed to obey the law require the least regulatory energy. The main thing is to make sure they know the correct course of action. Labeling, which tells them which activities are proscribed, may be enough in most cases to secure compliance. Rational actors, deterrence tells us, may need to be reminded that detection and punishment are available. When actors in the lower levels of the pyramid do break the rules, regulators initially can use relatively lighter sanctions—warnings, shaming, civil penalties—on the assumption that labeling or deterrence will be sufficient to get these actors back on the right track. If these base-of-the-pyramid strategies are not effective, then regulators can move up the pyramid to enforce more punitive strategies (license revocations, fines, and so on) with the ultimate and most severe deterrence strategy being at the peak of the pyramid (imprisonment or incapacitation). However, a synergistic process allows regulators to move up and down the pyramid with a number of enforcement options of varying degrees of punitiveness that theoretically would lead to favorable public health outcomes while avoiding deleterious effects of labeling and shaming.

Measuring Deterrence and Labeling in PHLR

Incorporating concepts from criminology when evaluating public health effects of law requires their measurement. In this section we review a few examples of how deterrence and labeling concepts have been measured for research.

Deterrence

There is little argument that drinking and driving and its related motor vehicle crashes and fatalities still remain a significant public health concern (Wagenaar, Maldonado-Molina, Erickson, et al., 2007). Therefore, it comes as no surprise that the application of legal sanctions for drinking and driving is widespread, and sanctions have been imposed for multiple purposes including deterrence, punishment, retribution, and incapacitation (Ross, 1982). As they relate to deterrence specifically, examples of legal sanctions for drinking and driving include fines, loss of license, jail time, and associated large-scale media campaigns publicizing the penalties and their enforcement (Freeman & Watson, 2006). Three studies in particular have examined the deterrent effects of penalties such as these at the individual level (specific deterrence) (Freeman & Watson, 2006; Piquero & Pogarsky, 2003) and aggregate level (general deterrence) (Wagenaar, Maldonado-Molina, Erickson, et al., 2007) that have relevance for PHLR (see also Paternoster & Piquero, 1995; Piquero & Paternoster, 1998).

Using the following hypothetical vignette scenario among a large sample of college students, Piquero and Pogarsky investigated the deterrent effects of varying penalties and other components of deterrence (such as certainty and severity):

> Suppose you drove by yourself one evening to meet some friends in a local bar. By the end of the evening, you've had enough drinks so that you're pretty sure your blood alcohol level is above the legal limit. Suppose that you live about 10 miles away and you have to be at work early the next morning. You can either drive home or find some other way home, but if you leave your car at the bar, you will have to return early the next morning to pick it up [Piquero & Pogarsky, 2003, pp. 162–163].

Regarding the certainty of punishment, the respondents answered the following question after being presented with the hypothetical scenario: "If you drove home under the circumstances described above, what is the chance (on a scale from 0 to 100) you would be pulled over by the police?" The severity of the punishment was assessed with the following question: "If you are convicted for drunk driving, you will not go to jail or receive a fine. However, your driver's license will be suspended for . . . [either one or twelve months]." Furthermore, Piquero and Pogarsky included measures of vicarious or indirect punishment experiences, which are also influential deterrence concepts (Stafford & Warr, 1993), by asking the respondents to report the percentage of people they knew who had ever been charged with drunk driving and the percentage of people they think had driven while intoxicated on at least several occasions. Finally, the likelihood of committing the crime was measured by asking the respondents to estimate on a scale of 1 to 100 the likelihood they would drive home under the circumstances provided in the scenario above.

Freeman and Watson (2006) provide a replication and extension of Piquero and Pogarsky's work, in which they recruited 166 recidivist drunk drivers who were all participants in a court-appointed probation order for a drinking and driving offense. These researchers collected a variety of deterrence-relevant information measuring perceptions of legal sanctions, experiences with direct and indirect punishment, and perceptions of the severity and celerity of punishment. Items in Freeman and Watson's deterrence questionnaire include

- My penalties for drunk driving have been severe.
- I drink and drive regularly without being caught.
- My friends often drink and drive without being caught.
- Out of the next hundred people who drink and drive in Brisbane, how many do you think will be caught?
- The time between getting caught for drunk driving and going to court was very short.
- My friends have been caught and punished for drunk driving.
- The penalties I received for drunk driving have caused a considerable impact on my life.
- When I drink and drive I am worried that I might get caught.
- The chances of me being caught for drunk driving are high.
- It took a long time after I was caught by the police before I lost my license.

In contrast to the studies reviewed on individual-level deterrence, Wagenaar, Maldonado-Molina, Erickson, et al. (2007) provided an empirical examination of the general deterrent effects of statutory changes in DUI fine and jail penalties (that is, severity) on alcohol-related crashes in the aggregate across states. Results indicated that mandatory fines appeared to have a general deterrent effect, while mandatory jail sentences generally did not. These studies illustrate evaluations of deterrence-theory-based laws at either the individual level (specific deterrence) or the aggregate level (general deterrence).

There are a number of examples of how deterrence applies in areas other than drinking and driving. For example, speed limit signs are posted to deter drivers from exceeding a safe traveling speed. Speed limits operate as a specific deterrent process as to drivers who have previously received a speeding ticket themselves, and as a general deterrent as to drivers who have heard of others being caught and punished for exceeding the posted speed limit. The certainty, severity, and celerity of the punishment and related fines, license suspensions, and so on all have an influence on the degree to which the public health benefits of posting speed limit signs is realized.

Electronic monitoring devices for convicted offenders also have an inherent deterrent element. These devices make it difficult or impossible for monitored individuals to leave their homes or workplaces in order to offend. Assuming that these devices are properly operating and being monitored, any departure from the permitted area would result in an immediate alarm to the authorities (certainty). Following this alarm, the probation or parole officer normally would swiftly respond to the alarm (celerity), document violation of the offender's probation or parole, and return the offender to jail (severity).

Researchers have also begun to study relative weights of certainty, severity, and celerity in effecting deterrence. A number of examples of reliable and valid measurement tools and scales can be found in the following sources (Durlauf & Nagin, 2011; Nagin, 2010; Nagin & Pogarsky, 2001). Furthermore, systematic reviews and meta-analyses provide helpful resources on how to measure elements of deterrence (Andrews, Zinger, Hoge, et al., 1990; Cullen, Pratt, Miceli, & Moon, 2002; Cullen, Wright, & Applegate, 1996; Howe & Brandau, 1988; Howe & Loftus, 1996; Klepper & Nagin, 1989; Nagin, 1998; Nagin & Pogarsky, 2001; Pratt & Cullen, 2005; Pratt, Cullen, Blevins, Daigle, & Madensen, 2006; Williams & Hawkins, 1986).

Labeling

There can be little argument that sex offender registration and community notification provides one of the most identifiable and current examples of labeling in criminology. Although sex offender registration is not necessarily a new idea (Logan, 2009), the universal requirement for convicted sex offenders to register with law enforcement, have their identifying information posted on publicly accessible, Internet-based registries, and (at least in some jurisdictions) have community organizations and residents notified of their identities and residential locations (Terry & Ackerman, 2009) has presented a real-world experiment on the effects of such laws on population-based public health outcomes such as sexual violence.

A growing number of studies have begun to question the effectiveness of universal application of sex offender registration and community notification policies due to their misperception regarding sex offender specialization and recidivism (Zimring, Jennings, Piquero, & Hays, 2009; Zimring, Piquero, & Jennings, 2007). Furthermore, research has identified a number of collateral consequences for sex offenders as a direct result of having been labeled a "sex offender" and experiencing the associated negative and stigmatizing effects of this label. For example, Tewksbury (2005) collected information from a mail-based survey administered to offenders listed on the Kentucky Sex Offender Registry and asked them about their experiences since becoming a registrant. There was a wide range of negative experiences reported, with the most common experiences including loss of job (43 percent); denial of promotion at work (23 percent); loss or denial of place to live (45 percent); treated rudely in a public place (39 percent); asked to leave a business (11 percent); lost a friend who found out about registration (55 percent); harassed in person (47 percent); assaulted (16 percent); received harassing or threatening telephone calls (28 percent); received harassing or threatening mail (25 percent).

Considering the prevalence of such negative experiences, reintegration and avoidance of long-term stigmatization among labeled and registered sex offenders might be difficult at best (Braithwaite, 1989). Furthermore, such negative experiences likely lead to a reduction in protective factors and a corresponding increase in risk factors for re-offending. Reducing re-offending probably requires creating conducive conditions for successful societal reintegration (McAlinden, 2006).

Laws on sex offender registration and community notification illustrate how a theoretically integrated model may be tested. The research question is whether these laws reduce rates of sexual violence (a population-based public health outcome) by providing a specific deterrent effect (preventing sexual violence recidivism among sex offenders) and a general deterrent effect (deterring would-be first-time sex offenders) while avoiding unduly stigmatizing labeling effects and preventing registrants' successful reintegration into society. Recent empirical evidence on sex offender registration and community notification laws suggests that deleterious consequences of the labeling effects of these laws may be exceeding the beneficial deterrence consequences (Sandler, Freeman, & Socia, 2008; Schramm & Milloy, 1995; Tewksbury, 2005; Tewksbury & Jennings, 2010; Vasquez, Maddan, & Walker, 2008; Zgoba, Veysey, & Dalessandro, 2010).

Public Health Law Research Challenges

Theory, as the term is used in all social sciences including criminology, should be viewed with modesty and constraint, because, unlike in many physical sciences, theoretical ideas of causation of crime and the quantitative and qualitative relationships between important concepts and constructs are not fully defined or measured. Operationalizing and measuring constructs related to human conduct are more controversial and ambiguous tasks than are usually encountered in studying constructs related to the physical world. Theory in criminology and the social sciences as a consequence is underdeveloped, suggesting cause-effect relationships without necessarily providing an ability to precisely predict prospectively.

There are inherent tensions between crime control and public health objectives that can present problems for public health law research. Consider the tug-of-war between harm-reduction strategies and political incentives to look tough on crime. "Get tough" measures such as drug crackdowns are often serious impediments to achieving beneficial crime control and public health objectives. Ultimately, academics, practitioners, and lawmakers should make a more concerted effort in developing partnerships to design research programs addressing shared crime and public health issues and draft and implement effective laws and policies that strike a balance between crime control and public health objectives.

Conclusion

This chapter described how theories and methods from the field of criminology, particularly deterrence and labeling theories, help explain how law influences behavior. Following a discussion of the effects of criminal and non-criminal laws and a review of theoretical frameworks for deterrence and labeling theories, we presented three causal diagrams that graphically depicted ways law can affect population health outcomes via the complex mediating mechanisms emerging from deterrence and labeling theories. Examples of ways to measure and empirically examine these concepts were also provided. Finally, we discussed the theoretical and methodological challenges that exist as well as offering a series of recommendations and directions for future research for those interested in examining public health effects of laws in light of prominent theories in criminology.

Relevant public health law and the research on its effects can both inform and be informed by criminology. This mutually beneficial relationship centers on how each discipline informs the theoretical thinking and empirical knowledge base upon which each relies to deepen their contributions to public life. For example, each discipline shares a concern for health in prospective thinking about policy. The very concept of deterrence in criminology is a prospective and preventive approach completely consistent with the public health concern with prevention. Ideally, policies directed at criminal behavior as well as unhealthy behaviors are most effective when they prevent negative effects rather than having to deal with corrective ex post facto actions. Furthermore, criminological ideas regarding labeling have important implications for generalized patterns of behavior that can be elements in prevention policies. This is well illustrated by the labeling efforts directed at tobacco use as a public health concern. Labeling unhealthy and antisocial behaviors as unhealthy and undesirable are common mechanisms for both disciplines.

It is clear that the nexus between criminology and public health law research extends beyond these abstract domains. Persons drawn into the criminal justice system bring with them serious public health issues. For instance, this population exhibits greater degrees of morbidity than the general population, and often is involved in higher rates of unhealthy behavior compared to the general public. They are also less likely to have any form of health insurance outside the general public assistance offered to the indigent. In sum, they offer special challenges to public health policy while simultaneously being potentially less tractable to the usual health delivery services available to citizens. In addition, offenders' motivation for a healthy lifestyle, perceptions of self-interest, and patterns of thought may be radically different from the typical population-wide patterns that public health practitioners often assume. Thus there are many ways in which criminological theory, data, and research help advance public health law and improve population health outcomes.

Summary

Criminology is the scientific study of the nature, extent, causes, and control of criminal behavior. Two theories—deterrence and labeling—are widely used by criminologists to explain the influence of criminal law on behavior. Public health law researchers investigating effects of regulations and sanctions on health behavior can draw on these theories and the research methods and tools criminologists have devised to test them.

- Deterrence posits that the choice to act out criminally is a product of the rational assessment of the anticipated rewards of criminality versus the potential costs imposed by law. Manipulating this calculation (through punishment and the perceived likelihood of detection) is the underlying basis of deterrence.

- Labeling theory explains crime and criminal law as products of a social process of meaning making. Certain behaviors, not necessarily intrinsically harmful, are labeled as "crimes" and those who commit them as "deviants." Labeling theory explains how these labels emerge and how people's identities and behaviors are influenced by them.

- The two theories can be integrated to explain how ideas about crime, fears of punishment, and expectations of detection work in relation to each other to shape individual and organizational behavior in response to law.

Further Reading

Braithwaite, J. (1989). *Crime, shame, and reintegration*. Cambridge: Cambridge University Press.

Nagin, D. S. (2010). Imprisonment and crime control: Building evidence-based policy. In R. Rosenfeld, K. Quinet, & C. Garcia (Eds.), *Contemporary issues in criminological theory and research: The role of social institutions* (Papers from the American Society of Criminology 2010 Conference). Belmont, CA: Wadsworth.

Nagin, D. S., & Pogarsky, G. (2001). Integrating celerity, impulsivity, and extralegal sanction threats into a model of general deterrence: Theory and evidence. *Criminology, 39*(4), 865–891.

Stafford, M., & Warr, M. (1993). A reconceptualization of general and specific deterrence. *Journal of Research in Crime and Delinquency, 30*(2), 123–135.

Wagenaar, A. C., Maldonado-Molina, M. M., Erickson, D. J., et al. (2007). General deterrence effects of U.S. statutory DUI fine and jail penalties: Long-term follow-up in 32 states. *Accident Analysis and Prevention, 39*(5), 982–994.

Chapter 6

Procedural Justice Theory

Tom R. Tyler   Avital Mentovich

Learning Objectives

- Define and describe the components of procedural justice.

- Illustrate the significance of legitimacy and self-regulatory behavior in developing, implementing, and enforcing public health law.

- Design a public health law research study that incorporates procedural justice in examining compliance to a public health law.

Law is a prominent intervention tool through which government can seek to achieve public health goals (Burris, Wagenaar, Swanson, et al., 2010). To take a straightforward example, governments have created regulations banning smoking in public places, and have provided penalties, typically a fine, for those who disobey those rules. The government similarly promotes public health by regulating the quality of drugs that are sold in America, again creating rules and enforcing them through a system of fines and, in extreme cases, criminal penalties. These regulations are an effort by government to improve public health by putting the force of law behind stopping unhealthy behaviors.

It might be initially imagined that the way these laws influence behavior is straightforward. If a law is passed and backed up by threats of fines, arrest, or incarceration, behavior will change. If wearing safety belts is mandated, people will wear belts to avoid getting a ticket. The threat of a sanction certainly can work, but obtaining a high level of compliance with the law is complex and can be difficult; the ability of law to shape public behavior is the result of many interacting factors that vary depending on local conditions, the behavior, and the target population. From a social psychological perspective, the effectiveness of the legal system depends at least in part on the willingness of citizens to voluntarily consent to the operation of legal authorities and to actively cooperate with them.

Social psychologists posit that behavior is determined by two main forces. The first is the pressure of the situation or the environment, and the second includes the motives and perceptions that the person brings to the situation. In Lewin's famous equation, behavior is understood to be a function of the person and the environment: $B = f(P, E)$. An expanded conception of the *person* term includes the set of social and moral values that shape the individual's thoughts and feelings about what is ethical or normatively appropriate to do. The *environment* includes the way legal officers and institutions behave in their creation and enforcement of rules.

Where compliance with the law is concerned, two values constituting what sociologist Max Weber called "legitimacy" are of particular importance to defining P: the individual's sense of obligation to obey authorities, and his or her sense of trust and confidence in legal authorities. These feelings of legitimacy, and the willingness to comply with law, are influenced by the legal environment. Research has made a compelling case for the positive effect of perceptions of procedural justice on an individual's sense of a rule's legitimacy and his or her compliance with it. This chapter will examine the complexity of compliance and propose an approach to studying health-related behavior that has been effective in other settings. This approach is known in the literatures on law, regulation, and social psychology as "procedural justice."

Complying with the Law

The problems involved in obtaining compliance with the law in everyday life involve a wide variety of regulations, ranging from traffic laws (Tyler, 2006b) to drug laws (MacCoun, 1993). While most people comply with the law most of the time, legal authorities are confronted with sufficient noncompliance to be challenging to regulatory resources. In situations such as the use of illicit or addictive substances, levels of noncompliance are high enough to suggest a substantial failure of current regulatory strategy (MacCoun, 1993). People do indeed comply with the law in the presence of a legal authority, but the same people often revert to their prior behavior once that authority is absent (McCluskey, 2003).

If citizens fail to sufficiently obey legal restrictions, further intervention by legal authorities eventually will be required to obtain the desired level of compliance. Continued surveillance and enforcement are sometimes feasible. For example, smoking bans in workplaces or restaurants are enforceable because these are inherently social settings and behavior is monitored. Similarly, smoking on airplanes can easily be monitored by smoke detectors and enforced by flight attendants. In other cases, ranging from speeding to substance abuse, consistent oversight and enforcement have been more difficult. The problem may be in developing strategies of monitoring or enforcement—hidden behaviors may be difficult to detect, for example—or we may know how to monitor the behavior—speeding for instance—but lack the resources to maintain enforcement at a sufficiently high level to achieve deterrence.

There are two principal models for compliance or rule adherence. The first is deterrence theory, also referred to as a sanction-based or command-and-control model. The assumption underlying this theory is that we shape behavior by varying the risks associated with breaking rules, the gains associated with adherence, or both (see Chapter 5). The legal system attempts to project credible risks for wrongdoing. As any driver knows who has stopped talking on a cell phone as a patrol car came into view, rule adherence can be influenced by whether people perceive that rule breaking will be detected and punished.

It is sometimes possible to motivate compliance by creating a risk of punishment for non-adherence (a fine for smoking) or incentives for adherence (payment for exercising at the gym). Studies demonstrate, however, that regulating behavior through the use of threat serves to undermine people's commitment to norms, rules, and authorities (Frey, 1997, 1998; Frey & Oberholzer-Gee, 1997). This is an important deleterious side effect of a deterrence-based regulatory approach. From a motivational perspective, instrumental approaches such as deterrence are not self-sustaining and require the maintenance of institutions and authorities that can keep the probability of detection for behavior that threatens public health at a sufficiently high level to constantly motivate the public through external means (that is, the threat of punishment or provision of incentives). Over time it becomes more and more important to have such external constraints in place, as whatever intrinsic motivation people originally had is gradually "crowded out" by external concerns. In other words, the very behavior of surveillance creates the conditions requiring future surveillance.

Self-regulation offers an alternative to the deterrence model. Here people are seen as motivated to follow rules because their own values suggest to them that doing so is the appropriate action to take. Voluntary healthy behavior that is motivated by a person's own attitudes and values is superior from a regulatory perspective to behavior that has to be coerced. When values are the driver of behavior, rule adherence does not need to be sustained either by enacting a credible system of surveillance and sanctioning or by developing a way to incentivize desired behaviors.

The general legal question is how to motivate everyday adherence to legal rules, or self-regulation. The key issue is how to create and maintain values that motivate people to take personal responsibility for behaviors that promote the public's health (Tyler, 2006a, 2006b). A good deal of research in the legal arena indicates that self-regulatory motivations are activated when people believe that legal authorities are legitimate and they therefore have an obligation to conform to the law (Tyler, 2007, 2008). Consequently, people who identify with legal authorities and imbue the legal system with legitimacy will voluntarily abide by laws and defer to authorities (Darley, Tyler, & Bilz, 2003; Jost & Major, 2001; Tyler, 2006a; Tyler & Blader, 2000).

In the designing of laws, two issues need to be dealt with—norms and sanctions. The first is the creation of conditions that encourage the development of values (or norms) that support following the laws. This involves recognizing public feelings and building upon them. Law can easily be used to solidify existing norms and may also push norms forward. However, there may well be limits to how far forward law can push norms. For example, with prohibition in an earlier era and drug laws more recently the law has had difficulty legitimizing laws that criminalize behavior widely viewed by the public as being acceptable. Second, laws shape behavior by creating sanctions, that is, fines, jail, and so on, for noncompliance. These laws may encourage compliance but can also undermine intrinsic motivations for compliance, such as legitimacy. And more severe sanctions that seem excessive and inappropriate may have an especially negative influence upon internal motivation to obey the law.

Legitimacy

The issue of legitimacy is widely studied in the arena of law, and it is clear both that the legitimacy of legal authorities (for example health officials, police officers) and of the law itself shapes law-related behavior (Tyler, 2006b). Modern discussions of legitimacy are usually traced to the writings of Weber (1968) on authority and the social dynamics of authority (for example, Zelditch, 2001). Weber, like Machiavelli and others before him, argued that successful leaders and institutions do not rely solely or even primarily on brute force to execute their will. Rather, they strive to win the consent of the governed so that their commands will be voluntarily obeyed (Tyler, 2006a). Legitimacy, according to this general view, is a quality that is possessed by an authority, a law, or an institution that leads others to feel obligated to accept its directives. When people ascribe legitimacy to the system that governs them, they become willing subjects whose behavior is strongly influenced by official (and unofficial) doctrine. They also internalize a set of moral values that is consonant with the aims of the system (Jost & Major, 2001). Although the concept of legitimacy has not featured prominently in recent discussions of social regulation with respect to law-abiding behavior, there is a strong intellectual tradition that emphasizes the significance of developing and maintaining positive social values toward cultural, political, and legal authorities (Easton, 1965, 1975; Krislov, Boyum, Clark, Shaefer, & White, 1966; Melton, 1986; Parsons, 1967; Tapp & Levine, 1977).

A values-based perspective on human motivation therefore suggests the importance of developing and sustaining a civic culture in which people abide by the law because they feel that legal authorities are legitimate and ought to be obeyed. For this model to work, society must create and maintain public values that are conducive to following behavioral norms. Political scientists refer to this set of values as a "reservoir of support" for government and society (Dahl, 1956). Studies indicate that values shape rule following (Sunshine & Tyler, 2003a, 2003b; Tyler, 2006a, 2006b; Tyler & Fagan, 2008), and that the influence of values is stronger than the effect of risk estimates (Sunshine & Tyler, 2003a).

Some laws merely facilitate social coordination—for example, making sure that everyone drives on the same side of the road. In these instances, the particular form of appropriate behavior is not the key issue. Rather, the important thing is that people agree upon what is appropriate and behave accordingly. While the law enforces such rules, enforcement is not a major societal issue because people have little or no motivation to undermine or disobey such rules. There is very little to be gained by driving on the wrong side of the road. Similarly, some laws are directed at rare acts that are deemed inherently wrongful, such as murder or the adulteration of food. Most people don't intend to break these rules, and have no objection to deterring the few who do through harsh punishment and surveillance.

Legitimacy becomes more contested when the function of the law is to restrict behavior that is not seen as inherently wrongful, and may even offer benefits to the actor. The case for legal intervention in matters like this is traditionally strongest, and therefore most likely to seem legitimate, in situations in which behavior harms others directly. For example, the case for restricting smoking via law became more compelling when smoking was recognized to have second-hand effects. This recognition of harm to non-smokers legitimated the introduction of smoking bans in public places in ways that the harm of smoking to smokers was never able to do. The public reasoning is that people have the right to choose to harm their own health but they are not entitled to choose to harm others.

Many public health measures address harm to people other than the actor, but just as many are partially or primarily paternalistic—aimed at encouraging people to avoid harming themselves by making healthier choices. Paternalistic public health restrictions present an interesting case for legitimacy-oriented approaches to compliance. They regulate everyday personal activities, promoting desirable health-related behavior (exercise, healthy diet, safe sex) or discouraging undesirable behavior (overeating, smoking, and drinking in excess). Sometimes the behavior—smoking, drunk driving, unsafe sex—threatens harm to others, but often the person most immediately at risk of harm is the actor him or herself.

There is vigorous debate as to whether it is proper for government to interfere with individual choices that do not pose a risk to others (Epstein, 2003; Thaler & Sunstein, 2008). A convinced anti-paternalist may regard any such law as illegitimate, regardless of its good intentions or the severity of the risk to the actors. But even those who are prepared to accept some paternalism as a matter of principle (or who don't even think about the issue) may not share the health policy maker's sense of the risks of the behavior or the advantages of giving it up. Smoking, drinking, and eating are all things that people enjoy doing. Convincing them to change gratifying behaviors voluntarily is no easy task. Indeed, forcing them to change their own behavior against their will risks undermining the legitimacy of legal authority.

Interventions that merely provide information have limited effects. Despite the fact that people are the primary beneficiaries of their own better health, studies make clear that people often fail to engage in practices that ensure that health. This is true in terms of everyday life, in which people drink too much, use unhealthy drugs, have sex without protection, become obese, and smoke. Even with the benefit of simple guidance, such as the food pyramid developed by the United States Department of Agriculture, people do not conform to eating regimes intended to prevent or minimize health problems that are prevalent across the population.

The threat of punishment seems also to work poorly. Both practically and politically, many important health-related behaviors, such as overeating of unhealthy foods, are going to be hard to directly address through laws that punish those who engage in the behavior. People like high-fat foods, for example, and the food industry deploys huge resources to retain that support and forestall regulation. Even if there were widespread popular support for punishing those with unhealthy lifestyles, it would be hard to devise or enforce any suitable regulations. Problems of surveillance are likely to be particularly important, given that activities such as being a couch potato, snacking, and having sex tend to happen in the privacy of the home.

These factors predict that public health efforts to regulate unhealthy behaviors are likely to look similar in the future to how they have looked in the past. Activities that are seen as innately bad and dangerous to others will be prohibited. Paternalistic public health regulations that seek to motivate an individual to forego a short-term benefit in return for a long-term one will continue to rely more on "soft" regulatory techniques. These include warning and informational labels or signs, official guidelines, and attempts to make healthy behavior a default option. In a few cases, involving products that have been perceived to have a risk-utility profile akin to cigarettes—trans fats, to take a recent example— bans may be enacted. Similarly, "sin taxes" may on occasion be extended to new products, like sugar-sweetened beverages, to increase the incentive to avoid them. Getting support for these measures, and getting the desired level of compliance and behavioral change, will depend to a great degree upon the extent to which people either trust that the government's view of the risks and safe behavior is correct, or take the view that they ought to obey the law because it is the law—in other words, on legitimacy.

It is trust in the motivations and character of both legal and non-legal authorities (the U.S. Food and Drug Administration, the Centers for Disease Control and Prevention, the Surgeon General) and others in the public health system of regulation that matters most when everyday people as well as organizations responsible for healthy behaviors (for example schools, corporations) are trying to decide whether to accept the decisions and guidance of such authorities. People should not need to feel obligation to obey decisions that are in their own interest, but mistrust of the motivations of public health authorities may lead to suspicion about their recommendations and may undermine the willingness to follow their directives and advice. Therefore, people can be motivated to engage in healthy behaviors and not to engage in unhealthy behaviors by their feelings of responsibility and obligation to authorities (that is, by legitimacy).

The extension of a value-based model to public health and public health law suggests that public health laws and behavioral guidelines are most likely to gain compliance if they are perceived as legitimate. It is therefore important for public health authorities and institutions to consider the factors that shape their legitimacy—and important for health researchers to study them. Further, the role of law can be a facilitative one. If desirable practices for creating and sustaining legitimacy are identified, the legal system can create and implement structures for mandating those practices.

Procedural Justice

If public health authorities know that they can benefit from being viewed as legitimate they need evidence-based guidance as to how they can facilitate such public views. Studies suggest that legitimacy can be built through procedural fairness. Authorities can gain a great deal in terms of legitimacy when they follow clear norms of procedural justice, including impartiality, transparency, and respect for human dignity (Tyler, 2003). Thus implementing fair procedures as well as providing favorable or fair outcomes can provide a solid basis for establishing system legitimacy with public health authorities. Questions about the extent to which procedural justice is enacted by health authorities, and the effects procedural justice has on health behaviors, constitute an important agenda for public health law research. This section discusses some theoretical and methodological aspects of this agenda.

Elements of Procedural Justice

Procedural justice is the study of people's subjective evaluations of the justice of procedures—whether they are fair or unfair, ethical or unethical, and otherwise in accord with people's standards of fair processes for social interaction and decision making. Subjective procedural justice judgments have been the focus of a great deal of research attention by psychologists because they have been found to be a key influence on a wide variety of important group attitudes and behavior (Lind & Tyler, 1988; Tyler, 2000).

Procedural justice has been especially important in studies of decision acceptance and rule following, which are core areas of legal regulation. A central point for legal authorities is that people are responsive to evaluations of the fairness of procedures, even if authorities do not provide the outcomes people hoped for. Tyler and Huo (2002) for example, studied people's experiences with the police and courts. In the case of the police they found that the primary way that people had personal experiences with the police was by calling them for help. However, when people called the police for help, approximately 30 percent of the time they reported a negative outcome (that is, a problem not solved). So, in situations in which the police might want to help they are not always able to do so. Yet, in studies of the general population, people are found to regard the police as legitimate if they believe that the police exercise their authority through fair and impartial means (Sunshine & Tyler, 2003a; Tyler, 2006a). Indeed, the evidence suggests that procedural justice judgments are more central to judgments of legitimacy than are such factors as the perceived effectiveness of the police in combating crime. To the extent that people perceive law enforcement officials as legitimate, they are significantly more willing to comply with the law in general (Sunshine & Tyler, 2003a; Tyler, 2006a).

When people indicate that authorities are or are not procedurally fair, what do they mean? Recent discussions identify two key dimensions of procedural fairness judgments: fairness of decision making (voice, neutrality) and fairness of interpersonal treatment (trust, respect) (Blader & Tyler, 2003a, 2003b). Studies suggest that people are influenced by both of these aspects of procedural justice.

Procedures are mechanisms for making decisions. When thinking about those mechanisms, people evaluate fairness along several dimensions. First, do they have opportunities for input before decisions are made? Second, are decisions made following understandable and transparent rules? Third, are decision-making bodies acting neutrally, basing their decisions upon objective information and appropriate criteria, rather than acting out of personal prejudices and biases? Fourth, are the rules applied consistently across people and over time?

Quality of interpersonal treatment is found to be equally important. It involves the manner in which people are treated during a decision-making process. First, are people's rights respected; for example, do authorities follow the rules consistently and correctly? Second, is their right as a person to be treated politely and with dignity acknowledged, and does such treatment occur? Third, do authorities consider people's input when making decisions, and are decision makers concerned about people's needs and concerns when they make decisions? Finally, do authorities account for their actions by giving honest explanations about what they have decided and why they made their decisions? Do they make clear that they have considered people's arguments and why they can or cannot do as people want? Judgments about the character and motivation of the decision maker—issues of trust in the intentions of others—are conceptualized in the procedural justice literature as a distinct aspect of interpersonal treatment. So in the procedural justice literature trust in intentions (motive-based trust) is usually framed as being a component of procedural justice.

If people view as legitimate only those authorities who make decisions with which they agree, it would be difficult for authorities to maintain their legitimacy, insofar as they are required to make unpopular decisions and to deliver unfavorable outcomes. With state and local health authorities, for example, the effective practice of reducing chronic and fatal illnesses resulting from smoking or second-hand exposure to smoke has involved prohibiting the sale of tobacco products to minors. Mandating people to take actions that require effort, willpower, and potentially enduring pain, or at least lack of benefit, requires that those individuals have a basis for viewing the authority involved as someone who ought to be deferred to and accepted.

Tyler, Mentovich, and Satyavada (2011) examined the role of procedural justice in promoting deference to doctor's recommendations by interviewing patients about their own doctors. They found that the procedural justice of the doctor was a strong predictor of both believing that the doctor had a competent treatment plan and accepting his or her treatment recommendations. The quality of interpersonal treatment was found to be especially important. Further, patients who believe their doctor acted fairly were less likely to indicate that they wanted to change doctors.

Procedural Justice in Organizations

Recent research in organizational settings suggests a very promising direction for law in motivating healthy behaviors. Such research shows that the manner in which authority is exercised in organizations influences the way people within them feel about themselves, including shaping their feelings of self-esteem and self-worth (Tyler & Blader, 2000). These findings have developed within the psychological literature on procedural justice, but are of obvious relevance to health given the increasing recognition of the effect of workplace hierarchy on the health outcomes of employees (Commission on Social Determinants of Health, 2008).

Studies show that creating procedurally just organizations enhances the physical health of people within those organizations. In a laboratory study, Vermunt and Steensma (2003) examined the influence of procedural justice upon the level of stress participants experienced when involved in a difficult mental task. They used physiological measures of stress and found that fairness mitigated stress levels. Schmitt and Dorfel (1999) studied factory workers and found that procedural justice lowered psychosomatic problems (for example, sick days taken; days at work when the worker "felt sick"). In a similar study of workers in health centers in Finland, Elovainio, Kivimäki, Eccles, & Sinervo (2002) found that procedural justice lowered occupational strain. Meier, Semmer, and Hupfeld (2009) found that procedural justice in a sample of employees was linked to depressive mood among those with high but unstable self-esteem. Suurd (2009) found that procedural injustice was related to psychological strain in a sample of military personnel.

This connection between the procedural justice of organizations and stress among their members is strongly supported by a series of epidemiological studies. Kivimäki, Elovainio, Vahtera, Virtanen, & Stansfield (2003) studied a sample of 1,786 female hospital employees and found that low procedural justice was linked to higher levels of psychiatric disorders. Kivimäki, Ferrie, Head, and others (2004) studied 10,308 civil servants and found that procedural justice was related to self-reported health. Similarly, Liljegren and Ekberg (2009) found that procedural justice was related to self-reported health in a sample of Swedish workers. Kivimäki, Ferrie, Brunner, and others (2005) found that in a study of 6,442 British civil servants procedural justice was related to coronary health disease. Further, it has been found that procedural justice is linked to smoking, with those who feel unfairly treated 1.4 times as likely to be heavy smokers (Kouvonen, Vahtera, Elovainio, et al., 2007); to drinking, with the unfairly treated 1.2 times more likely to be heavy drinkers (Kouvonen, Kivimäki, Elovainio, et al., 2008); and to problems with sleeping at night (Heponiemi, Kouvonen, Vèanskèa, et al., 2008).

In light of the findings above, important questions emerge for public health law researchers in relation to how organizations can best promote fair procedures, what particular effects such procedures can have, and whether law should mandate justice within organizations. In their study of mandated justice, for example, Feldman and Tyler (2010) use a combined survey and experimental design that examined the influence of whether fair procedures in a work organization are the choice of management or the result of government-mandated

rights. Their findings suggest that government-mandated fair workplace procedures have a more positive impact on employees in terms of attitudes toward
the company and behavior in the workplace. New research is needed to produce evidence on whether mandated procedures have a direct impact on
employee health.

Researchers can also explore the question of whether voluntary corporate
efforts yield better results than mandated efforts. Research on "new governance"
has revealed less of an emphasis on formal legal regulation and more on the
voluntary efforts of both civic groups and market-driven business organizations
to create and maintain internal procedures for enforcing, among other things,
standards of ethics and social responsibility (Braithwaite, 2008; Gunningham,
2007; Lehmkuhl, 2008; Parker, 2002; Shamir, 2008). These new forms of governance highlight the importance of reconsidering the degree to which the state
should intervene directly within work organizations by mandating appropriate
procedures.

The literature on governance also highlights the idea that procedural justice
can occur in two ways. First, people can experience fair procedures when
policies are being created. Here the emphasis has been on community participation and allowing community input when policies are being created. Second,
the authorities involved in implementing policies can act fairly. It is not enough,
for example, to implement a smoking ban using fair procedures. Procedural
justice also involves allowing affected parties to participate in discussions
about whether there should be rules regulating smoking and what those rules
should be.

Measuring Legitimacy and Compliance

Tyler's central work on the concept of legitimacy and compliance and how to
measure them is his book titled *Why People Obey the Law* (2006a), which
explored the question of why people comply with the law and, in particular, why people cooperate with legal authorities. The research for this book
employed a large-scale questionnaire that was subject to a repeated pretesting
process in which people were interviewed using the instrument and then it was
rewritten (Tyler, 2009). The questionnaire was administered via telephone in
two waves, the first with a random sample of 1,575 Chicago residents and
the second with a random sample of 804 citizens who were reinterviewed one
year later.

This research was focused empirically on peoples' experiences with and
attitudes toward the police and the courts as well as peoples' compliance with
the law (see Tyler, 2006a, Appendix A). Many questions were designed to
measure the concept of fairness, such as the following:

Overall, how fair were the procedures used by the police to handle the situation when they stopped you? Were they:

__ Very fair

__ Somewhat fair

__ Somewhat unfair, or

__ Very unfair

__ Do not know [Tyler, 2006a, p. 180].

What emerged both during and after the research for *Why People Obey the Law* is that while having a fixed set of responses is helpful, it is also important not to have yes-or-no questions but rather to use scales so that there is variation in the responses obtained. For example, instead of soliciting a "yes" or "no" answer to the question of "Were the police dishonest," it's more useful for analytical purposes to ask "Would you say you 'agree strongly,' 'agree,' 'disagree,' or 'disagree strongly'?" Breaking scales up into smaller questions can help simplify the response format. For instance, the researcher could ask a question with one of two possible answers (for example, "Is the person honest or dishonest"), and then depending on that answer, ask a follow-up question with scales that measure levels of dishonesty (for example, "very dishonest," "somewhat dishonest") (Tyler, 2009).

Measuring compliance is also challenging and requires appropriate scaling. During the first wave of the Chicago study it became clear that people did not want to admit to illegal behavior. For example, when asked, "Have you taken inexpensive items from stores without paying for them," all 1,575 respondents indicated "never," suggesting that shoplifting never occurs. Therefore, scaling was introduced to the questionnaire for the second wave in order to capture not simply whether someone did something wrong or not, but rather if they broke the law "almost never" or "practically almost never," and so on.

Overall, measuring peoples' compliance behaviors through self-reporting is limited, but it nonetheless remains useful if no direct evidence of behaviors is available. Evidence of compliance behaviors provided by others, including legal authorities, is one way of compensating for this limitation (Tyler, 2009). Tyler, Sherman, Strang, Barnes, and Woods (2007), for example, have used police arrest data in recent research on compliance. Another common, useful technique is asking about one's friends or peers—"How many of your friends use heroin (or shoplift, and so on)?"—and use that indirect measure as an index of the person's own behavior or to more accurately estimate population prevalence. The idea is that when estimating what others are doing they use their own behavior as a guide. And because they are not being asked directly about themselves, self-presentation issues are less salient and responses are more accurate.

Mechanisms Through Which Law Affects Public Health

The roles of procedural justice and legitimacy as mechanisms through which law influences public health are captured in Figure 6.1. Path A captures the behavior of public health authorities toward citizens and groups in terms of the core dimensions of procedural justice (impartiality, transparency, respect, fairness). Such authorities may be individual agency personnel tasked with law enforcement or organizations that have the authority and responsibility to create and sustain healthy corporate environments for workers. Path B represents the legitimacy (obligation, trust, and confidence) of legal authorities, which flows from their procedurally just character, and with the existence of system legitimacy, people are motivated to comply with the law (path C).

The type of motivation captured here is internally driven and value-based (as opposed to instrumentally driven and based on the threat of punishment or the receipt of incentives). On the basis of this motivation, people comply with the law (path E), thereby undertaking the prescribed healthy behaviors (path G) that affect different public health outcomes (fewer deaths, fewer injuries, lower rates of communicable disease) (path I) depending on the area of intervention. We also reviewed studies pointing to the role of procedural justice, trust, and ultimately legitimacy in reducing stress (path D). Less stress can yield direct health benefits such as fewer psychiatric disorders (path H), and it can also lead to healthier behaviors including drinking less often (path F), which in turn contributes to population-level health outcomes (path I) such as lower death rates from impaired driving.

The various paths in this causal diagram point to areas of needed empirical research in the field of public health law. While the mechanisms discussed here are theoretically grounded in a range of empirical contexts, including compliance with criminal laws and the associated outcome of public safety, attention should be placed more squarely on factors shaping compliance with public health directives. The diagram presented here provides a framework for conceptualizing research questions in this area, ones that will require the development of

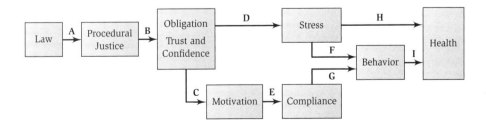

Figure 6.1. Procedural Justice Mechanisms Through Which Law Affects Public Health.

appropriate instruments for measuring peoples' experiences with, and attitudes toward, public health authorities.

Conclusion

This chapter has discussed the advantages of voluntary healthy behavior motivated by attitudes and values over behavior that has to be coerced. Self-regulation is activated when people believe that legal authorities are legitimate, but in public health law such legitimacy cannot be assumed. Many public health directives are paternalistic, asking individuals to change behaviors that are personally gratifying and that may pose no direct threat to the health of others. Regardless of the scientific evidence behind such directives, gaining compliance with them requires legitimacy. Therefore, failure to build legitimacy not only undermines compliance with a particular law but risks undermining the overall legitimacy of the public health system of regulation and advice.

Research on compliance has shown that legal authorities can gain a great deal in terms of legitimacy when they follow clear norms of procedural justice, including impartiality, transparency, and respect for human dignity (Tyler, 2003). Questions about the role of procedural justice in shaping system legitimacy warrant greater attention in public health law research, as do questions about the effects of legitimacy on health behaviors. Public health agencies can attend to procedural fairness and legitimacy not only in the actual enforcement of the law but also in the formulation of behavioral guidance (such as recommended vaccination schedules). The logic model presented here offers a framework for studying law's effect on public health through the mechanisms of procedural justice and legitimacy.

The most relevant empirical evidence on procedural justice as a mechanism for shaping health behaviors comes from organizational settings. A number of studies show that creating procedurally just organizations enhances the physical and mental health of people within those organizations. A key question for public health law research is whether government should mandate the use of fair procedures and the creation of a climate of ethicality in an effort to produce desirable health outcomes.

In summary, the law can shape health-related behavior through providing incentives for healthy behavior and punishments for unhealthy behavior. However, the argument we are making, drawing upon the literature on self-regulation, is that the best approach is to promote favorable attitudes and values, changing what people feel they should do with respect to their health behaviors. This involves creating trust and confidence in health authorities. How precisely this should be done in relation to various health behaviors is an important area of empirical inquiry.

Summary

The effectiveness of behavioral regulation depends in significant part on the willingness of citizens to consent to the commands of legal authorities and to actively cooperate with them. Two values constituting what sociologist Max Weber called "legitimacy" are of particular importance to compliance: the individual's sense of obligation to obey authorities, and his or her sense of trust and confidence in legal authorities. While it is sometimes possible to motivate compliance by creating a risk of punishment for non-compliance, regulating behavior through threats can undermine people's own commitment to norms, rules, and authorities. Voluntary healthy behavior that is motivated by a person's own attitudes and values is superior from a regulatory perspective to behavior that has to be coerced. When values are the driver of behavior, rule adherence does not need to be sustained either by enacting a credible system of surveillance and sanctioning or by developing a way to incentivize desired behaviors.

Legitimacy is a quality that is possessed by an authority, a law, or an institution that leads others to feel obligated to accept its directives. Self-regulatory motivations are activated when people believe that legal authorities are legitimate and they therefore have an obligation to conform to the law, and when people have trust and confidence in those authorities. People who identify with legal authorities and imbue the legal system with legitimacy will voluntarily abide by laws and defer to authorities. Legitimacy can be built through procedural fairness. Procedural justice is the study of people's subjective evaluations of the justice of procedures—whether they are fair or unfair, ethical or unethical, and otherwise in accord with people's standards of fair processes for social interaction and decision making. The two key dimensions of procedural fairness judgments are fairness of decision making (voice, neutrality) and fairness of interpersonal treatment (trust, respect). Robust tools have been developed to measure procedural justice and have been used in important health research.

Further Reading

Sunshine, J., & Tyler, T. R. (2003a). The role of procedural justice and legitimacy in shaping public support for policing. *Law & Society Review, 37*(3), 513–548.

Tyler, T. R. (2006a). *Why people obey the law*. Princeton, NJ: Princeton University Press.

Weber, M. (1968). *Economy and society*. Berkeley: University of California Press.

Chapter 7

Economic Theory

Frank J. Chaloupka

Learning Objectives

- Identify how economic theory intersects with public health law.
- Evaluate effects of economic incentives and disincentives on public health outcomes.
- Examine information failure, externalities, internalities, and market power as they affect a public health problem.

Economics is the study of how society allocates scarce resources. Economic players interact through the supply of and demand for various goods and services. A key assumption of modern economic theory is that individuals are seeking to maximize their own well-being subject to the constraints they face. Individual consumers aim to maximize the satisfaction ("utility," in the language of economics) they gain from consuming, subject to the prices they face for goods and services in the market, time constraints, and their own incomes and wealth. Producers aim to maximize the profits they receive from supplying goods and services to the market, subject to the costs of inputs into production, available production technologies, and demand for the products they produce. Under ideal conditions, the result of economic players acting to maximize their own well-being in freely operating markets will be an efficient allocation of scarce resources. When markets are not operating under ideal conditions, laws and regulations can change the relative costs and benefits that influence decisions consumers and producers make and, as a result, lead to an allocation of resources improved from that which would result from unregulated markets.

If the market is operating under ideal conditions, laws and regulations will result in a less optimal allocation of resources compared to that which would result from the free market.

Economics, law, and public health intersect because many markets do not operate under ideal conditions. Instead, there are a variety of "market failures" that lead to an inefficient allocation of resources in a way that creates public health consequences. Economic agents are assumed to have full information and to act rationally when making decisions. However, information about the short- and long-term costs and benefits of consuming or producing some products is often limited, and individuals make choices they later regret. The full costs of consuming or producing are often not borne by those making the consumption or production decisions (negative externalities). Conversely, consumption or production of some goods or services generates benefits that go beyond the individual consumer or producer (positive externalities). Producers facing limited competition will likely supply less of a good to the market and charge more for it than would be optimal from a societal perspective. When such market failures exist, the changes in consumption decisions, production decisions, or both that result from laws and regulations can lead to a more optimal allocation of resources than would result from the free market.

The public health consequences that result from market failures are enormous. Almost half of all deaths in the United States are the result of modifiable behaviors, including tobacco use, poor diets and physical inactivity, alcohol and other drug use, unhealthy sexual activity, and violence (Mokdad, Marks, Stroup, & Gerberding, 2004, 2005). Over the past few decades, health economists have made substantial contributions to our understanding of how laws, regulations, and other policies can address market failures in order to improve public health. This chapter provides an introduction to the concepts used by economists in this research. It begins by providing a discussion of the economic rationale for government intervention in a variety of markets in which individual behaviors lead to public health consequences. This is followed by a discussion of policy interventions that address these market failures, beginning with demand-side approaches to promoting public health through legal interventions and emphasizing the concept of the "full price" of consumption. Legal approaches to addressing the supply side of these markets are then briefly reviewed. The last section summarizes and provides some concluding comments. Examples of where economic theory and research has helped inform public health law are provided throughout.

Laws, Regulations, and Economic Behavior

Homo Economicus, the informed, rational, and self-interested "economic man," is at the heart of much of classical economic theory (Persky, 1995). By seeking to maximize his own self-interest subject to constraints around him, his interactions with other economic men will lead to the efficient allocation of society's scarce resources.

Laws and regulations will alter the conditions under which economic man makes these decisions, as illustrated in Figure 7.1. Law can change the information environment by mandating more information of a particular kind or by restricting the flow of other information. Laws can require that the contents of particular products are listed on product packaging, while others can require that packages include warnings about the consequences of consumption. Mass-media and other public education campaigns provide information that can alter consumers' perceptions of the relative costs and benefits they receive from consuming a given product, resulting in different consumption choices. Other policies can restrict producers from conveying information by limiting the content of or channels through which they advertise their products or how these products are labeled.

Laws and regulations can enhance or constrain the market power of producers or consumers. Antitrust laws aim to prevent producers from gaining

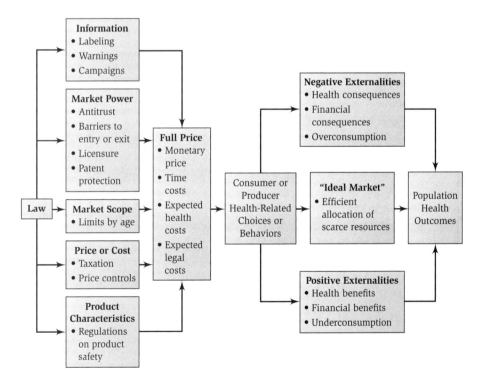

Figure 7.1. How Economic Factors Affect Population Health.

significant market power or abusing the market power that they do have. At the same time, collective bargaining laws allow unions to gain market power that enables them to offset the "monopsony" power that large firms have. By erecting entry barriers that reduce the number of firms in a given market, policies can increase market power for those that are operating in the market. Licensure requirements that establish density standards, for example, will limit the number of firms in a given market, reducing competition from potential entrants and generating market power for those with licenses. In many countries, governments monopolize a variety of product markets. Exclusive territory policies provide market power within a given geographic area while limiting the ability of firms to compete outside of that area.

The scope of a particular market is something else that can be changed by laws and regulations. Laws can prohibit some from participating in given markets by setting minimum age requirements for purchase or use of particular products. Likewise, labor laws may set minimum and maximum ages for workers in particular fields. Laws and regulations can also alter the characteristics of a product. Some may prohibit various ingredients, while others may mandate certain product safety features.

Finally, laws and regulations can directly alter the prices of a product or key inputs into the production of that product, or can affect the costs associated with consuming that product. Excise taxes add to the price consumers pay for particular products, while subsidies reduce prices. Minimum wage laws raise the labor costs faced by firms, while rent control laws limit the price received by property owners. Tax credits for education reduce the costs of schooling for students and their families. Minimum price laws or bans on quantity discounts raise consumer prices.

That resources will be optimally allocated by the interactions of unfettered supply and demand depends on several key assumptions: that individuals have the information that they need to make fully informed choices; that they fully understand and can adequately process this information; that they behave rationally, weighing the short- and the long-run costs and benefits of their decisions; that the individual consumer bears the full costs and receives the full benefits of his or her consumption; that the individual producer likewise bears the full costs and gains the full benefits of producing; and that neither the producer nor the consumer has market power that allows them to influence prices.

Market Failures

Economists refer to situations in which one or more of these key assumptions are violated as market failures, which result in an inefficient allocation of resources. This is where economics, law, and public health intersect. While laws and regulations are adopted for a variety of reasons, the existence of market failures provides an economic rationale for governments to adopt policies that change the outcomes that would result from a free market. Examples of these market failures and key legal mechanisms for addressing them are described in the following sections.

Information Failures

One market failure that generates considerable public health consequences is imperfect or asymmetric information regarding the health risks that result from consuming a variety of products. Perhaps the clearest example is cigarette smoking. Cigarette smoking in the United States rose rapidly in the first half of the twentieth century and, given the lags between onset of smoking and onset of lung cancer and other diseases caused by smoking, it wasn't until the 1950s that strong evidence linking cigarette smoking to lung cancer first appeared in the scientific literature. Consequently, individuals made decisions to smoke with far from full information about the health risks from smoking. In the decades since, the evidence linking cigarette smoking to an ever-increasing number of diseases has grown, but many individuals continue to underestimate this risk, particularly in low- and middle-income countries. Moreover, many of those who have a general appreciation of these population risks fail to adequately internalize the threat to their own health.

This information failure has been further complicated by information asymmetries among consumers and producers. The release of millions of pages of internal tobacco company documents in various lawsuits provided clear evidence that cigarette companies were aware of these risks and altered product design in a way that alleviated consumers' health concerns while failing to significantly reduce or eliminate these risks. Filtered low tar and nicotine cigarettes were marketed as less harmful but were, in fact, as deadly as the cigarettes that they replaced. Despite the increasing scientific evidence to this effect, many smokers continue to see these as less harmful than full-flavored cigarettes.

Market failures due to imperfect or asymmetric information are further complicated in many markets by the fact that initiation of use for many of these products begins in childhood or adolescence, a time when many are prone to heavily discount the short- and long-term health consequences that result from consumption. For example, despite the information provided in school-based substance abuse prevention classes and through other sources, significant proportions of U.S. eighth grade students do not report "great risk" from using marijuana regularly (32 percent), taking LSD regularly (61.4 percent), taking ecstasy occasionally (55.0 percent), having five or more drinks once or twice each weekend (42.8 percent), or smoking one or more packs of cigarettes daily (39.1 percent) (Meyer, 2010).

This discounting of risk among young people is even further complicated by an under-appreciation of the addictiveness or habitualness of the use of harmful products. Orphanides and Zervos (1995) provide a nice theoretical framework for how "imperfect foresight" can result in many youths experimenting with addictive substances, with some becoming addicted. In their model, the risk of becoming addicted varies among individuals, as do each individual's subjective beliefs about his or her potential to become addicted. As an individual experiments with substance use, this subjective belief is updated through a Bayesian learning process. Those who underestimate their potential for addiction can end up addicted. Thus, rather than the "happy addict" implied by economic models that assume well-informed individuals making rational decisions with perfect foresight (Winston, 1980), addicted individuals regret ever having started. Empirical evidence is consistent with this type of "learning and regret," with considerable majorities of adult smokers, for example, wishing that they had never started smoking (Fong, Hammond, Laux, et al., 2004). Similarly, while only 3 percent of those smoking daily as high school seniors thought that they would definitely be smoking in five years, almost two-thirds were still smoking seven to nine years later (Johnston, O'Malley, Bachman, & Schulenberg, 2011).

Externalities

Externalities occur when individual consumers or producers do not bear the full costs of their consumption or production (negative externalities) or when there are benefits from consumption or production that go beyond the individual consumer or producer (positive externalities). From a societal perspective, when externalities exist, economic agents left to their own devices will generate an inefficient allocation of resources. The inefficiencies that arise in the presence of various externalities create public health consequences.

When there are negative externalities in consumption, there are costs that result from consumption that are not borne by the individual consumer, resulting in greater-than-optimal consumption at a lower-than-optimal price. There are countless examples of negative externalities that generate sizable public health consequences, from lung cancers, cardiovascular diseases, and other adverse health effects non-smokers experience when exposed to tobacco smoke pollution to violence caused by alcohol and drug abuse that kills or injures innocent bystanders. Similarly, when there are negative externalities in production, there are costs to society that are not reflected in the costs paid by producers that result in overproduction and lower-than-optimal market prices. Perhaps the best example of a negative externality in production is the air and water pollution that results from emissions or discharges during production that causes numerous health consequences among those exposed to various toxins.

Alternatively, positive externalities in consumption imply that persons other than the individual consumer of a given good or service benefit from that consumption. Positive externalities in consumption lead to under-consumption of a product. One example of a positive externality in consumption is the reduction in the risk of infectious disease to others that results from an individual receiving a vaccination for that disease. Thus the benefits to society are considerably larger than those to the individual. Positive externalities in production occur when a producer does not receive the full benefit of production, resulting in less-than-optimal output at a higher-than-optimal price. Pharmaceutical drugs that reduce the public health burden caused by numerous diseases provide examples of positive externalities in production. A pharmaceutical company concerned that the substantial investment it needs to make in developing a new drug would not be recouped if its competitors could easily copy and market the drug once it hit the market will under-invest in research and development, leading to fewer such drugs being supplied.

Health behaviors that create significant public health consequences can also generate sizable financial externalities. There are many estimates of the economic costs of behaviors such as cigarette smoking, excessive alcohol use, and illicit drug use, as well as of the obesity that results from poor diets and physical inactivity. Centers for Disease Control and Prevention (2008), for example, estimates that cigarette smoking resulted in average annual health care costs of $96 billion over the period from 2001 through 2004, while smoking-attributable productivity losses amounted to an additional $96.8 billion each year.

While many in the public health community focus on the overall economic costs that result from various health behaviors, economists generally distinguish between internal costs (those borne by individual consumers) and external costs (those borne by others). This distinction has important implications for policy. For example, smokers' higher health insurance premiums, greater out-of-pocket costs, and lower wages, at least for the most part, do not constitute a market failure but rather reflect the increased health risks they incur by smoking, their greater use of health care, and the lost productivity that results from the increased absences resulting from diseases caused by smoking. Financial externalities are limited to the lost productivity and costs of treating the consequences of exposure to tobacco smoke pollution among non-smokers and the costs of treating smoking-attributable diseases in smokers that are paid for through public health insurance programs. Some economists have gone further to look at net external costs, offsetting the increased costs at a point in time with the reductions in social security payments and Medicare spending that result from smokers dying younger than non-smokers (for example, Manning, 1991).

Internalities

More recent economic models have incorporated the experimental evidence from behavioral economics in models that imply that much of what have traditionally been considered internal costs are more appropriately treated as external costs (for example, Gruber & Kőszegi, 2008). These "internalities" result from the time inconsistency inherent in individual's preferences. Traditional models assume that individuals exponentially discount the future costs and benefits of their consumption decisions, implying that their decisions will be consistent over time. Behavioral economic experiments, however, demonstrate that preferences are not consistent over time and that individuals are conflicted between their desire for short-run gratification and their recognition of long-term consequences. These more recent models allow for hyperbolic discounting of future costs and benefits, producing a more accurate depiction of how individuals actually behave and capturing the conflict between short-run gratification and long-run regret reflected in many health behaviors. In these models, the long-run consequences to the individual that result from unhealthy choices in the short run can be viewed as external to that individual's future self. This new approach has significant implications for public health policies in that it implies greater scope for government intervention than implied by traditional models. For example, Gruber and Kőszegi (2008) show that on the basis of this approach optimal cigarette taxes could be twenty or more times higher than they would be using traditional economic models.

Market Power

Economists consider perfectly competitive markets to be optimal in that these lead to the most efficient allocation of resources—one in which the marginal benefits from consuming are equated to the marginal costs of producing. When producers are faced with more limited competition, they are said to have market power. This market power allows them to charge higher prices than would result in a more competitive market, while less is produced and consumed.

While ideal in theory, perfectly competitive markets rarely exist in the real world; some degree of market power is inevitable, and the extent of this market power can have public health implications. For example, in the pharmaceutical industry, some have argued that the branding of prescription drugs and the extensive direct-to-consumer marketing of these drugs results in a market failure by creating perceptions among consumers that comparable, less costly generic drugs are not a good substitute for the branded drug (for example, Institute of Medicine Committee on the Assessment of the U. S. Drug Safety System, Baciu, Stratton, & Burke, 2007).

Policy Interventions to Address Market Failures

When considering laws and other policies that would reduce the public health consequences of market failures such as those just described, economists distinguish between "first best" and "second best" interventions (Jha, Musgrove, Chaloupka, & Yurekli, 2000). First-best interventions are those that narrowly target the market failure at issue and do not have broader effects. For example, mandating nutrition labeling on packaged foods and beverages is a way of providing consumers with information to make better, informed choices on the basis of a product's caloric, fat, and nutrient content.

However, a one-to-one correspondence between market failures and interventions does not always exist, or sometimes the first-best intervention that does exist fails to reach key populations. In these cases, second-best interventions, which typically take a blunter approach and have broader impact, may be more effective. Policies such as taxes and subsidies that alter prices of healthier and less healthy options are perhaps the best examples of a highly effective, second-best intervention.

Laws, regulations, and other policies targeting market failures that generate significant public health consequences address failures that occur on both the demand side and the supply side of the market. This section provides an overview of key policy domains and provides examples in which economic research has played an important role in policy development and implementation.

Demand-Side Policies

When it comes to public health laws that target the demand side of the market, economists emphasize the concept of full price as the mechanism through which these policies influence health-related behaviors and their consequences. Full price includes not just the monetary cost of a product but also the other costs associated with obtaining and using that product. Particularly important among these other costs are time costs and the potential health and legal consequences of consumption.

Excise Taxes

In *An Inquiry into the Nature and Causes of the Wealth of Nations*, the father of modern economics Adam Smith (1776) wrote, "Sugar, rum, and tobacco are commodities which are nowhere necessaries of life, which are become objects of almost universal consumption, and which are therefore extremely proper subjects of taxation." Smith was focused on the revenue-generating potential of taxes, but in recent years it has become clear that taxes are also a highly effective policy for improving public health. Pigou (1962) was the first to suggest that levying taxes on products that generated negative externalities in consumption would improve economic efficiency. However, conventional wisdom long held that consumption of harmful, addictive substances such as tobacco, alcohol, and other drugs would be unresponsive to the changes in prices resulting from taxes and other factors. Extensive economic research conducted over the past few decades, however, clearly demonstrates that higher taxes and prices lead to significant improvements in public health by reducing the use of harmful products. Given the huge public health burden it causes, much of the economic research has focused on cigarette smoking and other tobacco use, showing that higher tobacco product taxes and prices lead adult tobacco users to quit, keep former users from restarting, prevent initiation and uptake among young people, and lead to reductions in consumption by those who continue to consume (International Agency for Research on Cancer [IARC] & World Health Organization, 2011). The impact of higher taxes and prices on overall cigarette smoking in the United States over the past several decades is illustrated in Figure 7.2.

Several studies go further in showing that higher tobacco taxes, because of declines in tobacco use that result from them, lead to reductions in the public health and economic consequences of tobacco use (IARC & World Health Organization, 2011). The extensive evidence base demonstrating the effectiveness of tobacco taxes in reducing tobacco use has contributed to nearly every state and the federal government increasing their cigarette and other tobacco taxes over the past two decades, with average state cigarette taxes rising nearly fivefold since 1990, while the federal tax has increased more than sixfold.

Similarly, numerous studies have found that increases in alcoholic beverage prices that result from higher alcoholic beverage excise taxes reduce the prevalence, frequency, and intensity of drinking (Cook, 2007; Wagenaar, Salois, & Komro, 2009). Additional research shows that higher taxes and prices improve public health by reducing the consequences of excessive alcohol use, including motor vehicle traffic crashes and other injuries, liver cirrhosis and other alcohol-attributable mortality, violence and other crime, and risky sex and sexually transmitted disease rates (Wagenaar, Tobler, & Komro, 2010; Xu & Chaloupka, 2011). Despite this evidence and in contrast to the sharp rise in tobacco taxes observed over the past two decades, average alcoholic beverage taxes have declined after accounting for inflation, contributing to increases in drinking and its consequences (Xu & Chaloupka, 2011).

The public health success with tobacco excise taxes, coupled with increased recognition of the obesity epidemic in the United States, has increased interest in using taxes as a policy tool for improving diet by reducing consumption of high-calorie, low-nutrient-density foods and beverages. Much of the debate to date has focused on sugar-sweetened beverages, given their relatively high levels of consumption, evidence that their consumption contributes to weight

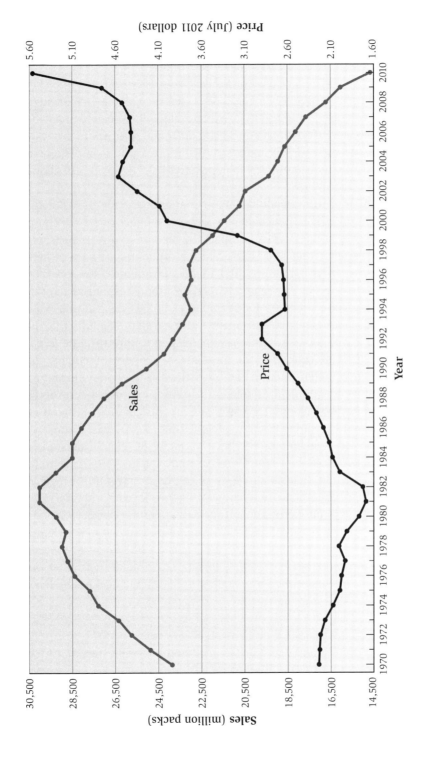

Figure 7.2. Cigarette Prices and Cigarette Sales, United States, 1970–2010.

Source: Tax Burden on Tobacco, Bureau of Labor Statistics, and author's calculations.

gain, their low or no nutritional value, and economic research demonstrating that beverage consumption responds to price (Chaloupka, Powell, & Chriqui, 2011). Currently, most states tax these beverages under their sales tax systems, with a few states levying small excise or similar taxes. However, existing taxes are small, and sugar-sweetened beverages are taxed the same as artificially or unsweetened beverages. As a result, existing economic research finds that existing taxes have little to no impact on weight outcomes; estimates from some studies, however, do indicate that more significant taxes (for example, one or two cents per ounce) would likely lead to population-level reductions in obesity (Powell & Chriqui, 2011).

Studies of tobacco and alcohol demand that account for the addictive aspects of consumption conclude that the long-run impact of tax and price increases is greater than the short-run impact. In general, and consistent with economic theory, studies that have looked at the differential impact of taxes and prices on population subgroups find that young people, less-educated populations, and those on low incomes are relatively more responsive to price. With respect to cigarette smoking, for example, estimates suggest that youth smoking is two to three times more sensitive to price than is adult smoking. The finding that lower socioeconomic groups respond more to price is particularly important in the context of the more recent economic modeling that allows for time-inconsistent preferences described earlier. Specifically, it implies that low-income populations benefit the most from the self-control that results from higher taxes so that these taxes are progressive, rather than regressive as implied by conventional models (Gruber & Kőszegi, 2008).

Finally, nearly all estimates of the price elasticity of overall demand for tobacco products, alcoholic beverages, and sugar-sweetened beverages indicate that demand is in the inelastic range, implying that a given price increase leads to a less-than-proportional reduction in aggregate consumption. This, combined with the fact that taxes account for only a portion of prices, implies that increases in taxes on these products will generate significant new revenues in the short-to-medium term. Some states, particularly with respect to tobacco, have earmarked a portion of tax revenues to support some of their other prevention, treatment, and control efforts, adding to the public health benefits of higher taxes.

SUBSIDIES

Increasing the consumption of products that improve public health can be accomplished by reducing prices of these products through subsidies. Given costs associated with their implementation however, subsidies to promote healthier behaviors have not been as widely used as taxes have been to discourage unhealthy consumption. Nevertheless, some governments do use subsidies in an effort to promote public health, typically targeting them to narrow segments of the population. Perhaps the best examples are the various food assistance programs run by the U.S. Department of Agriculture aimed at preventing food insecurity and its consequences, including the Supplemental Nutrition Assistance Program (SNAP); the Special Supplemental Nutrition Program for Women, Infants, and Children (WIC); and the National School Lunch and Breakfast Programs. More recently, in efforts to promote healthier diets and curb obesity, some states and localities have begun experimenting with additional subsidies within these programs that further lower the prices of fruits, vegetables, and other healthier options. Limited economic research indicates that reductions in the prices of fruits and vegetables lead to increases in their consumption and at the same time result in healthier weight outcomes in at least some populations, suggesting that efforts to expand these subsidies may be an effective approach for reducing obesity (Powell & Chriqui, 2011).

Experimental evidence, however, raises some questions about the effectiveness of subsidies, particularly relative to taxation, as a means to improve diet and reduce obesity. Using an experimental grocery store selling widely purchased foods and beverages, Epstein and colleagues (2010) found that taxing less-healthy products led to reductions in purchases of these products, overall calories purchased, and proportion of fat purchased. In contrast, subsidies on healthier products, while increasing purchases of these products, led to increased purchases of less-healthy products as well, resulting in an increase in overall calories purchased while not improving the overall nutrient composition of foods purchased, suggesting that subsidies would be ineffective in reducing obesity. While a clearly artificial setting that forced participants to spend the savings they accrued on the subsidized product on other items in the experimental store rather than on other necessities, this does suggest that subsidies will likely have a smaller overall effect than taxes, given the income effect created by the subsidy.

Tax Credits and Deductions

Income tax credits and deductions are another tax policy that can be used to reduce the price of healthy behaviors in a way that promotes public health. For example, a recent paper by von Tigerstrom and colleagues (2011) describes the national and provincial income tax credits introduced in Canada that are designed to promote physical activity. Credits are provided that offset the costs of enrolling in various organized physical fitness, sports, and other recreational programs, as well as for the costs of public transit. While little empirical evidence exists on effects of these credits, the authors nicely describe why such credits are unlikely to have population-level effects on activity and obesity. Among the factors they note are the lag of a year or more between the time when costs are incurred and the benefit is received, the modest size of the credit relative to the costs of the programs it covers, the likelihood that it will be largely taken advantage of by those already enrolled in programs rather than increasing participation in these programs, and the likelihood that many new program participants will simply be substituting from other forms of physical activity to activity in programs covered by the tax credit.

OTHER PRICING POLICIES

Governments have a variety of other policy options for manipulating prices in a way that promotes public health. Many states, for example, have adopted laws setting a minimum retail price for cigarettes (Centers for Disease Control and Prevention, 2010). If the minimum price were set higher than the prices that would otherwise result from a freely operating market, cigarette smoking and its consequences could be reduced. In practice, however, these laws appear to have little impact on cigarette prices, with prices in the states that have adopted them similar to prices in states without them, after accounting for differences in state cigarette taxes. The one exception is in the handful of states that include price promotions in their policies, keeping price-reducing promotions from lowering the price below the minimum.

Similarly, as a part of the three-tier system states adopted for alcohol distribution following the repeal of prohibition, a number of states implemented policies setting minimum prices or requiring minimum markups on alcoholic beverages at various points in the distribution chain, while others banned quantity discounts at the wholesale level. One result of these policies is higher retail prices for alcoholic beverages which, given the evidence discussed, will result in reductions in harmful drinking and its consequences (Chaloupka, 2004). These policies, however, have come under increasing attack in recent years, given the limits they place on competition, with some states repealing them and court rulings in others invalidating them.

Policies like these, while indirectly raising prices and reducing consumption of targeted products, are likely to have less of an impact than tax policies that directly increase prices. The revenue generated from tax increases goes to governments, some of which use these revenues to support programs that add to the public health benefits of the tax. In contrast, policies that set higher-than-free-market-level prices generate additional profits for those involved in manufacturing and distribution of those products. These additional profits can be used to support increased marketing and other efforts that increase demand, partially offsetting the reductions in consumption that result from the higher prices.

TIME COSTS

Policies that raise the full price of consumption by adding time or inconvenience can similarly reduce consumption in a way that improves public health. For example, comprehensive smoke-free policies that ban smoking in private workplaces increase the cost of smoking by requiring smokers to leave their workplace and go outdoors to smoke, adding both time and inconvenience, particularly in inclement weather. Growing evidence clearly shows that comprehensive smoke-free policies are effective in reducing both adult and youth smoking, while at the same time reducing non-smokers' exposure to tobacco smoke pollution, directly addressing one of the externalities caused by smoking (IARC & World Health Organization, 2009).

PERCEIVED HEALTH COSTS

As discussed earlier, imperfect or asymmetric information creates a market failure that can have a negative affect on public health. Governments can address information failures by adopting policies that disseminate information on the health impact of various products or behaviors or by limiting producers' ability to spread such information. Some of these options are highly cost-effective, given their low cost of implementation and broad reach. Others are costly but still cost-effective, given the impact of the information on behavior. Still others have proven to be relatively cost-ineffective, given their high costs and lack of demonstrated effect. How effective and cost-effective these information interventions are depends on the type of information provided, the channels used to provide that information, and the audience being targeted.

Mandating the provision of information on product packaging, advertising, or elsewhere is one relatively low-cost approach to addressing information failures. For example, requiring health warning labels on all cigarette packages provides information about the harms that can result from smoking. In the United States, however, these labels have had little or no impact on smoking, given that the labels are not that visible and the information provided on them is relatively well known. International experiences, however, provide more support for the potential of pack warnings to reduce smoking. The International Tobacco Control Policy Evaluation Project's (ITCPEP) (2009) recent review of the evidence on warning labels produced several clear conclusions, including that pictorial warning labels are more effective than text-only warnings in raising and sustaining awareness about the risks of tobacco use; larger and more comprehensive (for example, more rotating messages) warning labels increase knowledge about the harms from tobacco use; and pictorial warnings increase motivation to quit, including strengthening quit intentions and increasing the likelihood of a quit attempt. Larger, graphic warning labels of this type will soon be coming to the United States as a result of a mandate by the Food and Drug Administration (FDA).

Alternatively, governments can limit the provision of potentially misleading information that leads to reduced risk perceptions. For example, there is considerable evidence that the use of misleading descriptors on tobacco product packaging and advertising (for example, light, low tar, mild) leads some users to perceive some products as less harmful to health or less addictive than others, and to view these products as alternatives to quitting. The FDA recently implemented a ban on the use of these descriptors in the United States. However, such bans may not go far enough, as tobacco companies have adapted to the ban on descriptors by using colors in their product names or packaging to suggest similar concepts, leading some tobacco control professionals to call for "plain" or "generic" packaging that would eliminate all brand-related imagery.

Governments can go further and limit or prohibit a variety of advertising and other marketing efforts that can similarly distort risk perceptions, although how far such policies can go is questionable, given First Amendment protections of free speech, which have been expanded by the courts in recent years to include commercial speech. To date, most such efforts have been voluntary, industry-initiated limits that aim to reduce children's exposure, such as the Children's Food and Beverage Advertising Initiative (CFBAI) that aims to reduce television advertising of less healthy foods and beverages during children's programming. Given the narrow focus of the CFBAI on children's programming, there has been little improvement in the nutritional quality of the products youth are seeing advertised on television, suggesting that such voluntary initiatives have little public health impact (Powell, Schermbeck, Szczypka, Chaloupka, & Braunschweig, 2011).

Alternatively, public education campaigns can be implemented to raise awareness of the harms from consumption of tobacco, alcohol, other drugs, and other products, or to raise awareness of the benefits of healthier behaviors such as physical activity. These can take many forms, from school-based education programs aimed at influencing youth behavior to large-scale, mass-media campaigns that target broader audiences and that can influence social norms. A mix of such efforts has been widely implemented for tobacco, with comparable, albeit more limited efforts targeting other health behaviors. Evidence is mixed with respect to the effectiveness of school-based programs in promoting healthier youth behavior. For example, Thomas and Perera's (2006) comprehensive review of school-based tobacco education programs found that some programs had short-term but not sustained effects and that the largest and most rigorous intervention reviewed produced no evidence of a long-term impact on smoking behavior. School-based programs that have been found to be successful in the short term tend to emphasize the role of social influences and to develop skills to resist these influences; such programs are most effective when implemented as part of a more comprehensive strategy that includes control policies and broader education efforts. In contrast, mass-media campaigns that use a variety of communications channels (including television, radio, print, billboards, and the Internet) have repeatedly been shown to reduce tobacco use (National Cancer Institute [NCI], 2008).

EXPECTED LEGAL COSTS

Policies that raise the expected legal costs of engaging in a particular behavior will add to full price, reducing the likelihood and frequency of engaging in that behavior. Economic theories of crime emphasize two key factors that influence expected legal costs: the probability of being caught and convicted and the swiftness and severity of the penalty imposed. Increasing either factor raises the expected legal costs and, as a result, reduces targeted behaviors and their public health consequences.

Policies targeting drinking and driving are good examples of laws that raise anticipated legal costs in a way that promotes public health and that addresses the related negative externalities. Policies implementing sobriety checkpoints and breath testing and other efforts to detect drunk drivers raise the probability of detection, while lowered *per se* illegal blood alcohol content laws increase the probability of conviction. Policies that specify mandatory minimum fines or jail terms can raise expected penalties, while administrative license revocations increase the swiftness of the penalty. Extensive research by economists and other social scientists has demonstrated that these types of laws have reduced the likelihood of drinking and driving and the traffic crashes that result from it, and, as a result, have improved public health.

Supply-Side Policies

Laws, regulations, and other policies targeting the supply side of the market also have considerable potential to influence public health. These policies work to increase supply and to reduce the monetary and time costs of a given product, leading to increased consumption, while those that restrict supply work in the opposite direction, resulting in a higher full price and reduced consumption.

SUPPLY CONSTRAINTS

Policies that constrain supply can take many forms, from outright prohibition to efforts to control distribution through licensing, legal sanctions, and other approaches. Some such efforts are broad-based, such as the short-lived Eighteenth Amendment, which banned the manufacture, distribution, and transportation of alcoholic beverages or the current policies that make sale and distribution of a wide variety of drugs illegal. Others can be more narrowly focused, such as bans on the sale of alcohol to those under twenty-one years of age and the increasingly prevalent restrictions on the sale of at least some sugar-sweetened beverages in schools. The number of outlets selling a particular product can be restricted by requiring a license to operate and restricting the number of licenses available, as many jurisdictions do with alcoholic beverages. Similarly, the location of outlets can be limited through zoning laws that prohibit certain types of establishments in residential areas or near schools. In the case of alcoholic beverages, some states further constrain supply by monopolizing the wholesale and, in some cases, retail distribution of some beverages.

These types of supply constraints ultimately affect consumption of targeted products through their effects on several aspects of full price. Those that limit the number or location of outlets raise the time costs associated with consumption by reducing physical access. Those that prohibit the sale or distribution of various products can add to the expected legal costs. By reducing competition, constraints on supply result in higher prices. Numerous studies by economists, social scientists, public health researchers, and others have shown that constraints on supply, by increasing full price, reduce consumption and associated public health consequences.

However, at least some policies that constrain supply can create other health, social, and economic problems, in addition to the desired impact in reducing demand and its public health benefits. These consequences result from the profit opportunities created by supply constraints. This is most apparent in the markets for illicit drugs, in which high profits from the sale and distribution of these drugs result in considerable violence as existing suppliers try to protect their position and new players try to gain a foothold. Whether or not the benefits in reduced use and its consequences are worth the additional costs is much debated.

Supply Stimuli

Similarly, there are a variety of laws that seek to increase the supply of some goods and services in order to improve public health. By increasing supply, time costs are reduced and increased competition can lower prices, thereby increasing use. Various supply-side policies are being employed, for example, in efforts to promote healthier eating and increased activity in order to reduce obesity. Communities are offering tax incentives and changing zoning policies to attract supermarkets and other stores offering a greater variety of higher-quality, lower-priced fruits, vegetables, and other healthier foods and beverages in food deserts—neighborhoods where residents have little or no access to healthier options. Similar approaches are being used to attract physical fitness clubs and other establishments offering sport and recreational opportunities. Others are requiring or investing in changes to the built environment that increase the venues in which their residents can be active, from local park and recreation facilities to increased presence of sidewalks and trails.

Other laws aim to stimulate the supply of new drugs to promote public health by treating a variety of non-infectious diseases and preventing the spread of infectious diseases. Particularly important is patent protection afforded to producers who develop new drugs in exchange for disclosing the science behind it. By granting monopoly control over the distribution of a drug for a limited period of time, patents generate profits that offset the research and development costs that led to the new discovery. At the same time, the information disclosed as part of the patent increases the likelihood of additional advances.

Measurement Issues

Much of the economic analysis of public health law focuses on how law alters the full price of health-related behaviors. Consequently, developing measures of full price is central to economic analysis of these behaviors. Some aspects of full price are relatively easy to measure, while others can be more challenging.

Monetary prices of products that are legally consumed are readily available in various databases. Particularly useful are the scanner-based databases that record the monetary prices of all transactions, along with detailed information on characteristics of products and various price-reducing promotions. Prices for some products can also be derived from consumer expenditure survey data, directly obtained in surveys of individuals or collected observationally at the point of sale. For products subjected to excise taxes, the taxes themselves can be a good proxy for price in the absence of significant geographic differences in the costs of production and distribution, as in the case of cigarettes or alcoholic beverages. Prices for illegal products are more challenging to collect and are subject to considerable variation depending on the quantity and quality of the product. Nevertheless, economists have tried to develop price measures for illegal products, most notably illicit drugs, on the basis of information collected from undercover purchases and seizures, as well as from individual self-reporting.

The time costs of consuming are another key component of full price. For legally available products, economists often use measures of outlet density as a proxy for time costs, with greater physical density reflecting lower costs of obtaining a given product. For example, many economic analyses of drinking and its consequences control for alcohol outlet density, which can vary considerably across jurisdictions depending on differences in alcohol control policies. Others will use measures derived from questions about perceived availability collected in surveys, particularly for illegal products.

Expected health costs are a more challenging component of full price to measure. Economic time-series studies of health behaviors often use indicators of health "shocks" as proxies for new information about the health consequences of a particular behavior. Many economic time-series studies of cigarette demand, for example, included indicators for things such as the release of the 1964 Surgeon General's report and televised advertising about the health consequences of smoking broadcast under the Fairness Doctrine in the late 1960s. More recent studies have tried to capture exposure to mass-media counter-advertising campaigns and other public education campaigns, with exposure varying both cross-sectionally and over time. For example, exposure to campaigns that highlight the consequences of illicit drug use is assessed using Nielsen data on gross or targeted rating points measuring potential exposure to the televised advertising that is a key part of these campaigns. Still others use measures of perceived harm obtained from various surveys.

Economic theories of crime provide a nice foundation for developing measures of expected legal costs (see Chapter 5). These theories emphasize the importance of the risks of being caught and convicted, along with the swiftness and severity of the sanctions levied upon conviction. Economic analysis of the impact of drunk driving policies, for example, capture these multiple dimensions of expected legal costs with indicators for policies such as preliminary breath test laws (that increase the probability of arrest), *per se* illegal BAC laws (that raise the probability of conviction), administrative license sanctions (that impose relatively swift sanctions), and mandatory minimum penalty laws (that can increase the severity of the sanctions).

Conclusion

Economic theory provides a helpful framework for assessing effects of a number of public health laws. It highlights market failures that exist in the markets for a variety of goods and services, the use of which have considerable implications for population health. Information failures lead to overconsumption of products such as tobacco, alcohol, and sugar-sweetened beverages, resulting in many health, economic, and social consequences. Other information failures result in under-consumption of products such as fruits and vegetables, condoms, and smoking cessation services that, if consumption were increased, would improve public health. Similarly, use of many products can have harmful effects on others, while use of other products can create benefits among those that go beyond the individual consumer. Market failures create a clear economic rationale for governments to intervene through the use of laws, regulations, and other policies so as to minimize the inefficiencies that result and, by doing so, to improve public health.

Economic theory provides guidance on the types of policies likely to be effective in addressing market failures and in improving public health. The key economic mechanism through which these policies work is by affecting the full price of a behavior. Policies that increase the full price of unhealthy behaviors or reduce the "full price" of healthier behaviors have the potential to significantly improve public health. Particularly important are policies that directly influence prices of various goods and services, such as taxes on unhealthy products and subsidies for healthier options. Other interventions that raise time costs associated with obtaining and consuming, alter perceived health consequences and benefits of consumption, and raise the expected legal costs of consuming can also change behaviors in a way that improves public health. Laws that create incentives for increased supply of goods or services with public health benefits, thereby lowering the prices and the time costs of using them, can similarly improve the public's health.

Summary

Economics is the study of how society allocates scarce resources. Modern economic theory rests on the assumption that individuals seek to maximize their own well-being, subject to the constraints they face. Under ideal conditions, in freely operating markets, this will result in an efficient allocation of scarce resources. Economics, law, and public health intersect because many markets do not operate under ideal conditions. Instead, there are a variety of "market failures" leading to an inefficient allocation of resources—and negative public health consequences.

Market failures include imperfect information and informational asymmetries, negative and positive externalities, time inconsistencies in individual preferences (internalities), and excessive market power. Law can address market failures by changing the relative costs and benefits that influence the decisions consumers and producers make. Law can also

- Change the information environment by mandating or restricting information

- Create or constrain the market power of producers or consumers

- Change the scope of a market by prohibiting participation by certain purchasers or producers

- Alter the characteristics of a product, the prices of a product, key inputs into the production of that product, or the costs associated with consuming that product

Laws targeting market failures that generate significant public health consequences address failures that occur on both the demand side and the supply side of the market. On the demand side of the market, economists emphasize the concept of full price as the mechanism through which these policies influence health-related behaviors and their consequences. Full price includes not just the monetary cost but other costs associated with obtaining and using a product. The experience of excise taxes on cigarettes and alcohol illustrates the potential for impact. Subsidies, tax credits and tax deductions, and various other mechanisms may also be used to influence consumption decisions. Policies that raise the full price of consumption by adding time, inconvenience, or expected legal costs associated with the behavior can similarly reduce consumption in a way that improves public health.

Supply-side policies use economic levers to increase the supply of healthy products and decrease the supply of unhealthy ones. Policies that constrain supply can take many forms, from prohibition to efforts to control distribution through licensing, legal sanctions, and other approaches. Supply stimuli used in public health include tax incentives and zoning changes. These types of supply constraints or stimuli ultimately affect consumption of targeted products through their impact on several aspects of full price. Measures of full price are essential to economic analysis of legal interventions in public health.

Further Reading

Chaloupka, F. J., Tauras, J. A., & Grossman, M. (2000). The economics of addiction. In P. Jha & F. J. Chaloupka (Eds.), *Tobacco control in developing countries* (pp. 106–130). Oxford: Oxford University Press.

Cook, P. J. (2007). *Paying the tab: The costs and benefits of alcohol control*. Princeton, NJ: Princeton University Press.

Gruber, J., & Kőszegi, B. (2008). *A modern economic view of tobacco taxation*. Paris: International Union Against Tuberculosis and Lung Disease.

Jha, P., Musgrove, P., Chaloupka, F. J., & Yurekli, A. (2000). The economic rationale for intervention in the tobacco market. In P. Jha & F. J. Chaloupka (Eds.), *Tobacco control in developing countries* (pp. 153–174). Oxford: Oxford University Press.

Chapter 8

The Theory of Triadic Influence

Brian R. Flay   Marc B. Schure

Learning Objectives

- Identify and describe diverse behavioral mechanisms by which public health laws and regulations influence population behavior.

- Illustrate, using the theory of triadic influence, how a specific public health law may influence institutional, social, and personal behavior.

- Apply measures of social psychological and sociological constructs in evaluations of public health laws.

Social psychology has played a central role in both describing and predicting health behaviors, and those behaviors are related to a range of important health outcomes (Flay, Snyder, & Petraitis, 2009; Glass & McAtee, 2006; Jolls, Sunstein, & Thaler, 1998; Petraitis, Flay, & Miller, 1995). Public health increasingly has acknowledged the important effects of laws and regulations in improving population health (Burris, Wagenaar, Swanson, et al., 2010). Laws and regulations affecting sanitation infrastructure, food safety, and immunizations historically have had dramatic positive effects on reducing communicable diseases (Cutler & Miller, 2004; Gostin, Burris, & Lazzarini, 1999; Sperling, 2010; Stern & Markel, 2005). With the rise of chronic diseases as major public health issues (Anderson & Horvath, 2004), population behavior and sociocultural environmental exposures are crucial targets for prevention efforts (Brownson & Bright, 2004). The behavioral sciences have made enormous contributions in guiding public health efforts to address these modern-day issues, and social psychology is likely to play an increasingly important function in understanding the mechanisms by which legal systems influence health behaviors and outcomes.

This chapter first classifies laws and regulations according to the specific types of causal mechanisms by which they are believed to effect behavior change. We present relevant theories from the field of social psychology to illustrate how various behavioral mechanisms might facilitate specific behavioral changes. We offer the theory of triadic influence (Flay & Petraitis, 1994; Flay, Snyder, & Petraitis, 2009) as a comprehensive and integrative model for understanding the inter-connections between many social psychological and sociological theories. Finally, we discuss measurement of relevant constructs.

Health-Behavior Laws and Regulations from a Social Psychological Perspective

From a social psychological perspective, laws and regulations that influence health behaviors can be differentiated by the distinctive mechanisms involved in changing specific behaviors. While the nature of laws and regulations may be different, the behavioral mechanisms will often be similar.

Prevention and Safety Laws

Prevention and safety laws are some of the most common "interventional public health laws." Immunization laws are aimed at preventing the spread of communicable diseases. Driver safety regulations aim to reduce death and disability among motorists and pedestrians. Safety regulations are also an important component of occupational health, intended to reduce harmful exposures and injuries in work settings. From a social psychological perspective, the most likely mechanism of action of safety laws is that they provide people with the information they need to understand the benefits (reduced chances of injury or death) of complying with a particular law and the costs (penalties or possibility of litigation or tort) if they choose to not comply.

Environmental Exposure Regulations

Historically, environmental exposure regulation has been one of the legal foundations of public health. For example, sanitation laws ensured a standard for clean water and proper disposal of waste products. Such feats were accomplished by substantial funding for proper urban infrastructure (Perdue, Gostin, & Stone, 2003). In modern times, emergence of evidence that exposure to lead, historically used in many home and industrial products, was harmful to health led regulators to set standards to ensure that lead would no longer be used in the manufacturing of most products (Lewis, 1985). Most recently, laws that prohibit smoking in public buildings have reduced toxic exposures and altered specific behaviors of those affected (Fichtenberg & Glantz, 2002).

Intuitively, most environmental regulations would seem to influence organizational or individual behavior through the same informational and motivational mechanisms described above for prevention and safety laws. For example, motivations to comply with regulatory standards may be seen in light of the desire to avoid penalties or litigation. As information and awareness of environmental toxins increases, causal pathways are also likely to occur through changing social norms, thereby affecting the behavioral patterns of whole populations. For example, notable shifts in adults' attitudes and practices regarding childhood exposure to tobacco smoke have occurred with increased awareness of the harmful effects of second-hand smoke (McMillen, Winickoff, Klein, & Weitzman, 2003).

Access and Availability Laws

Laws and regulations affect access to and the availability of health-enhancing and health-inhibiting products and resources in multiple ways. For example, Wagenaar and Perry (1994) demonstrated how legal availability laws (that is, age limits), economic availability laws (alcohol tax), and physical availability regulations (zoning for liquor businesses) all affect youth access to and consumption of alcohol. Similar types of laws influence access to health care (that is, health insurance parity laws), food choices (school and workplace vending rules), and exercise opportunities (land use laws promoting parks and trails). Laws against possession of tobacco or illicit drugs also come with penalties that are intended to deter the behavior itself.

From a social psychological perspective, access, availability, and possession laws have their effects through two mechanisms. First, they change people's perceptions of the availability of, and expectancies about, the *personal* costs and benefits of using a product or service. Second, they influence people's motivation to comply or cooperate and one's expectancies about the *social* costs and benefits of adopting the behavior or not. Although personal versus social costs and benefits are considered as two separate causal pathways in social psychological theories (Fishbein & Ajzen, 1975), they have been considered as one pathway by other social scientists such as economists, as components of subjective expected utility theories (Bauman & Fisher, 1985; Savage, 1954; Starmer, 2000; Stigler, 1950). According to Tyler (1999), perception processes also involve evaluations that reflect pride and respect within the organizational (or cultural) system, and those evaluations become strong influences of motivation to cooperate.

"Soft" Laws (Information and Labeling)

"Soft" regulatory strategies rely on choice architecture, education, and the provision of information without legal penalty to the ultimate targets of individual behavior change (although they are typically mandatory and penalty-based with respect to the parties providing the product or service to the consumer). These laws are used in many areas, including food nutrition and calorie labeling, alcohol and tobacco warning labeling, and other product contents labeling. Laws and regulations are often linked to or require the dissemination of messages encouraging individuals to adopt a healthier behavior or to comply with a particular law. From a social psychological perspective, the causal pathway from regulation to behaviors passes through attitudes and norms. The ideas of "libertarian paternalism" (Jolls, Sunstein, & Thaler, 1998) and soft regulatory strategies "nudging" people to make the "right" decisions (Thaler & Sunstein, 2008) are interesting perspectives on this.

Social Psychological Causal Mechanisms

This chapter focuses on the "changes in behavior" mediator in the Burris and associates (2010) model of public health law research (see Figure 1.1). Some effects of laws and legal practices on behavior are mediated by changes in environment (the physical environment as well as social structures and institutions). We also describe theory-based mediators of effects of laws and legal practices on behavior and effects of changes in environments on behavior. There are many possible mediators, as we will describe.

To this point, we have suggested only two primary causal pathways by which laws related to prevention and safety, environmental exposure, access and availability, and possession may have their effects. First, information about required behaviors and the costs of non-compliance informs attitudes toward a behavior, and, second, compliance requires consideration of social norms (even those with a legal basis) and the motivation to comply or cooperate with them. We now introduce two more. To the extent that laws change the behavior of specific individuals, we may also observe a secondary effect on the behavior of others that arises from people learning by observing others (Akers, 1977; Bandura, 1977b). A final causal pathway involves self-efficacy, or the confidence one has of being able to successfully engage in a specific behavior (Bandura, 1977a).

Theories That Explain How Costs and Benefits Predict Behavior

The idea of the consequences of a behavior having costs and benefits is common to multiple social psychological theories, including expectancy-value, subjective-utility, and decision-making theories. Expectancy-value theories posit that people's choices are influenced by their beliefs and values regarding a specific behavior or activity (Feather, 1982; Wigfield, 1994; Wigfield & Eccles, 2000). For example, applied to alcohol consumption behavior, the positive expectations of feeling good and enhanced social interactions act as behavioral motivators, and the negative expectations of acting stupid or having a hangover the next day act as behavioral restraints (Jones, Corbin, & Fromme, 2001). The value placed on the positive or negative expectations determines how strong the motivators or restraints will be. If one anticipates negative consequences, such as being fined for underage drinking, and sees that negative consequence as being serious, then that anticipation (expectation or expectancy) will play a key role in deciding whether or not to engage in that behavior.

Subjective-expected utility theory is a particular version of expectancy-value theory, developed to test probabilities of risky economic decision making (Fishburn, 1981; Savage, 1954). *Utility* refers to one's satisfaction (or evaluation). Utility is combined with one's knowledge or belief in the likelihood (in statistical terms, probability) that an expected event will occur. In essence, much like expectancy-value theories, decisions regarding a behavior ultimately will depend on the relative evaluations and expectancies of the perceived consequences of a behavior (Bauman & Fisher, 1985).

Theories of decision making formalize the use of utilities and their evaluations in reaching decisions (Simon, 1959). Heuristics theory is a relevant approach to understand how problem-solving and decision-making processes occur with experience-based information. In terms of behavioral mechanisms, this approach helps explain how previous experiences can feed back into and "inform" other determinants of health behavior. In everyday human contexts, trial-and-error experiences help to inform future behavioral choices. Heuristics theory posits that hardwired or learned heuristic "rules" guide individual judgments, regardless of available relevant information or certainty (Kahnemann, Slovic, & Tversky, 1982; Tversky & Kahneman, 1974).

Perhaps the most well-known social psychological theories that have applied expectancy-value concepts to health behaviors are the theory of reasoned action (Fishbein & Ajzen, 1975) and its derivative, the theory of planned behavior (Ajzen, 1985). In these theories, *information* influences one's *beliefs* about the consequences of a behavior (*expectancies* or expectations) together with one's *evaluation* (or valuing) of that behavior. Thus expectancies and evaluations are derived from information and values, respectively. Information can be provided through laws and regulations (or, more accurately, by the publicity about them). Values are derived from one's religious background, the educational system, one's family and childhood socialization, and other broader sociocultural factors (politics, laws, mass media, and so on). Laws and regulations may or may not be consistent with one's values—and this judgment of their fairness or legitimacy has some effect on the resulting motivation to comply with them (Tyler, 2006a). In the theories of reasoned action and of planned behavior, expectancies and evaluations combine to become *attitudes* toward the behavior (Fishbein & Ajzen, 1975). Aside from the costs or penalties of non-compliance, people's motivation to comply with authority (here a component of social normative beliefs) also plays a role in their choices.

Interpersonal Theories of Social Control

Theories of compliance with law derived from social psychology also help explain the effects of prevention and safety laws (Tyler, 1999) (see Chapter 6). Compliance theories assume that people comply with laws because of the risk and fear of punishment. Recent research, however, suggests that perceived legitimacy of laws is a more important determinant of whether or not people obey laws (Tyler, 2006a). Studies reviewed by Tyler support the argument that people's motivation to cooperate with others, in this case legal authorities, is rooted in social relationships and ethical judgments, and does not flow only (or primarily) from the desire to avoid punishments or gain rewards.

One approach to how social relationships drive behavior, social attachment theory, suggests that individuals have an inherent need for close relations with others whether it is a child-parent relationship or an intimate or romantic relationship (Ainsworth & Bowlby, 1991). These close relationships almost always rely on a set of expectations whereby individuals within that relationship have varying expectations of each other and varying motivations to comply. Ryan and Deci's (2000) work on intrinsic and extrinsic motivational factors is also relevant for understanding compliance. For example, a child may be rewarded for good behavior or punished for bad behavior, or a child may wish to please her or his parents by performing a desirable behavior. Indeed, research has demonstrated that prosocial attachment and commitment is a strong predictor of behavior (Hirschi, 2002). Compliance motivations are directly affected by the degree and quality of attachment (interpersonal bonding)—people who are attached to conventional societal norms are more likely to be motivated to comply with laws and regulations that limit their behavioral choices (Gottfredson & Hirschi, 1990). Police and other authorities benefit from the more active cooperation of such people in the community (Sampson, Raudenbush, & Earles, 1997; Sunshine & Tyler, 2003a; Tyler & Huo, 2002). Willingness to cooperate with authorities or comply with laws develops from the experience of fairness when dealing with authorities. This fairness leads to evaluations of legitimacy, a key precursor of motivation to comply or consent and results in voluntary acceptance (Tyler, 2006a).

To the extent that laws change the behavior of some people, the behavior of others might follow. Social learning theories from both psychology (Bandura, 1977b) and sociology (Akers, 1977) describe this process. According to these theories, social learning is seen to take place in the context of social structures, whereby individuals learn through interactions with different people in multiple social contexts. Application of social learning theories for understanding deviant behavior (criminal or unhealthy) emphasizes how social influences serve as either protective or risk factors (Akers, 1998; Akers & Jensen, 2007). Social situations provide the contexts for social interactions, whereby perceived norms and compliance motivations mediate legal effects. This is more likely to be true when the others who change their behavior include individuals within one's close social circle or family, as motivations to please or comply with them are much stronger.

An extension of social learning and other theories, social cognitive theory (Bandura, 1986b) describes how learning from social role models has multiple results. First, it can influence one's beliefs (expectancies) about the consequences of a behavior together with one's evaluation of the value of that behavior. As noted earlier, expectancies and evaluations combine to become attitudes (Fishbein & Ajzen, 1975). A second result is that role models help one learn new skills, which then influence self-efficacy. Third, to the extent that role models are important to you, you will be motivated to please them (or comply with them). Motivation to comply, combined with normative beliefs (how you think others want you to behave), produces social normative beliefs (Fishbein & Ajzen, 1975), which in turn influence intentions (one's decision whether or not to engage in the behavior).

Social relationships and networks clearly play an important role in determining people's behaviors, including their reactions to the law. Social network theories constitute a broad set of theories describing structural characteristics, functions, and types of social support that exist in an individual's social network (Borgatti, Mehra, Brass, & Labianca, 2009). Peer cluster theory demonstrates how small groups of peers share similar beliefs, values, and behaviors (Oetting & Beauvais, 1986). Similarly, from sociology, differential association theory (Sutherland, 1942) proposes that individuals learn values, attitudes, and motivations for behavior within small groups. Therefore any behavior is more probable for those with intimate exposure to others performing that behavior. Observational learning illustrates how the adoption of a new behavior is facilitated through seeing others performing that behavior reinforced by reward systems within one's social system (Bandura, 1986a; Unger, Cruz, Baezconde-Garbanati, et al., 2003).

Intrapersonal Theories

Individual predispositions and personality traits guide one's self-determination (will), skill development, and decision making regarding a specific behavior. Important concepts within the intrapersonal dimension include self-regulation or control, social skills, and self-efficacy. One causal pathway suggested earlier involves self-efficacy—the confidence one has to engage in a specific behavior successfully. According to self-efficacy theory (Bandura, 1977a, 1986a), compliance with a law or regulation about a specific behavior will improve to the extent the rule is accompanied with information about how to accomplish that behavior or, better still, training in how to do the new behavior. As people's skill to do the behavior (and, therefore, their confidence or self-efficacy about doing it) improves, they will be more likely to perform that specific behavior.

According to the theory of planned behavior, self-efficacy is the third leg directly affecting one's decision making or intentions toward performing a behavior. Those with low self-efficacy are easily discouraged and less likely to trust their ability to perform a behavior, and therefore are less likely to actually perform that behavior. In contrast, those with high self-efficacy regarding a specific behavior will likely utilize great effort to ensure that they achieve their expected behavioral outcomes. Theoretically, self-efficacy facilitates or buffers against compliance with laws and regulations. Self-efficacy could represent either confidence in one's ability to obey the law or confidence in one's ability to disregard or elude the law.

According to Bandura (1986a, 1986b), self-regulation is achieved by acquiring self-management skills and can be manifested in a number of ways, including goal setting, seeking social support, and self-rewards (to name a few). Self-control theory (Akers, 1991) posits that one's relative self-control forms during childhood and tends to remain stable throughout adulthood. Lower levels of self-control are associated with ineffective or incomplete socialization. Those with low self-control are more likely to engage in delinquent behaviors, including health-related behaviors such as drug use (Gottfredson & Hirschi, 1990). Therefore legal penalties or punishments have varying degrees of effect, depending on one's level of self-control, and one's level of self-control thereby mediates effects of public health laws. In short, people with high levels of self-control are more likely to comply with legal restrictions than those with lower levels of self-control.

Self-esteem has been thought of as a component of self-concept by which individuals evaluate their competence and worth in their social environment (Cast & Burke, 2002). Thus social competence and social skills are closely related to the concept of self-esteem. In general, research has shown associations of higher self-esteem with more positive outcomes, and a similar correlation of lower self-esteem with negative outcomes. Self-esteem has been conceptualized as outcome; as self-motivating; and as a buffer from negative experiences. Cast and Burke attempted to integrate these three conceptualizations within the context of identity theory. DuBois, Flay, and Fagen (2009) presented the self-esteem enhancement theory to help guide interventions related to self-esteem, in which self-esteem and esteem formation and maintenance processes are depicted as moderators of well-being. In the context of legal effects, self-esteem likely plays a mediating role, whereby improved self-esteem strengthens one's capacity for appropriately handling negative pressures in a manner compliant with laws and regulations.

The self-motivation conceptualization of self-esteem is related to Deci and Ryan's (1985) self-determination theory, by which intrinsic and extrinsic motivations vary in degrees according to one's goals or reasons. Intrinsic motivation is enhanced when three psychological needs—competence, autonomy, and relatedness—are met (Ryan & Deci, 2000). Levels of self-determination likely both moderate and mediate effects of laws. Those with higher levels of self-determination are more likely to comply with laws and regulations—unless such laws and regulations are regarded as illegitimate, in which case, self-determination may act as a buffer to compliance. Those with higher levels of self-determination are also more likely to vote and be otherwise engaged in their community, leading to a feedback effect on the development of laws and regulations and their perceived legitimacy.

Summary Comments on Social Psychological Theories

We have described numerous theories explaining various dimensions of behavior. These are listed in Table 8.1. These accounts of behavior can be organized within a *social ecological model* (Bronfrenbrenner, 2005). In this model, behavior is influenced at three main levels: within people themselves (that is, the individual's personality and predispositions), with respect to the social relationships surrounding the individual, and in the broad sociocultural environment. Laws and regulations, of course, are part of the sociocultural environment, along with economic and political systems, the mass media, religions, and other cultural systems.

Table 8.1. Social Psychological Theories Informing Mechanisms of Legal Effect.

Evaluative Theories	Interpersonal Theories	Intrapersonal Theories
Value-expectancy theories: Subjective-expected utility theory Theory of reasoned action Theory of planned behavior Theories of decision making: Heuristics theory	Compliance theories: Deterrence Procedural justice Social attachment theory Intrinsic and extrinsic motivation Social learning theories Social cognitive theory Social network theories Peer cluster theory Differential association theory	Self-efficacy theory Self-control theory Self-esteem theory Self-esteem enhancement theory Self-determination theory Bounded rationality

We have described four major pathways through which laws and regulations can affect behavior, and summarized social psychological theories that elaborate those pathways. The first is that laws and regulations provide information that, in turn, informs expectancies or expectations about consequences that together form attitudes toward the behavior targeted by the law or regulation (laws and regulations → information → expectancies and evaluations → attitudes). A second causal path suggests that laws and regulations have their effects through the interpersonal pathway of influencing attachment to conventional norms leading to motivation to comply (laws and regulations → attachment to conventional norms → motivation to comply). Third, we described pathways through changes in the behavior of initial compliers, thereby changing social norms (laws and regulations → change behavioral norms → normative beliefs). A fourth pathway is through people learning new behaviors from others (laws and regulations → modeling or training → self-efficacy).

Note how each of these pathways moved from the ultimate (or root) cause of behavior, here the laws and regulations, to a cause closer to behavior but still somewhat distal (for example, information, attachment to conventional norms, social norms, behavioral models), to causes even closer to or very proximal to behavior (that is, attitudes, social normative beliefs, and self-efficacy). It is immediately obvious that the proximal predictors of behavior are consistent with social cognitive theory (Bandura, 1986b) and the theories of reasoned action (Fishbein & Ajzen, 1975) and planned behavior (Ajzen, 1985)—all of these pathways are mediated by intentions or decisions to do the behavior. That is, changes in any one or all of attitudes (the result of expectancies and their value), social normative beliefs (the result of motivation to comply and normative beliefs) and self-efficacy (the result of will or opportunity and skill) related to a specific behavior are likely to lead to changes in one's intentions or decisions to perform that behavior; and intentions are a good predictor of actually doing (or at least initiating) the behavior. In the theory of planned behavior, behavioral control (one's perceived control over a specific behavior) replaces self-efficacy (one's actual or perceived ability to perform a specific behavior). Finally, note that the use of intentions to predict behavior has a practical advantage in public health law research: survey methods can be used to reliably measure intentions in those situations in which direct observation of actual behavior is impossible.

All of these pathways sound rational, but there is wide recognition that rationality is limited. People exhibit bounded rationality, bounded self-interest, and bounded willpower (Jolls, Sunstein, & Thaler, 1998). Bounded rationality refers to cognitive limitations, so that information may be forgotten or habits have formed that limit the acceptance of new information. Bounded self-interest refers to the fact that people care about others and what those others think about them, so they may act to please others or avoid negative judgments from others, rather than act in their own self-interests. Bounded willpower refers to the limited self-control or self-determination that we all experience with some behaviors such as smoking or eating. Notice the parallel of these three kinds of bounded rationality with the social-ecological levels in which the causes of behavior operate.

Many theories rely on intrapersonal concepts for understanding behavior, while social psychological theories posit that social contexts (interpersonal relationships) are just as important. Furthermore, social-ecological models suggest that behaviors must be understood in the broader sociocultural contexts in which they occur (Bronfrenbrenner, 2005). Clearly, none of the proposed causal pathways toward behavior operate in a vacuum—all three are strongly affected by individual (intrapersonal) and social (interpersonal) factors. Each of these types of theories has offered important insights regarding the emergence of specific health behaviors. However, their contributions are limited to the extent that the scope of any specific single theory accounts for a limited set of influences on behavior. The theory of triadic influence was developed to integrate many of the theories above and others, and to provide a comprehensive explanation of the many causes of behavior. As will be seen, each of the major pathways just described, and other related ones, can be unified in this integrated, comprehensive theory (Flay & Petraitis, 1994; Flay, Snyder, & Petraitis, 2009).

The Theory of Triadic Influence

The theory of triadic influence (TTI) represents an integration of many of the theories discussed in the previous section, as well as others. It organizes them in a coherent way that explains health-related behaviors and guides interventions for health-behavior change. We find the framework useful for explaining the effects of laws and regulations on people's health behaviors and population-level public health. As a broad ecological model, the TTI provides a meta-theoretical approach both to explaining health-related behaviors and for guiding health behavior change. The TTI posits that theories and variables can be organized along two dimensions: social-ecological streams of influence and levels of causation (Petraitis, Flay, & Miller, 1995).

The Basic Elements of the TTI

The TTI proposes that causes of behavior operate through multiple pathways from ultimate to distal to proximal levels of causation; that these pathways flow through three ecological streams, each of which has two substreams; and that experience with a behavior feeds back to change the initial causes (Figure 8.1). We discuss each of these elements in turn.

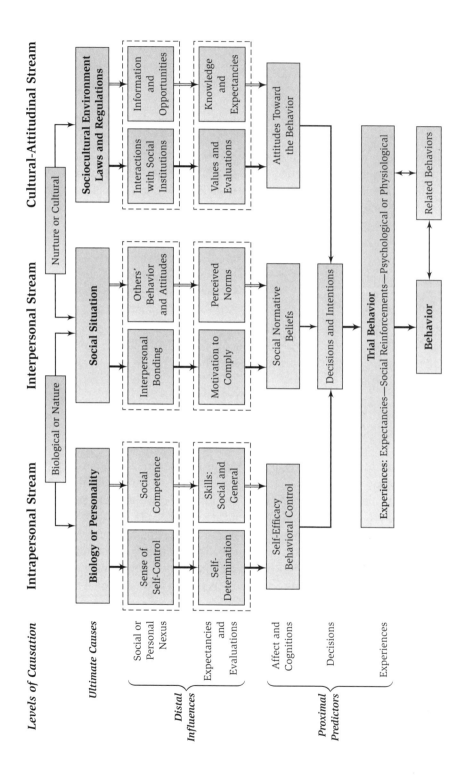

Figure 8.1. The Theory of Triadic Influence.

STREAMS OF INFLUENCE

The TTI proposes that causes emanate from and flow through three streams of influence. The intrapersonal stream flows from genetic predispositions and personality through self-determination (will) and skills to self-efficacy. The interpersonal, or social-normative, stream flows from one's social contexts and relationships (community, peer networks, family) through others' behaviors and one's level of attachment to those others, to social normative beliefs. It includes perceived norms about others' behaviors and one's motivation to comply with or please those others. The cultural-attitudinal, or sociocultural, stream flows from broad sociocultural factors (politics, economics, the law, mass media, religion) through one's interactions with these social systems and how those interactions determine one's attitudes toward a specific behavior. It includes how the social systems influence one's values and evaluations of consequences. It also considers how the information provided by these institutions influences one's expectations (or expectancies) about the consequences of a behavior. All three streams end at one's intentions (or decisions), which ideally provide a reliable prediction of actual behavior.

As shown in Figure 8.1, within each of the three main streams, two substreams represent distinct processes leading to decisions, one that is more cognitive and rational (the right-hand, or multilined, substream within each stream) and one that is more affective or emotional (the left-hand or solid substream within each stream). Psychologists tend to emphasize the affective or emotional aspect of the second substream; sociologists are more likely to emphasize the self- or social-control aspect (Gottfredson & Hirschi, 1990).

LEVELS OF CAUSATION

The TTI arranges these variables affecting behavior along multiple levels of causation—from ultimate causes to distal influences to proximal predictors (Flay, Snyder, & Petraitis, 2009). Some variables, such as attitudes toward the behavior, social normative beliefs about the behavior, and self-efficacy or behavioral control (confidence in doing a specific behavior), can have direct effects on intentions about that specific behavior and therefore are proximal causes of that behavior. Other variables are causally distal, influencing factors that can be mediated by other variables. These include the individual's social competence, attitudes and behaviors of others, and the individual's interactions with social institutions. Finally, many variables—such as law, poverty, neighborhood characteristics, and personality—represent underlying or ultimate causes of behavior over which individuals generally have little control.

The TTI proposes that causal mechanisms generally flow from ultimate to proximal causes within each of the three streams of influence. Yet while the general flow of causation occurs predominantly within each stream, variables may also interact across streams. Thus multiple ultimate and distal moderating and mediating factors may work together to increase or decrease the probability of a behavior occurring. For example, one's personality may moderate the effects of a law on one's values.

FEEDBACK AND RECIPROCAL DETERMINISM

Experience with a behavior may produce physiological, social, or psychological reinforcements that feed back into many of the upstream variables that originally led to the behavior. Systems theories (Leischow, Best, Trochim, et al., 2008; Sterman, 2006; Wiese, Vallacher, & Strawinska, 2010) describe this as forming feedback loops, while social cognitive theory (Bandura, 1986b) describes it as reciprocal determinism. The key concept of reciprocal determinism suggests that any type of environmental influence may affect the behavior of individuals and groups, *and* that the behavior of individuals and groups may, in turn, affect the environment.

Application to Public Health Laws

The TTI cultural-attitudinal stream illustrates how public policies and laws affect individual health behaviors primarily by shaping social and institutional practices and structures. Institutional structures and practices influence one's opportunities and access to products and information, and affects capacities for interacting with that institution. Drawing on theories reviewed earlier, the TTI proposes that attitudes toward a specific behavior are determined by expectancies and evaluations about that specific behavior. One's attitudes toward a specific behavior are one of the key proximal predictors affecting intentions and behavioral adoption.

Besides interactions of individuals with institutions and popular cultural milieu, social psychologists also recognize the important role of interactions that occur within one's social context. Core concepts in the interpersonal stream of the TTI include bonding with or attachment to important others (Ainsworth & Bowlby, 1991), other's behaviors (role modeling) (Bandura, 1977a, 1986a), motivation to comply (or desire to please), and social normative beliefs (Fishbein & Ajzen, 1975). The TTI suggests that family structures and dynamics and peer relations are ultimate causes within social contexts that lead to one's social normative beliefs. Laws and policies may influence individual perceptions and decisions about behavioral adoption or restraint by affecting one's beliefs about social norms.

Intrapersonal concepts are also important to consider when evaluating laws and policies. Individual predispositions and traits guide one's decision making regarding a specific behavior. Important concepts within the intrapersonal dimension include social skills, self-control or regulation, and self-efficacy.

In the intrapersonal stream of the TTI, one's personality determines one's levels of self-control or regulation, which, in turn, moderate the influence of policies or laws. One's levels of self-esteem and self-determination not only moderate effects of existing policies and laws but also may help in the development of new policies and laws.

The TTI takes a step beyond other integrative theories, such as social cognitive theory, in that it integrates a wider range of psychological and sociological theories of behavioral development and change. The TTI organizes many of the key concepts from these theories, and others, in a coherent way that explains health-related behaviors and guides interventions for health behavior change. Furthermore, the TTI provides a systems perspective that includes development, feedback, control systems, and a systematic view of how multiple causes influence multiple behaviors either directly, through mediated pathways, by moderating other causes, or through feedback systems.

Feedback from behavior can be to any causal level, proximal, distal, or ultimate. A developmental perspective is incorporated into the TTI, in that all of the causal paths may be moderated by different developmental stages (ages), and changes in behavior may influence developmental trajectories. The TTI also makes it clear that distal and ultimate causes influence multiple behaviors (for example, one's personality influences all manner of behaviors).

PATHWAYS OF INFLUENCE

We propose that public health laws have their primary causal action through the cultural-attitudinal stream. Laws primarily alter access to or availability of goods and information related to knowledge or expectancies of consequences. Laws give rise to and structure interactions with government institutions; these experiences in turn influence one's view of the legitimacy of authorities or one's evaluations of the expected consequences of a specific behavior. Both of these paths influence attitudes toward the behavior, which, in turn, influences decisions and trial behavior. A positive experience with the behavior will feed back to influence expectancies and evaluations (and information and relationships with social institutions, including the legal system) to determine future behavior. Ultimately, repeated trial behavior that is repeatedly reinforced will lead to regular (habitual) behavior.

The paths through the cultural-attitudinal stream are similar to many rational theories of decision making and utility theories in economics (Starmer, 2000; Stigler, 1950) and to procedural justice and deterrence theories of compliance (see Chapters 5 and 6). Public health laws may also have their effects through less rational pathways that involve social relationships and emotions. For example, laws may have mediating influences on social and intrapersonal factors. For example, a law may lead others to change their behavior or attitudes (interpersonal stream). This will lead to changes in perceived norms. Then, to the extent that one is bonded with and desires to please (comply or cooperate with) others, one's social normative beliefs will be altered, leading to changed intentions and behavior. Laws may also have a direct influence on one's sense of control or social competence in the intrapersonal stream. Disability discrimination law, for example, may validate a person with a disability in her efforts to get accommodations at work (Engel & Munger, 2003), which will lead to changes through the intrapersonal stream down to self-efficacy and from there to intentions.

Aspects of the other streams may affect (moderate) how one responds to laws. Poor self-regulation or impulsiveness (sense of self or self-control), for example, may reduce the effects of a law on one's behavior by moderating the pathway from information to attitudes, or the path to values. Or, if everyone in one's immediate social context is not following a new rule, then one's perceived norm will be that the new behavior the regulation is intended to influence is not expected by one's associates; the resulting social normative belief will be against the new regulation as will the resulting intentions and behavior and attitudes toward the behavior—at least until enforcement imposes some costs, changes the norms, or both.

Tyler (1999, 2006a) suggests that innate human desire to cooperate is the product of an array of inter- and intra-personal components, including trust, legitimacy, emotions, attitudes, and norms. De Cremer and Tyler (2005) have posited the importance of the "sense of social self" to the production of cooperative behavior. These views actually combine aspects from all three streams of the TTI: self-esteem and sense of self-control from the intrapersonal stream; social bonding (attachment) and motivation to comply from the interpersonal stream; and interactions with or involvement in social institutions and attitudes from the cultural-attitudinal stream. If compliance with law is seen as a form of social cooperation, sense of social self will determine, to a large degree, one's degree of compliance with a new law or regulation. If the law is seen as having legitimacy, as having been created in a fair way by trustworthy authorities, then compliance will be high among those with a strong sense of social self. In contrast, if the law lacks legitimacy in the eyes of the public, then compliance will be low, especially by those with a strong sense of social self.

Practical Measures

The TTI helps identify key constructs that explain variance in behavior that can be measured to inform how laws change health-related behavior. We discuss measures of eleven variables that are central to understanding how legal institutions and practices affect behavior. Many resources exist for measurement development besides those we reference here (Dillman, 1991, 2007), including government resources (General Accounting Office, 1993; Houston,

1997). We provide brief considerations for measurement development and identify some examples of measures of constructs from the TTI and other theories that have demonstrated good reliability and validity.

The Cultural-Attitudinal or Sociocultural Stream

In this section, we discuss measures of knowledge and beliefs, values, and attitudes toward behavior.

KNOWLEDGE AND BELIEFS ABOUT EXPECTED CONSEQUENCES

Knowledge of laws and beliefs about expected consequences is a distal factor in the cognitive substream of the cultural-attitudinal stream of the TTI. Knowledge about laws includes the important issue of comprehension of those laws and their intent. Opinion polls often contain items to assess such knowledge or beliefs. Tidwell and Doyle (1995) developed a survey to assess driver and pedestrian comprehension of pedestrian law and traffic control devices. An example of a survey to assess beliefs is a sixteen-item measure of beliefs regarding physical activity that has shown good internal consistency (Saunders, Pate, Felton, et al., 1997). Leading from an item stem of "If I were to be physically active most days it would . . .", sample items include "Get or keep me in shape," "Make me tired," "Be fun," and "Be boring."

VALUES

Values are a distal component of the TTI's cultural-attitudinal stream flowing directly toward one's attitudes about a behavior. A popular measure of general values is the Rokeach Value Survey (Rokeach, 1973; Rokeach & Ball-Rokeach, 1989). This self-administered value inventory is divided into two parts, with each part measuring different but complementary types of personal values. The first part consists of eighteen terminal value items, which are designed to measure the relative importance of end states of existence (that is, personal goals such as freedom, equality, health, national security, a world at peace). The second part consists of eighteen instrumental value items, which measure basic characteristics an individual might see as helpful to reaching end-state values (for example, ambitious, responsible, honest, obedient). The scale has been used widely with Likert scales (for example, a five-point agreement scale) so that conventional statistical tests can be performed (Rokeach, 1973; Rokeach & Ball-Rokeach, 1989). Many other measures of specialized values are available (Gibbins & Walker, 1993). The Culture and Media Institute (http://www .mrc.org/cmi/default.aspx) conducts the National Cultural Values Survey (Fitzpatrick, 2007), which assesses cultural values such as morality, thrift, charity, and honesty or integrity (including willingness to break the law, cheat on unemployment benefits, or tolerate illegal drug use).

ATTITUDES TOWARD THE BEHAVIOR

This is the proximal predictor of behavior within TTI's cultural-attitudinal stream of influence. Ajzen (2003) provides guidance on the construction of attitude scale items specific to any particular behavior. The simplest attitude items are of the form "It would be bad for me to drive after drinking" answered on a scale of "completely agree" to "completely disagree." Fishbein and colleagues (2001) also suggest utilizing an expectancy-value index to indirectly measure attitudes. For example, two questions would be asked regarding a specific consequence of a particular behavior: one about one's beliefs about the probability of the consequence (expectancy), the other about one's values about (evaluation of) the consequence. The product of those two items could be summed with other paired items to create the attitude index.

Examples of valid and reliable attitude scales include Brand and Anastasio's (2006) fifty-item Violence-Related Attitudes and Beliefs Scale (V-RABS) and Polaschek and colleagues' (2004) twenty-item Criminal Attitudes to Violence Scale (CAVS). Using a seven-point agreement scale, sample items from the V-RABS include "Trying to prevent violent behavior is a waste of time and money"; "People become violent because of their family environment"; and "The majority of violent crimes are committed by people who have mental illness."

The Interpersonal or Social-Normative Stream

In this section, we discuss measures of social attachment (bonding), observed (modeled) behaviors, and social normative beliefs.

SOCIAL ATTACHMENT (BONDING) WITH FAMILY, FRIENDS, AND SCHOOL

The interpersonal bonding component of the TTI's interpersonal stream is suggestive of Hirschi's (2002) theoretical constructs of attachment, commitment, and belief. Libbey (2004) provides a review of school attachment, bonding, and connectedness measures and items used to assess student attachment. Another example of a somewhat reliable measure of bonding (Jenkins, 1997) includes items such as "Do you care a lot about what your teachers think of you?" "Do most of your teachers like you?" and "Most teachers are not interested in anything I say or do."

OBSERVED (MODELED) BEHAVIOR AND ATTITUDES

Others' behavior and attitudes is also a distal component of TTI's interpersonal stream, directly influencing perceived norms. An eight-item measure that has shown good reliability was tested by Saunders and colleagues (1997) to measure social modeling for physical activity. Using the item stem "A friend or someone in the family . . .", sample items include "Thinks I should be physically active"; "Encourages me to be physically active"; and "Has been physically active with me."

SOCIAL NORMATIVE BELIEFS

As a proximal predictor of behavior, social normative beliefs concern one's perception of the social influences on one's behavior. Consensus among theorists suggests that, because this measure is concerned with judging the degree to which one is motivated to comply with a particular person or social group, specific behaviors should be measured in paired items assessing both perceptions of norms (what others expect of one) and motivation to comply with those others. Ajzen (2003) provides guidelines for constructing such scales.

We could not identify any developed and tested scales for social normative beliefs using the paired-item format. However, Huesmann & Guerra (1997) provide an example of a reliable twenty-item scale measuring normative beliefs about aggression. We found an eight-item version of this scale (Huesmann & Guerra, 1997), which has high reliability with elementary and middle school students (Schure, Lewis, Bavarian, et al., 2011). Using a four-point response scale, example items include "It is wrong to hit other people"; "If you're angry, it is OK to say mean things to other people"; and "It is wrong to get into physical fights with others." Another example concerns normative beliefs about water conservation laws (Corral-Verdugo & Frías-Armenta, 2006). Items include "The government should pass laws banning the settlement of industries around dams, rivers, lakes, and aquifers" and "The state should impose fines on people who waste water."

The Intrapersonal Stream

In this section, we discuss measures of self-control or regulation, social competence and skills, and self-efficacy.

SELF-CONTROL OR REGULATION

In the TTI framework, self-control or regulation is seen as a distal-level variable within the intrapersonal stream. Two measures demonstrating good reliability assessing self-control are the thirty-six-item Self-Control Schedule (Facione & Facione, 1992) and the Total and Brief Self-Control Scales (Rosenbaum, 1980), with thirty-six and thirteen items, respectively. Sample items from the Self-Control Schedule include "When I have to do something that is anxiety arousing for me, I try to visualize how I will overcome my anxieties while doing it"; "When I am depressed, I try to keep myself busy with things that I like"; and "When I plan to work, I remove all the things that are not relevant to my work." Response items are on a six-point scale indicating the degree to which each statement is characteristic of the respondent.

Social Competence and Skills

In the framework of the TTI, skills are the distal cognitive component that flows directly into self-efficacy. This variable is important to assess, as the development of general and behavior-specific skills can be instrumental in determining one's likelihood of adopting a behavior. The 131-item Conners Teacher Rating Scale (CTRS-R), measuring six behavioral domains (Conners, Sitarenios, Parker, & Epstein, 1998), is a reliable social skills scale. Teachers rate specific behavioral items related to cognition (forgets things, avoids mental effort), perfectionism (neat, over-focused), and impulsivity (restless, excitable).

Critical thinking is an important skill domain that can affect many types of behavior. The eighty-item Watson-Glaser Critical Thinking Appraisal (Watson & Glaser, 1980) and the forty-item California Critical Thinking Skills Test (Facione & Facione, 1992) have both shown good internal reliability. Subscale items measure five specific constructs: the ability to make inferences, recognize assumptions, make deductions, evaluate arguments, and make interpretations (Gadzella, Stacks, Stephens, & Masten, 2005).

Self-Efficacy

Self-efficacy derives from self-control or regulation (through self-determination or will) and social competence (through skills) in the intrapersonal stream. Fishbein and colleagues (2001) recommend that items measuring self-efficacy should be behavior-specific, be phrased in the present tense, and utilize wording from identified internal or external demands that may impose difficulty on one's ability to perform the behavior. For example, Resnick and Jenkin's Self-Efficacy for Exercise (SEE) Scale is a nine-item scale, developed for adults, and measures perceived confidence that one could continue to exercise despite various barriers. Items were prefaced with "How confident are you right now that you could exercise three times per week for 20 minutes if . . .", followed by items such as "the weather was bothering you"; "you were bored by the program or activity"; and "you felt pain when exercising." Usually, these measures use a 0 to 100 scale, suggesting the degree to which a person feels confident enough to perform that behavior. Bandura (2006) offers a clear guide on how to construct domain-specific self-efficacy scales depending on the context of research.

Decisions, Intentions, and Feedback from Experiences with the Behavior

In this section, we discuss measures of intentions and responses to feedback from experiences with the behavior.

DECISIONS AND INTENTIONS

As the key proximal mediating variable of the TTI, behavioral decisions and intentions provides the most strongly correlated predictor of a future behavior and can be assessed with measures of likelihood or probability of occurrence. For the development of a fixed measure, it is recommended that it be treated as a continuous variable along a response scale of likely to unlikely (Polaschek, Collie, & Walkey, 2004), although there have been issues raised as to how many points should be included for a validated measure (Davis & Warshaw, 1992). It is recommended that if respondents' answers are more reliable with a shorter response scale that they then be offered a two-part question (Fishbein, Triandis, Kanfer, et al., 2001). Thus, as should be noted for all types of measures, it is important to take into consideration the specific population for which the measure is being developed. The nineteen-item Scale for Suicide Ideation (SSI) designed to measure suicidal intention has shown high internal consistency and construct validity (Beck, Kovacs, & Weissman, 1979). A developed and tested intention measure for physical activity (Godin & Shephard, 1986) was used by Saunders and colleagues (1997) and includes a selection of five response items indicating a range of intention to be physically active during one's free time. Such statements range from "I am sure I will *not* be physically active" to "I am sure I *will* be physically active."

TRIAL BEHAVIOR PRODUCES FEEDBACK

Feedback from experience with a behavior is mostly captured through emotional reactions to the behavior. Hedonic theory focuses on affective responses to behavior as determinants of future behavior (Kahneman, 1999). Hedonic responses or emotional reactions (that is, good or pleasure versus bad or displeasure) can provide an index of the usefulness of behavior and its immediate outcomes that may influence decisions regarding whether or not to repeat the behavior (Cabanac, 1992; Kahneman, Frederickson, Schreiber, & Redelmeier, 1993). This tendency for humans to maximize pleasure and minimize displeasure has been examined extensively as a mechanism for various behaviors. It is a basic underlying mechanism of learning (Bandura, 1986a, 1986b).

Emotional reactions could be related to any stream of influence: in the cultural-attitudinal stream it would feed back to attitudes, particularly evaluation of consequences and values; in the interpersonal stream it would feed back to normative beliefs, particularly motivation to comply or social bonding or attachment; and in the intrapersonal stream, it would feed back to self-efficacy, particularly self-control or regulation and competence or skills. Fishbein and colleagues (2001) suggest that while no standardized measures have yet been developed, one could explore potential semantic differential terms that elicit more gut-like emotional reactions. Another approach would be to assess changes in attitudes, social normative beliefs, and self-efficacy after experiencing a behavior. For example, after first trying an illegal substance, an adolescent might have more positive or negative attitudes about drug use, depending on his or her physiological reactions; the adolescent's relationship with peers, parents, or the law or authority is likely to change, as is, therefore, his or her motivation to comply with (or please) them; and the adolescent's sense of self-efficacy to do the behavior (or to resist it) will have changed.

Conclusion

Many social psychological theories inform our understanding of the effects of public health laws and regulations on behavior. In this chapter, we provided a review of many of these theories that contribute to understanding the effects of public health laws. We also provided an integrative theoretical framework, the theory of triadic influence, to help guide future research on effects of public health laws. These theoretical perspectives make clear that laws have their effects on behavior through many pathways. The most obvious path is knowledge and values → expectancies and how they are evaluated → attitudes toward the behavior. However, many other pathways through social contexts or interpersonal relationships are also possible, involving role models (social learning) and perceived norms → attachment to or bonding with conventional values or others and motivation to comply with them → social normative beliefs. Yet other pathways occur through intrapersonal constructs, including social competence and sense of self control → skill plus will (self-determination) → self-efficacy. Attitudes, social normative beliefs, and self-efficacy each have cognitive and affective (control) components, and each contributes to the prediction of intentions to try or to adopt a particular behavior. Once a behavior is tried, the experience with that behavior can feed back in the personal, social, and cultural domains and change the original causes or predictors. All of this occurs during life-long human development over time. Clearly, the prediction of behavior is complex, and any new law or regulation should be evaluated rigorously to assess both expected and unexpected (positive or negative) effects.

Summary

Social psychology plays an important role in explicating mechanisms of legal effect. Social psychological theories offer theoretical constructs that help explain the web of psychological and social causes and mediators of intentions and behaviors that legal processes seek to modify. Social psychology pertains primarily to the "changes in behavior" mediator in the model of public health law research (see Figure 1.1), positing a number of possible causal pathways by which legal systems and policies may influence behavior. From a social psychological perspective, laws and regulations can be classified according to the type of causal pathway by which behaviors are modified, for example, through changing attitudes, normative beliefs, or self-efficacy concerning a specific behavior. We outline plausible pathways for many types of laws and regulations, including prevention and safety laws; environmental exposure regulations; laws regulating availability of health-enhancing and health-inhibiting products and resources; and "soft" laws that prompt or inform rather than command the ultimate actor (for example, labeling laws).

Given the large number of social psychological theories and the need to structure disparate theories in relation to each other, the theory of triadic influence (TTI) is a comprehensive and integrative model that we use for describing relationships among various theoretical constructs. The TTI posits that laws and regulations influence behavior through multiple causal pathways, from ultimate causes, through distal influences and proximal predictors, all mediated by the proximal influences of attitudes toward, social normative beliefs about, and self-efficacy regarding a particular behavior. Reliable measures for these and other constructs are readily available.

Further Reading

Flay, B. R., Snyder, F. J., & Petraitis, J. (2009). The theory of triadic influence. In R. J. DiClemente, M. C. Kegler, & R. A. Crosby (Eds.), *Emerging theories in health promotion practice and research* (2nd ed., pp. 451–510). San Francisco: Jossey-Bass.

Petraitis, J., Flay, B. R., & Miller, T. Q. (1995). Reviewing theories of adolescent substance use: Organizing pieces in the puzzle. *Psychological Bulletin, 117*(1), 67–86.

Tyler, T. R. (2006a). *Why people obey the law*. Princeton, NJ: Princeton University Press.

Chapter 9

Integrating Diverse Theories for Public Health Law Evaluation

Scott Burris   Alexander C. Wagenaar

Learning Objectives

- Recognize how theory on mechanisms of effect can support causal inference.

- Use evidence on the mechanisms of legal effect to explain the basis for legal reform and innovation to others.

- Combine concepts from various theories of how laws operate to illustrate specific hypotheses regarding legal effects on population health.

The preceding chapters have introduced a variety of theoretical frameworks and practical tools for studying *how* laws and legal practices influence behavior, environments, and, ultimately, health outcomes in a population. Theoretically grounded research illuminating mechanisms of legal effect has at least three important benefits for public health law research and practice:

- *Defining the Phenomena to Be Observed.* Theories of how law influences structures, behaviors, and environments help identify effects to measure—tell us where to look, at what point in time we might expect to see effects, how effects might evolve over time, and what sort of intended and unintended effects to look for.

- *Supporting Causal Inference.* Study of how law works provides evidence of plausible mechanisms that can be used to assess causation. Theory helps unpack a law into regulatory components that may have varying contributions to the overall effect, and helps identify dose-response relationships between specific legal components or dimensions and health-related outcomes.

- *Guiding Reform and Implementation.* Assuming confidence that law is causing an effect, research on how it does so provides important guidance on ways to influence the magnitude of the effect, reduce unintended consequences, or produce the effect more efficiently.

As the preceding chapters show, we draw on a rich and diverse literature to understand mechanisms of law. There is no single correct theory, and therefore no need to make an exclusive choice. Rather, the choice of what theory or theories to draw upon is a practical one based on research questions and designs, types of law or regulatory approach under study, and state of current knowledge about the matter being investigated. This chapter first elaborates on why it is so important to investigate *how*, as well as *whether*, law is having an effect on health, using safety-belt laws as one example. It then uses a second example in greater detail—the health effects of criminal laws regulating HIV exposure through sex—to illustrate how diverse theories of legal effect can be productively used.

The Value of Opening the Black Box

The stick-figure picture of law is that lawmakers issue a rule, and people obey it. A causal diagram for a public health law evaluation study based on this simple equation might start with no more than three boxes: one for law, one for the required behavior, and one for the health outcome. If the behavior is an established, good-enough proxy for a health outcome (such as safety-belt use in relation to crash morbidity and mortality), we could even dispense with a box for health outcome. Or, if we were correlating the law with crash outcomes, we could use the health outcome as a proxy for the required behavior. In studies so conceived, the chain of events between issuance of a rule, compliance, and its health outcomes is hidden within a black box. For some laws, and for some research purposes, this may be fine: the news of a law may be rapidly and widely disseminated, the rate of compliance may be quite high, or the relationship between the required behavior and a health outcome may be very strong. In some cases, local differences in the event unfolding in the black box (for example, the level of enforcement) may be small, or have little impact, so that with enough data points they do not significantly influence the result in the aggregate. Or perhaps there is no empirical research on a particular new law, and an initial "black box" study linking the law to an important health outcome represents an important contribution. Thus it is not always essential to know what is happening within the black box to accurately measure effects of a law on health. But the black box in which law unfolds is, at best, a placeholder for further development in a causal model, and at worst a sign of theoretical imprecision and a source of potential causal misattribution.

Defining the Phenomena to Be Observed

Law is just one of many factors that shape health outcomes. Although we often speak of a "chain" of causation, in which one event leads to another, a more apt metaphor is a causal web. As Swanson and Ibrahim explain in Chapter 10, one way to open the black box is to place the law within a causal diagram that depicts the process through which law is expected to have its effect, and the relation of law to *other* potential causes. In quantitative studies, measurement decisions and data interpretation may depend upon assumptions concerning how quickly or evenly a law will have an effect. In these processes, the researcher necessarily states hypotheses—falsifiable propositions about legal effects—and identifies candidate variables for observation and measurement. Generating testable hypotheses is greatly facilitated by an underlying theory of how law works. And, articulating a theory of the mechanism of effect makes clear underlying (and often hidden or imprecise) assumptions regarding why a given law is expected to have an effect or expected to have no effect.

Consider a mandatory safety-belt law. A change in safety-belt use after the passage of a law could be conceptualized as the result of deterrence: the causal diagram begins with the law, then proceeds through rational choices by drivers to compliance or non-compliance based on the likelihood and cost of detection. This theory would direct researchers toward an inquiry into drivers' risk aversion, or their perceptions of the likelihood and cost of detection. It is also plausible, however, that the law works by signaling the official adoption of an existing social norm of safety-belt use. On this theory, the causal diagram would highlight variables related to drivers' beliefs about the legitimacy of government authority or their beliefs about what people whose regard they value would expect them to do. A researcher could then test multiple theories, by, for example, surveying drivers about both their perceptions of punishment risk and their beliefs relevant to a normative theory. Or the researcher may make a reasoned choice about which theory to investigate further. For example, if the researcher is aware that the law has a trivial fine and is not being enforced, she may elect not to prioritize deterrence as a subject of investigation. In this way, theory makes it possible to systematically generate and test explanations of how law is working.

In a quasi-experimental study of the impact of a new safety-belt law, the researcher will need to decide how long to observe crash outcomes before and after the law, and at what interval (daily, weekly, monthly, annually; see Chapter 14). If we theorize that the law works solely via deterrence, we might predict a lag between the effective date of the law and increased compliance due to the time it takes for enforcement to ramp up and word to naturally spread. The expected pattern of gradual effect would shape study decisions about length of follow-up data collection and width of observation intervals. A slowly evolving effect might suggest a wider time resolution and a longer period of observation. If, on the other hand, we theorize that the law works largely by publicizing and reinforcing a social norm, and if it includes funds for a substantial publicity campaign that begins even before the effective date, we might use a narrower time interval and a shorter period of observation after the law takes effect.

Supporting Causal Inference

Causal inference is both empirically and philosophically challenging. Much of the research on how law influences health is observational. It may demonstrate a correlation between a law and a health outcome, but has a limited capacity to demonstrate that law *caused* the outcome. In making causal inferences about law, we typically are confronted with a complex system, only some of the elements and outcomes of which have been or can be observed, and in which law is just one element. As we discuss elsewhere in this volume, experimental and quasi-experimental research designs can help us attain a high degree of confidence in causal inference, but in any sort of study of causation in a complex system, both observational and experimental evidence of causation is bolstered by evidence that reveals more of the system's elements. Evidence of the mechanism through which law might have caused the effects—defining a demonstrable chain of events between the law and the effect—can help us decide whether an inference of causation is warranted and how confident we should be. Filling in the black box is, in PHLR, closely analogous to the "evidence of biological plausibility" criterion that is a widely accepted heuristic for assessing causation in epidemiology (Hill, 1965; for a discussion of criteria approaches to causal inference, see Ward, 2009). If one has a robust association between the proposed cause and the observed effect, an inference of causation is bolstered by evidence documenting the links in a causal web between them. And understanding the causal web requires good theorizing.

We return to the safety-belt question. There are many possible explanations for a correlation between safety-belt use and a law requiring it. A safety-belt law may have caused a change in use, but it is also possible that increasing use of safety belts changed social norms, leading to legislation as a sort of endorsement or signal of what had already occurred. Or both the rise in use and the law could be independent results of some other factor, such as a privately funded educational campaign to increase safety-belt use. Research that showed that drivers who feared detection and punishment were significantly more likely to use safety belts would support the inference that law was having an effect via deterrence. By contrast, a finding that there was no connection between wearing a safety belt and knowing about the law or regarding safety-belt use as the right thing would undermine the inference that law was driving the change in behavior. In neither case is the mechanism research conclusive, but in connection with other data it supports better judgments by researchers and policy actors.

Guiding Reform and Implementation

Having confidence that a law is having an effect on health outcomes is not the end of the PHLR inquiry. Logically we should desire that law have the largest positive effect it can possibly have, with the fewest negative side effects. Lawmakers will want to know not just whether the law works but at what cost. Along with cost-benefit and cost-effectiveness analysis, research that documents the mechanisms of legal effect can make a valuable contribution to making law work better. Documentation of implementation can identify practices that enhance or reduce the law's impact. Some enforcement strategies may be better than others, or may cost more than others that are equally effective. Negative side effects may be largely the result of how the law is enforced or implemented, rather than an inevitable consequence of the law's terms or design.

Safety-belt law again offers an example. As states began to pass these laws, two different enforcement strategies were used. In some states, failure to wear a safety belt was deemed a *primary* traffic violation, giving police officers the authority to stop and ticket drivers for that reason alone. In other states, the enforcement was "secondary," meaning that police officers could only issue a ticket for a safety-belt violation if the driver was being stopped for some other violation. We would not expect the difference in enforcement to make much difference in compliance if what drove compliance was normative agreement with the rule, or the legitimacy of the government. All states had better outcomes with safety-belt laws than without. Over time, however, researchers showed that compliance was significantly higher, and crash outcomes better, in states that adopted primary enforcement. In this instance, the deterrent impact of primary enforcement seems to have made a difference to a sufficiently large number of drivers. Knowing this allowed lawmakers to make a change in enforcement provisions that improved the beneficial effects of the rule.

Also important is that different segments of the population may be differentially affected by particular legal mechanisms, and effects of particular mechanisms likely vary over time as society changes. Differential effects across groups and time reinforce the importance of theory and illustrate how selecting a single theory is often unnecessary and possibly inappropriate. In the case of safety-belt laws, about 15 percent of drivers used belts voluntarily when they were made available in cars (after some educational campaigns). Compulsory use (even with only secondary enforcement) then increased belt use to the majority of drivers. Once the prevalence leveled off at approximately 60 to 70 percent, more active primary enforcement was needed to reach the remaining non-users. Apparently, normative effects of the law achieved a large part of the first major improvement in belt use and associated safety gains, while deterrence effects increased in importance for those starting to use belts later.

Keep in mind that the field of public health has firmly found that it is almost always easier and more effective to eliminate the need for individual (especially repetitive) behavior change (see Chapter 3). In the case of safety belts, public health professionals also worked on a parallel strategy to help protect car occupants from injuries without requiring individuals to engage in the behavior of using a safety belt every day—advocating for and achieving the mandatory installation of air bags in all automobiles sold in the United States. The design of airbag technology drew strongly on the sciences of physics and biomechanics, and advocacy caused regulatory tools to then be used to ensure the devices were universally installed in cars. This change in the environment around occupants of vehicles automatically protected all people in cars every day, advancing safety beyond that afforded by belts alone and providing significant protection also to those who remained non-users of belts despite the normative and deterrence effects of compulsory belt use laws.

Integrating Diverse Theories in Public Health Law Research

As the preceding chapters have shown, there are many tools available for opening the black box. PHLR researchers can draw upon a variety of theories developed by sociolegal scholars to explain how laws are put into practice and how they influence environments and behaviors. Similarly, it is possible to integrate laws within general social and behavioral theories. And it is in fact possible to do both at the same time. These methods make it possible to substantially improve the validity, utility, and credibility of health research on effects of laws and legal practices. There is no simple single theory, no easy way to integrate all theories into a single grand theory, and no prescribed way to use theory. We now illustrate this diversity by applying multiple theories to a single example.

Thirty-four states in the United States have statutes that explicitly criminalize sexual behavior of people with HIV under at least some circumstances (Bennett-Carlson, Faria, & Hanssens, 2010). In the remaining states, people with HIV have been prosecuted under various general criminal laws for exposing others to HIV or transmitting the virus (Lazzarini, Bray, & Burris, 2002). "Criminalization of HIV," as this phenomenon is known, has been criticized on a number of grounds (Burris & Cameron, 2008; Csete, Pearshouse, & Symington, 2009). There are many cases of the criminal law being used to severely punish assaultive behavior by people with HIV—spitting or biting, for example—that does not pose a significant risk of transmitting HIV. Similarly, many of the statutes are written broadly (or poorly) enough to cover sexual behavior, such as kissing, that has no realistic prospect of transmitting the virus (Galletly & Pinkerton, 2004; Wolf & Vezina, 2004). As applied to sexual behavior that does pose a significant risk of HIV, the laws generally require disclosure, safer sex (for example, condom use), or both. Here we focus on the main question for public health law research: whether criminal laws requiring disclosure of HIV status to partners lead to fewer instances of sexual HIV exposure and a reduction in the incidence of HIV in the population.

This is a difficult question to answer, for many reasons. There is no way to randomize exposure to the treatment (law). And in this case, quasi-experimental designs are also difficult or impossible. To begin with, we lack an objective measure of the outcome. Data on HIV incidence are lacking. Incidence is estimated on the basis of statistical analysis of HIV tests, which may come months or years after infection. Although technologies now exist that make it possible from a test to determine whether the person being tested was recently infected or not, generally we cannot attribute HIV infection events to specific times or places. Studies of the impact of criminal law on HIV therefore use self-reported sexual behavior as the main outcome measure (Burris, Beletsky, Burleson, Case, & Lazzarini, 2007; Delavande, Goldman, & Sood, 2007; Horvath, Weinmeyer, & Rosser, 2010). Even if a better outcome measure were available, we would be faced with the problem that many factors influence HIV infection and HIV risk behavior aside from the law. These range from population prevalence of HIV (the higher the prevalence the greater the likelihood that a given partner will have HIV) to availability and use of antiretroviral treatment (which reduces infectivity) to local norms of condom use to perceptions of risk about HIV. Widespread treatment could reduce HIV incidence even if no one practiced safer sex or disclosed infection; people in a low-prevalence population could practice unsafe sex against the law yet incidence would not change.

There are also challenges in defining the exposure to law across many jurisdictions. The laws differ from state to state, sometimes substantially; places without statutes are not places where law is absent—everywhere the same behavior may be charged as a crime under a general heading such as assault. Finally, accurately measuring whether people even know what the law is can be difficult to do in a way that does not bias later responses by prompting people to think about law. Moreover, because of the overlap between beliefs about law and preexisting social norms and beliefs, people may know about the law without knowing about it—a person who states correctly what the law is may have actual knowledge of the law, or merely assume that the law exists because of beliefs about what is the right thing to do. We end up with observational research that can correlate attitudes about what is right and legal with self-reported behavior and various demographic characteristics, but that has very limited ability to explain whether or how law is causing behavior change (Horvath, Weinmeyer, & Rosser, 2010). Or we resort to mathematical modeling that can test logical hypotheses but ultimately relies on unverifiable assumptions about behavior (Galletly & Pinkerton, 2008). This is precisely the sort of case in which theory about how law could lead to changes in health and health behavior can help us design studies that can shed credible light on the impact of law.

Compliance Models

Since we are interested in whether a law is influencing behavior, it makes sense to start with theories that explain why people obey the law. We will use the theories canvassed in the preceding chapters to generate testable hypotheses that will allow researchers to fill in the black box between an HIV-specific criminal law and sexual behavior.

KNOWLEDGE OF LAW

The threshold question in any compliance theory is whether people actually know what the law is. If they are not aware of the law at all, then their behavior can hardly be said to entail "complying" with it. The first hypothesis follows:

1. Sexually active people are aware of the law regulating the sexual behavior of people with HIV.

Generally speaking, evidence suggests that specific knowledge of the law in the general population is low. That is, most people are not lawyers and could not locate a specific provision in the code or define the elements of a crime. At the same time, people may have a pretty good idea of what is "against the law" simply on the assumption that behavior they regard as bad is also illegal. Applying this heuristic to HIV works pretty well, in that most people (including most people with HIV) seem to believe that it is right to protect or disclose to a partner (Horvath, Weinmeyer, & Rosser, 2010), and failure to do so under at least some circumstances could be prosecuted in every state in the union. Burris and colleagues used two measures in their study: the belief of the respondent that the law prohibited sexual behavior without disclosure of sero-positive status or use of a condom, and the actual law in the state of residence (Burris, Beletsky, Burleson, Case, & Lazzarini, 2007). That approach allowed the researchers to explore both objective and subjective pathways for legal effect. In contrast, Galletly and colleagues surveyed people with HIV in one state to find out not only whether they were aware of a specific law but also how well they understood its provisions and where they had learned of it (Galletly,

DiFranceisco, & Pinkerton, 2008). Armed with a reasonable measure of legal knowledge or belief, we can explore compliance.

CRIMINOLOGY: DETERRENCE

In Chapter 5, Jennings and Mieczkowski explain that criminological theories of compliance—deterrence and labeling—begin with the assumption of rationality. The individual, aware of the law and having some beliefs about its enforcement, will make behavioral choices on the basis of a "utilitarian assessment of pain and pleasure." In our case, the law proposes to punish people with HIV who have sex without disclosing their status or using a condom. The deterrence hypothesis holds that a person will comply with the law if he or she believes that detection and punishment are sufficiently likely and severe enough that the prospect of future pain outweighs the attraction of current pleasure. For example, in Klitzman's qualitative study of attitudes toward these laws, one participant described "how the threat of such a law had altered his own actions after he made 'a fatal mistake' by not disclosing to a woman who later said that he was trying to kill her and that she could report him to the police. He explained that this legal threat motivated him to alter his behavior with future partners" (Klitzman, Kirshenbaum, Kittel, et al., 2004).

In this model, rational choice is not a hypothesis but a premise. We assume that people who know about the law will make a rational choice. The causal diagram (see Figure 5.1) posits that these beliefs will be influenced by "direct and indirect exposure" to law—some combination of personal experience with law enforcement, such as being warned about unsafe behavior, and indirect experience, such as reading about prosecutions in the news. These experiences contribute to core beliefs about the certainty, celerity, severity, and equity of punishment for violating the law. This in turn produces two hypotheses to test:

2. People who have had more experience with the law are less likely to report sexual behavior inconsistent with the law.

3. People with positive beliefs about certainty, celerity, severity, and equity will be less likely to report sexual behavior inconsistent with the law.

Chapter 5 discusses both scenario-based and survey methods for assessing these elements. In the case of HIV criminalization, the latter are illustrated by Burris and colleagues (2007). To measure experience with law, subjects were asked whether they were aware of people being arrested for various acts covered by the law, and how much they knew about these cases. The perceived likelihood of being caught was measured by a set of Likert-scaled items about the likelihood of being caught for activities such as unprotected sex. The perceived severity of the sanction was measured with a set of Likert-scaled items such as "I'm not worrying about jail when I have sex or shoot drugs." The responses were then scaled to create variables for each concept. No significant relationship was found between experience and compliance, and finding as to certainty or severity was intriguing: people who scored higher on the severity and certainty scales were more likely to report compliance with the law, but with some minor exceptions knowledge of the law was not associated with compliance. Thus people who were generally more concerned about being punished for a variety of actions were more likely to practice safer sex or disclose HIV to a partner, but this was not apparently a product of the specific law at issue.

ECONOMICS

Criminological deterrence theory is virtually identical to standard economic analysis of why people obey criminal law. Like criminology, economics assumes a rational person who will seek pleasure and avoid pain (that is, maximize utility) on the basis of an objective assessment of the probabilities. Following the theory, people who are "risk-neutral"—that is, who treat the value of punishment as equal to the benefit to be gained from the behavior—will comply with the law if the punishment is set higher than the value of benefit gained divided by the probability of detection (Polinsky & Shavell, 2007).

Delavande, Goldman, and Sood (2007) used this assumption in a paper that also tried to account for the chances of a person actually getting into trouble. Their basic formula illustrates how economics can be used to state a set of deterrence hypotheses:

> Consider a representative risk-neutral HIV+ person who resides in a state that prosecutes HIV-infected individuals for exposing others to the virus through sexual contact. Let $\Pi > 0$ denote the disutility from being prosecuted and P (pros) be the probability of being prosecuted. The probability of being prosecuted in turn depends on the likelihood that a potential partner would report the sex act to the state and the probability that the state would prosecute conditional on receiving a report:
>
> $$P(Pros) = P(reported) \times P(presecuted\ reported) = P(reported) \times \rho$$
>
> The parameter ρ is a key policy of interest—states with higher values of ρ have more stringent law enforcement against HIV+ individuals [Delavande, Goldman, & Sood, 2007, p. 5].

Using this formulation of deterrence, they applied data on sexual behavior to test whether more stringent law enforcement increases safe sex, decreases disclosure of HIV-positive status, and decreases the probability of a sexual encounter. (Unlike other studies discussed here, this one found that aggressive prosecution had all these effects, which, if nothing else, reminds us that methodological and theoretical choices matter.)

CRIMINOLOGY: LABELING

Deterrence in criminology and economics assumes a rational actor calculating risks and benefits. There are plausible reasons for applying this rationality assumption to sexual behavior, but sex can also be seen as the product of social forces. Labeling theory has immediate plausibility in analyzing the effect of criminal laws governing sex because of the basic question of whether having unsafe sex or failing to disclose should be considered "wrong," or whether people who engage in unsafe sex should be considered "criminals." The labeling theory causal diagram (see Figure 5.2) suggests that some individuals with HIV may respond to the label of criminal by defining themselves as rebels or deviants, or that a social-level view of people with HIV (or gay men or sexually active people) as criminal may feed the development of an offender subculture or may deter people from disclosing their HIV status or seeking behavioral health services. Labeling theory suggests a number of interesting hypotheses, including the following:

4. People who internalize the label of criminal will be more likely to report sexual behavior inconsistent with the law.

5. People who perceive that society regards their behavior as deviant will be more likely to report sexual behavior inconsistent with the law.

6. The more people are aware of prosecutions or other negative societal reactions to the "deviant subculture," the stronger the effect of the label.

Although studies of HIV criminalization have not yet explicitly deployed labeling theory, a number of studies suggest ways these hypotheses could be tested. Dodds, Bourne, and Weait (2009) used semistructured interviews with sexually active gay men in Britain to investigate the effects of criminalization on attitudes and behaviors. Some men, they found, reacted to the labeling of sexual behavior as a crime by, as it were, acting more like criminals, "maximizing their anonymity, and being less open about their HIV status, avoiding disclosure" (p. 141). Also using interviews, Mykhalovskiy (2011) found that the labeling of sexual behavior as criminal might influence behavior along another, unexpected pathway: HIV risk-reduction counselors reported concerns about openly discussing questions of disclosure and condom use out of fear their records might be subpoenaed in a criminal case. Social attitudes toward unsafe HIV sexual behavior, or people with HIV generally, may be measured through survey research, such as Herek's studies of HIV-related stigma (Herek, 1988, 1993; Herek, Capitanio, & Widaman, 2002).

PROCEDURAL JUSTICE

The challenge with sex is that it is usually conducted in private. Likewise, only an extremely small percentage of sexually active people with HIV are arrested or prosecuted (Lazzarini, Bray, & Burris, 2002), so the objective chance of detection and punishment is small. Moreover, as labeling theory suggests, people's views on the "rightness" of the law or the fairness of its implementation could also influence compliance. Procedural justice offers a way to get to at least two important subjects: internal motivation to comply, which matters a good deal when we are talking about what is in essence an uncontrolled social behavior, and the fact that government regulation of sex, not least gay sex, is highly contentious. It is possible that compliance of people subject to the law will be influenced by their views about whether the government should even be making these rules, or by their experiences with the "system." Procedural justice theory provides a way to understand and study these possible effects (Tyler, 1990).

Figure 6.1 is a causal diagram of the effect of procedural justice on compliance with law. For our purposes, we focus on the segment of the pathway linking the experience of procedural fairness, "legitimacy" (defined in terms of "obligation" and "trust and confidence"), and compliance. Chapter 6 explains that "[w]hen people ascribe legitimacy to the system that governs them, they become willing subjects whose behavior is strongly influenced by official (and unofficial) doctrine. They also internalize a set of moral values that is consonant with the aims of the system." Perceptions of procedural fairness—"fairness of decision making (voice, neutrality) and fairness of interpersonal treatment (trust, respect)"—are strong predictors of people's sense of governmental legitimacy.

Both legitimacy and fairness resonate in interesting ways when it comes to criminalization of HIV. It is easy to fall into the error of assuming that people at elevated risk of HIV—people who use drugs, men who have sex with men, or people who sell sex—are, by virtue of those behaviors, fundamentally different from other people in society. At the same time, it is plausible that people engaging in illegal acts such as drug use or prostitution may be more likely to have experienced what they feel is unfair treatment at the hands of authorities, and that they may not be as willing as others to accept an official view that drug use or prostitution is wrong. Similarly, gay men as a group may be more likely than others to reject a role for government in regulating sexual behavior, and to perceive laws that do so as a product of an unfair political system. The procedural justice perspective supports a number of interesting hypotheses about compliance with HIV-specific criminal laws, including the following:

7. People who have had positive experiences of procedural justice in their encounters with authority will be more likely to regard the law regulating the sexual behavior of people with HIV as legitimate.

8. People who regard the government as legitimate will be more likely to comply with laws regulating sexual behavior among people with HIV.

Qualitative research suggests that concerns about intentions behind these laws and fairness of their implementation resonate with gay men. Klitzman's interviewees had complex feelings about these laws. Some endorsed the mandate for responsibility, while others were concerned about effects on safer sex and testing. Others feared unfair prosecutions and believed that bedroom behavior was properly a private, not governmental, domain (Klitzman, Kirshenbaum, Kittel, et al., 2004). And perceived fairness may interact with perceived effectiveness of the law—if the law does not reduce HIV transmission, it is not fair to burden certain people with obligations or restrictions that do not apply to others. The closest thing to a test of these hypotheses in the literature can be found in the study by Burris and colleagues (2007). The study adapted items from Tyler (1990) to investigate both the experience of procedural justice and the extent to which respondents regarded the government as a legitimate regulator of sexual behavior. As a group, respondents (a convenience sample of people recruited at high-risk sex and drug-use venues) did not have strong feelings on either issue. Most of them did believe that it was morally right for people with HIV to disclose or practice safer sex, and this belief was consistent with their self-reported behavior—but expressing these beliefs was not related to beliefs about the law or whether a specific law actually applied to the respondent. The authors inferred from these results that norms did matter to sexual behavior, but that they were operating independently of the law. Law, in other words, was not playing a major role in sexual choices (Burris, Beletsky, Burleson, Case, & Lazzarini, 2007).

PUBLIC HEALTH

There are many examples of public health laws directed at individual behavior such as wearing safety belts. In public health, however, changing the environment is often seen as a more expeditious and effective way to promote health than intervening directly with individuals to change their behavior. Law can be a means of inducing changes in social, physical, and economic environments that change people's behavior or reduce individuals' exposure to unhealthy products or conditions (see Figure 3.1). Because law may also be a factor in exacerbating risk—for example by causing high levels of incarceration in some communities that expose many people to higher-prevalence prison environments and disrupt sexual networks—removing a law can be an important environmental intervention. A public health model of legal intervention suggests many hypotheses, including the following:

9. Laws and regulations that reduce the cost to consumers and increase ease of access to condoms will increase condom use and decrease rates of unprotected sex, unplanned pregnancy, STDs, and HIV transmission.

10. Laws that alter the physical layout and operating rules for public sex venues will reduce unsafe sex.

11. Laws that improve employment among young African American men will reduce incarceration rates, reduce HIV among this population, and reduce subsequent transmission to others.

Law might be used to require specific locations to provide condoms at no cost to the user, for example, requiring condoms be readily available in bathhouses. Regularly seeing condoms in a sex venue could change social norms around condoms and their acceptability, as well as increasing their use simply because of ease of physical access to them at a moment when they might be needed. Such an intervention in New York City bathhouses was associated with a significantly greater likelihood of consistent condom use during anal sex in venues receiving the intervention compared to control venues (Ko, Lee, Hung, et al., 2009). The basic logic applies to other locations, with regulations potentially requiring condom vending machines in rest rooms at high schools, colleges, gas stations, convenience stores, and so on. Ending legal practices that discourage condom use could also be effective. For example, police implementing laws against prostitution in some places reportedly treat a woman's possession of a condom as evidence of illegal activity, discouraging sex workers and other women from possessing them (Blankenship & Koester, 2002).

Law may also promote safer sex by requiring changes in the layout or operating rules of establishments that cater to people looking for sexual encounters. Courts and city councils have taken this approach over the course of the HIV epidemic, issuing orders and ordinances variously requiring public sex venues to remove doors from cubicles, enhance lighting, post safe-sex rules or warnings, and eject patrons having unsafe sex (Burris, 2003). William Woods and colleagues (Woods, Binson, Pollack, et al., 2003; Woods, Euren, Pollack, & Binson, 2010) surveyed seventy-seven gay bathhouses and sex clubs across the United States and reported that all were engaged to some degree in offering HIV prevention, and that most clubs that allowed sexual behavior among patrons had instituted one or more environmental interventions. Unfortunately, there are no published studies of the effectiveness of these efforts.

Thinking about how environments influence behavior tends to shift the focus from the way individuals cope with a given set of stimuli (that is, promoting "good choices") to promoting environments that maximize good options. Thus, in a public health framework, a researcher might be less likely to ask whether criminal law encourages safer sex than to investigate the "social determinants" of HIV transmission. For example, unemployment and lack of opportunities for full participation in society (along with other related factors) result in very high incarceration rates among U.S. black young men. In prison, many of those men acquire HIV—prisons appear to be a major "hot spot" for HIV transmission (World Health Organization, United Nations Office on Drugs and Crime, & UNAIDS, 2007). Social networks are important factors in the spread of HIV (Ward, 2007). Incarceration disrupts networks as those left behind in the community form new relationships (Khan, Wohl, Weir, et al., 2008). A variety of laws and regulations affect employment, business investment, and education and skills development in ways that increase or decrease employment opportunities for this population. These policies, rather than a specific prohibition of unsafe sex, may be the most important focus of public health law research.

Modeling Law Within Broader Social and Behavioral Theory

Our discussion thus far applies well-developed theories about how law works. They are quite rich, and provide many insights for public health law researchers. At this point, however, the reader may notice the bias in the foregoing inquiry: we have implicitly assumed that law is a significant, or at least detectable, driver of behavior. Rather than construct the question in a framework of how law influences behavior, a researcher could start with a general behavioral theory in which law is simply added as one of many factors and not treated as the preeminent effect to study.

The Theory of Triadic Influences

The theory of triadic influences (TTI) presents a detailed scheme for understanding the many factors that produce an intention to behave in a certain way and, ultimately, the behavior itself (see Chapter 8). It integrates and expands upon other theories that have shown the importance of three proximal factors to a behavior intention: the individual's attitudes toward the behavior, the individual's perception of social norms and beliefs concerning the behavior; and the actor's sense of self-efficacy or behavioral control in reference to the behavior. Figure 8.1 highlights main pathways along which law may be hypothesized to influence these constructs.

A law can influence an individual's attitudes toward a behavior along two substreams. In the "cognitive-rational" substream, law provides information about the behavior society expects or regards as desirable. This information may also be experienced more emotionally or affectively in interactions with social institutions. In both instances, the streams lead to an attitude toward the behavior composed of both conscious and rational elements, and more affective ones. And of course the legal inputs in this process are interacting with other ones as well, such as information about safe sex and HIV.

Law may influence behavior via self-efficacy or behavioral control if it makes a behavior easier to adopt. In our example, a law requiring universal condom use the first time people have sex with one another, as Ayres and Baker have proposed (Ayres & Baker, 2004), could in theory reduce the emotional and social barriers to proposing condom use when approaching sexual relations. Here, too, the broader behavioral science framework easily accommodates other possible influences on condom use, such as sex education or the provision of condoms in sex venues.

Finally, law can work via the social-normative stream. The theory posits that people will be influenced by how others perceive their behavior. We are sensitive to general social norms and the values of our important associates. Law may be taken as a reflection or reinforcement of social disapproval of unsafe sex, bolstering the norm of safer sex or disclosure. The innate desire to please others in relationships and to avoid conflict may promote safer behavior or disclosure, though of course the social milieu may send quite contradictory signals. A perceived norm of disclosure may be blunted in its effect on behavior by the perception that people with HIV are not considered desirable sex partners.

A great variety of hypotheses about HIV criminalization and sexual behavior can be generated and tested within this framework. One strategy is to embed standard compliance theory within the TTI. For example, one can conceptualize deterrence as operating via knowledge and expectancies; certainty, celerity, severity, and equity become variables within the pathway of rational responses to the environment. Or one can treat law as a distal influence on the social-normative stream, influencing others' behaviors and attitudes and the actor's perceived norms. The richness of the model makes it possible to test hypotheses about direct legal effects or to link tests of law to broader behavioral questions. Examples include the following:

12. People who know about the law are more likely to perceive a norm against having sex without disclosing HIV status or using a condom.

13. People who perceive a norm requiring safer sex or disclosure of HIV status are more likely to disclose or practice safer sex.

Hypotheses of this sort can be explored in interviews. Several of the respondents in the study conducted by Dodds and colleagues

> feared condemnation from their local gay community should it become known that they had engaged in unprotected sex as a diagnosed man. . . . A criminal prosecution case had the potential to make public such behaviour and raised the fear of judgment from peers and the negative social consequences of being identified as morally reprehensible. As a result they were particularly cautious about avoiding the circumstances that might lead to such an accusation. "I'm very, very acutely aware of kind of where the law is on it, you know? And although I could say that he knew I were positive there, [pause] I could

possibly still be ostracized if it came out in the community that I was the one who infected him and all of this sort of stuff. I didn't want that really and I didn't fancy being prosecuted" (Late 30s, diagnosed 18 years) [Dodds, Bourne, & Weait, 2009, p. 140].

An advantage of the TTI and several of the theories it integrates is that there are well-developed measurement approaches to eliciting information, scaling, and quantifying the results for purposes of predicting behavioral intentions and behavior. The survey designed by Burris and colleagues drew on the theory of planned behavior (Burris, Beletsky, Burleson, Case, & Lazzarini, 2007). In addition to a variety of items that explored people's own attitudes toward safer sex and disclosure, perceived behavioral control used true-false statements such as "If I am sexually aroused I can stop before sex to use a condom." Perceived social norms were investigated with true-false statements such as "People I know best expect that I will always discuss my HIV status with partners before having sex." The integration of behavioral theory and legal compliance avoids the assumption that law is a primary driver of behavior while at the same time allowing law to be investigated along the many plausible pathways of effect.

ECONOMICS

Economic theory rests on "rational actors" who seek to maximize utility as they see it. That bedrock explanation for how law influences behavior has already been discussed. Chapter 7 offers a more complex account of the operation of law in an economic framework. For most economists, a fully free market is by definition optimum, and the sole (or at least predominant) rationale for legal intervention in the market is to ameliorate market failures that prevent a truly free market. Some might feel uneasy about applying market language to choices and actions involving intimate encounters between individuals, but a long-standing closely related theory in sociology does exactly that. Social exchange theory (Blau, 1964; Homans, 1958) deems all social interactions (not just economic transactions) to be characterized by persons attempting to maximize their gain for a given investment, and has long been applied to human mate selection processes (Goode, 1970, 1971). The theory is not without its critics (Rosenfeld, 2005), but our purpose here is merely to illustrate application of such theory to the example before us.

Assuming that individuals seeking sex and other dimensions of an intimate relationship attempt to maximize their return on investment, for this "market" to work well everyone must have full information about the relevant dimensions under consideration in the transaction. Information on HIV status of potential partners is one such relevant data element, and laws requiring disclosure of sero-positivity are attempting to improve the operation of this market by improving information availability. The objective could be furthered by related regulations, such as requirements for regular automatic HIV testing at all preventive health care visits. As always, possible side effects of such efforts to improve information in this market must be considered, such as the risk that disclosure of HIV status, and reliance on that (potentially incorrect) disclosure by others might increase risk of HIV spread by reducing condom use, an outcome suggested by some recent studies (Butler & Smith, 2007).

"LAW AND SOCIETY" RESEARCH

The theories we have seen so far all tend to treat law as a distinct thing, a piece of information with an objective set of characteristics that acts, in a causal chain, on environments and people that are separate and distinct from the law. The law and society tradition moves beyond how people "use" or "obey" law to bring critical empirical attention to how the rule of law is socially constructed, enacted, contested, and perpetuated in social fields (Cooper, 1995). While there is certainly a body of evaluation research in the law and society literature, "the unique contribution of the law and society approach," Robin Stryker writes in Chapter 4, "is to suggest mechanisms of legal effect emphasizing *meaning-making*." This literature provides powerful theoretical and research methods for getting at how both legal agents and legal subjects understand their roles, their ability to act within a legal framework, and indeed the nature of that legal framework itself (Yngvesson, 1988).

The law and society approach doesn't just allow researchers to ask about the effect of laws in different ways, it suggests different questions. If law is within society and inside people's heads—a way of thinking, a form of meaning—the question is not so much how law influences individual behavior as how law shapes the meaning of acts and the identities of people, from which behavior flows. Law isn't just a set of expressed rules that instruct people specifically how to act in particular situations. "Law" is a repertoire of strategies for getting by, or an alien intrusion to be contested, or just one possible script for understanding one's situation (Ewick & Silbey, 1998). Laws more broadly contribute to the social structuring of expectations of what should and will happen, and how all that can be explained. So, for example, Musheno used case studies of people with HIV at the margins of society—welfare beneficiaries, drug users—to show how "[p]revailing ideologies and belief systems serve to codify what a person in a given position is likely to perceive or expect to accomplish when confronted with trouble. . . ." (Musheno, 1997).

Law and society research, with its focus on meaning, often draws upon qualitative methods, including interviews and participant observation, that allow people the opportunity not simply to explain law in their own words but to come to law when they are ready to see it. The concern that the researcher not define the law for the subject has produced some interesting methodological refinement. In their work on how law was influencing the lives of people with disabilities, for example, Engel and Munger (1996) used an "autobiographical" approach in which subjects told and repeatedly edited their life stories. Rather than starting with knowledge of law, or even asking specific questions about law, the researchers waited for the law to emerge on its own in the stories. Law, they found, was not just important when a formal claim or command was made. "Rights may be interwoven with individual lives and with particular social or cultural settings even when no formal claim is lodged. Rights can emerge in day-to-day talk among friends and co-workers; their very enactment can subtly change the terms of discussion or the images and conceptual categories that are used in everyday life. Such subtle yet profound effects may be overlooked in traditional studies of legal impact, yet they can be detected through the analysis in depth of life stories" (Engel & Munger, 1996, p. 14).

Law and society methods are well-suited to understanding how law operates as a meaning-making and meaning-expressing social activity. Public health generally has had its greatest success in interventions that work by changing the social and physical environment, which can both influence individual behavior and reduce exposure to toxic unhealthy conditions (see Figure 3.1). A sociolegal perspective could be deployed to investigate how the legal classification of homosexual behavior as a crime, or the long exclusion of gay people from marriage, might be shaping sexual relationships and the risk of HIV (Burris, 1998a; Chauncey, 1994). Here we consider two narrower hypotheses in the law and society vein:

14. The meaning and implementation of HIV criminalization laws and court decisions will be mediated by how HIV service organizations interpret them and integrate their interpretations into behavioral counseling.

15. Court proceedings and decisions in HIV criminalization cases will be shaped by underlying beliefs about race, nationality, class, and gender.

Working in an interpretive tradition, law and society research often is not framed in terms of testing a specific hypothesis. Nonetheless, researchers pursue specific questions within clearly stated theoretical parameters. Mykhalovskiy studied HIV criminalization as a case of "the social organization of knowledge," focusing on how criminal law shaped the environment of HIV testing and counseling organizations and the people within that environment. He used interviews and focus groups "designed to elicit experiential narratives in which participants reflected on the topic of criminalizing HIV nondisclosure in ways grounded in their actual, day-to-day experiences" (2011, p. 3). His "[a]nalysis of interview data was focused on bringing into view how an abstract criminal law obligation is made meaningful and expresses itself in people's lives through multiple social and institutional channels" (p. 3).

The work added insights into compliance. Mykhalovskiy found a great deal of confusion among his subjects about the meaning of the legal concept of "significant risk," which the courts in Canada used to create the dividing line for criminal liability in a sexual encounter. People with HIV seemed to have fairly precise knowledge of the rule—but didn't understand what it meant for actual behavior. For their part, counselors interviewed were equally confused, and for them the problem was compounded by having to offer guidance based on some resolution of the legal and public health advice on risks. Many felt that what they would endorse from a public health point of view as "safer sex" might be criminal under the "significant risk" approach used by courts. But beyond the difficulties of "counseling with an eye on the law" (2011, p. 5), Mykhalovskiy found signs of a process in which law changed the purpose and contents of risk reduction counseling, which in turn seemed to be changing the law: counselors were starting to promote disclosure as a way to avoid legal trouble, beyond its utility as a risk-reduction strategy, and in turn lawyers were noting that pro- secutors and judges were "citing to the fact that this person was counseled by public health nurse X on these three occasions to disclose and use a condom and then that becomes used to sort of bootstrap the criminal law obligation into you have an obligation to disclose and to use condoms, which in fact is not what the Supreme Court said. . . ." (p. 7). In this instance, law was not just influencing compliance—compliance was influencing law.

Law and society approaches can be used to explore in a richer way how law is shaping meaning and behavior. It can also be deployed to understand how a variety of social factors and processes influence how law is made and used. Matthew Weait, who conducted close textual analysis of court opinions, found that notions of risk and responsibility interacted with gender roles, race, and nationality to shape how judges applied legal rules in HIV exposure cases (Weait, 2007). His work illustrates how a public health law may actually be doing very different kinds of work, policing moral and ethnic boundaries. Many of the most influential social analyses of HIV have explored law's role in the mediation of HIV's shame, stigma, and inter-group conflict (Altman, 1986; Bayer, 1989; Patton, 1990). Social theory can help researchers explore the many legal influences on health and health behavior that do not work through specific behavioral rules directed at individuals.

Conclusion

This chapter illustrates the use of theory and tools from a range of social and behavioral sciences and legal research traditions to study mechanisms of legal effect in public health law research. Such theory largely addresses how law shapes health-relevant behaviors, but theory also guides investigation of legal mechanisms that influence health by changing institutions and environments. Scientists and legal scholars can and should draw upon theory to clarify and guide research questions, shape the design of studies, and increase specificity of hypotheses to investigate. Results from such studies then can better illuminate what happens between the passage of a law and changes in institutions, environments, and behaviors that enhance the health of the population. Better understanding of mechanisms of effect in any specific case, that is, confirming a theory in one situation, also substantially improves the generalizability of a successful public health law in one area to other times, places, settings, and other public health problems.

Summary

Theoretically grounded research illuminating mechanisms of legal effect has at least three important benefits for public health law research and practice: defining the phenomena to be observed, supporting causal inference, and guiding reform and implementation. The choice of what theory or theories to draw upon is a practical one based on research questions and designs, types of law or regulatory approach under study, and state of current knowledge about the matter being investigated. PHLR researchers can draw upon a variety of theories developed by sociolegal scholars to explain how laws are put into practice and how they influence environments and behaviors. Similarly, it is possible to integrate laws within general social and behavioral theories. And it is in fact possible to do both at the same time. These methods make it possible to substantially improve the validity, utility, and credibility of health research on effects of laws and legal practices.

Compliance theories explain why people obey the law. The threshold question in any compliance theory is whether people actually know what the law is. Both deterrence theorists and economic theorists posit that people will behave rationally given what they know about the law and the consequences of disobedience. Labeling theory posits that criminal law works by defining proscribed behaviors as "wrong" and people who engage in it as "criminals." Procedural justice theory focuses on the internal motivation to comply, and how it is influenced by the perceived fairness of legal authorities. In the public health tradition, law is often used to change social and physical environments to reduce exposure to risks, rather than to directly regulate individual behavior itself.

Rather than construct the question in a framework of how law influences behavior, a researcher also could start with a general behavioral theory in which law is simply added as one of many factors, and not treated as the preeminent effect to study. The theory of triadic influences (TTI) presents a detailed scheme for understanding the many factors that produce an intention to behave in a certain way and, ultimately, the behavior itself. Economics places the law and the phenomena it regulates within a framework of markets. Finally, research in the law and society tradition provides powerful theoretical and research methods for getting at how both legal agents and legal subjects understand their roles, their ability to act within a legal framework, and the nature of that legal framework itself.

Further Reading

Dean, K. (1996). Using theory to guide policy relevant health promotion research. *Health Promotion International, 11*(1), 19–26.

Hedstrom, P., & Ylikoski, P. (2010). Causal mechanisms in the social sciences. *Annual Review of Sociology, 36*(1), 49–67.

Hill, A. B. (1965). The environment and disease: Association or causation? *Proceedings of the Royal Society of Medicine, 58*, 295–300.

Part Three

Identifying and Measuring Legal Variables

Now that we have seen the wide range of theory that can be applied to public health law research, and perhaps gained a vision of hundreds of specific research questions, representing studies waiting to be done, we turn to the steps necessary to conducting high-quality PHLR studies. Before collecting and analyzing data, there is an intermediate step that involves drawing on theories of how law affects population health to specify the exact causal paths that will be the focus of a particular study. No single research project can study all possible causal links—all the ways that a law can affect health. Each study of necessity pulls out a few of those links for evaluation, on the basis of current state of knowledge regarding theory; particular laws that have been changed in substantial ways and thus present opportunities for study; types of data available; and resource constraints.

Swanson and Ibrahim begin this section with a practical guide to using causal diagrams. Causal diagrams clarify the specific theories and concepts that are the focus of the study; make explicit often implicit hypotheses about how the law works; shape the ways laws are measured for a particular study; reveal key implementation characteristics, mediators, and moderators that need to be measured; and point to the set of health outcome indicators best suited for the study. The causal diagram for a particular study illuminates expected patterns of legal effect over space and time, and therefore guides more than the measurement and data-collection features of the study. It also shapes the basic design of the study, the number and time spans of baseline and follow-up observations, and the composition of experimental and comparison groups.

The second and third chapters of Part Three focus on identifying and measuring characteristics of law. Measuring law for evaluation research is quite different from the way lawyers measure law in traditional legal research. Legal research typically is focused on assessing the idiosyncrasies of each particular law and how it can be applied to a single, particular situation, and usually is focused on current law. In contrast, scientific research is focused on measuring underlying theory-based dimensions or components of law, and relating those dimensions to broader events and outcomes in society. And, to more validly assess legal effects, scientists usually study effects of changes in law over time. Lawyers tend to be particularistic—each law is different from all the others (in other jurisdictions or other times). Scientists tend to be more generalist—similar laws need to be lumped into larger groups of laws for research on how they affect society. The complexities of coding laws into categories and assigning numeric values to register the amounts of various dimensions are addressed for statutory law and regulations by Anderson, Tremper, Thomas, and Wagenaar in Chapter 11, and the distinct issues that arise with coding case law are discussed by Hall in Chapter 12.

Chapter 10

Picturing Public Health Law Research

The Value of Causal Diagrams

Jeffrey W. Swanson   Jennifer K. Ibrahim

Learning Objectives

- Describe ways that conceptual models can be used to understand a phenomenon in public health law and translate that understanding into research designs.

- Construct a causal diagram, including inputs, mediators, moderators, outputs, and outcomes.

- Compare and contrast different applications of a basic causal diagram across a range of disciplines.

In 1927, New York publicist Frederick Barnard published a misattributed "Chinese proverb" that captured an obvious, yet profound idea: "One picture is worth ten thousand words." Barnard was trying to sell advertising space on streetcars, but the phrase aptly expressed a core truth about human cognition and learning: that we naturally use symbolic pictures to apprehend, organize, summarize, remember, and convey complex information.

Whether it is worth ten thousand or one thousand words (as today's shortened version of Barnard's adage has it), the reason we can trade all that language for "a picture" is that we understand the world around us largely through a process of simplifying representation (Dansereau & Simpson, 2009). We organize complex information into small chunks that can be visualized and recalled. We build mental models of the world—of what the chunks stand for and how they fit together and causally affect each other—and we unconsciously test and adapt such models to accommodate new, corresponding observations and experiences over a lifetime.

These images of our surroundings and of "how things work" are useful for what they include, but also for what they leave out; they enable us to ignore a vast amount of distracting information and to focus our attention on what is most relevant for a particular purpose. Models also allow us to understand a larger context, as they provide an overall orientation and a "place to stand," from which we can focus in on smaller sections of the picture.

Given the multidisciplinary perspectives of public health law research and the wide range of topics included in PHLR, the use of commonly understood pictures to illustrate ways in which law and health interact can be invaluable (Burris, Wagenaar, Swanson, et al., 2010). Ranging from laws that prohibit individual behaviors to laws that provide authority to act to laws that regulate organizational practices, PHLR seeks to understand the mechanisms by which laws can improve health; visualizing these mechanisms in diagrams is an important tool for achieving such an understanding. The purpose of this chapter is to review some basic conventions used to create visual models, evaluate relevant examples of models in published PHLR studies, and offer recommendations for constructing clear and informative models.

Varieties of Visual Representation

Academic disciplines—from the sciences to medicine, law, engineering, business management, and education—have long used formal schematic pictures to efficiently represent complex processes and to articulate theories about phenomena of interest (Coryn & Scriven, 2008; Ellermann, Kataoka-Yahiro, & Wong, 2006; Hamilton, Bronte-Tinkew, & Child Trends Inc., 2007; Jordan, 2010; Misue, Eades, Lai, & Sugiyama, 1995; Recker, Rosemann, Indulska, & Green, 2009; Wright, 1934). Various knowledge enterprises have given many names to their pet graphic images, as schematic pictures have become a key currency of technical information. Molecular diagrams depict basic structures of matter in chemistry (Daudel & Daudel, 1948). System flow charts illustrate how computer programs, court proceedings, and organizations work (U.S. Bureau of Justice, 2011). A business process model can show how a particular firm produces goods and services, sells a product, and makes a profit (Recker, Rosemann, Indulska, & Green, 2009). Logic models illustrate plans for public health or policy interventions and lay out criteria for evaluating whether these interventions function as designed and produce desired outcomes

(W. K. Kellogg Foundation, 2004). Concept mapping or concept webbing can elicit and clarify culturally divergent views of health and disease (Novak & Cañas, 2008). Statistical path analysis schematizes and guides empirical testing of theories of the component causes of social-behavioral phenomena in populations, drawing out ways in which causal factors sometimes interact or may take meandering detours in route to their effect (Duncan, 1966; Land, 1969; Wright, 1934). Regardless of the specific type of model and the associated discipline, all of these approaches are working to do the same thing: tell a story in a single image.

For their part, public health law researchers can use representational diagrams to derive specific research questions and hypotheses from a relevant theoretical framework and then design an appropriate study to test such hypotheses. An overarching model may encompass a broad agenda for research on a PHLR topic, thus allowing the investigator to locate and sequence particular research questions and projects while understanding how they fit into a "big picture." Diagrams can also be used to help policy makers and the general public understand a complex PHLR topic. By viewing a diagram that clearly depicts a law's effect in, for example, modifying individual health behaviors or risks in the environment, stakeholders can understand how law is supposed to work.

Our purpose in this chapter is not to comprehensively review all of the various graphical devices that have been used to corral knowledge across fields of human inquiry. Neither is it our purpose to endorse one discipline's particular modeling conventions or to propose some new iconography unique to PHLR. Rather, in what follows, we set forth a few general principles—suggest modest guidelines—for drafting graphic models that are likely to prove useful in conceptualizing, implementing, and critically evaluating innovative PHLR projects. We describe and illustrate several specific purposes that causal diagrams may serve, as they guide research on the effects of law and legal practices on population health.

What do we call these pictures for PHLR? Without taking it too seriously, we use the term *causal diagram* (CD). We suppose that *causal* is a key element, insofar as the depiction of determining relationships between variables is a main point of these devices; if nothing else, they show how one thing leads (or could lead) predictably to another. Second, *diagram* seems to work because its Greek meaning is, roughly, "to mark out by lines."

Elements and Conventions of Causal Diagrams

What are the basic components and rules of causal diagrams? Novak and Cañas (2008) provide a useful description of "concept maps" that applies generally to CDs at the simplest level: "graphical tools for organizing and representing knowledge. They include concepts, usually enclosed in circles or boxes of some type, and relationships between concepts indicated by a connecting line linking two concepts. . . . We define concept as a perceived regularity in events or objects, or records of events or objects, designated by a label" (p. 1).

For the most part, the concepts represented in CDs are variables—characteristics or quantities with changeable values, which may be either observed, observable in principle, or theoretically postulated. CDs have a dynamic quality, using arrows to depict temporal processes, relationships, and sequences of events. Figure 10.1 adapts the main ideas of traditional statistical path analysis (Duncan, 1966; Land, 1969; Wright, 1934) to illustrate some of the key components and representational conventions that are common to many CDs.

CDs of this kind can be read "chronologically" from left to right in the manner that one might read a complex grammatical sentence. The diagrams "tell a story" with a beginning, middle, and end; there are things that happen first (causes, inputs), things that happen last (effects, outcomes), and a variety of things that happen in the middle (mediators, pathways, interactions, arguments.) The "middle" involves a sequence of smaller steps or stages. Thus, depending on the focus of a particular study or analysis, the "dependent variable" may also function as an intervening output in the overarching PHLR model.

In Figure 10.1, the boxes labeled X1 through X4 could be considered antecedents or hypothesized component causes of Y. In turn, Y is the consequence, the thing to be explained, or the problem to be solved by an intervention. Boxes depicted on the left edge of the diagram are often referred to as "exogenous" or independent variables, meaning "of outside origin" and not affected by anything internal to the system. Variables configured to the right, within the system, are termed "endogenous." In some CDs, a double-headed

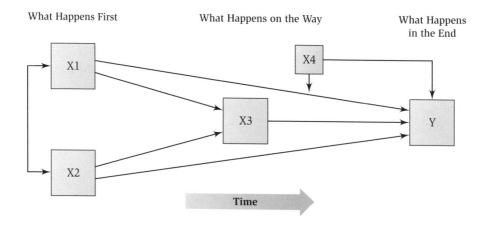

Figure 10.1. Some Conventions of Causal Diagrams.

arrow is drawn between two independent variables, as with the arrow connecting X1 and X2 in Figure 10.1. Here the arrow represents a preexisting correlation—a reciprocal association between two exogenous causes.

To put some flesh on the skeleton, let us consider a hypothetical CD depicting the effects of state firearms laws on the rate of gun-related fatalities. If we were to assign relevant labels to the boxes in Figure 10.1, variable X1 might represent the household gun ownership rate while variable X2 might stand for the restrictiveness of a state's gun laws. In a test of a PHLR theory of gun control effectiveness, these two variables predictably would be correlated with each other, as indicated by the arrow connecting X1 and X2, and both would be expected ultimately to affect the risk of gun violence in the community (Y).

The box labeled X3 in the diagram is a *mediator*—a variable that comes between the main cause(s) and the effect in question (Edwards & Lambert, 2007). To qualify as a true mediator, a variable must be related significantly both to the preceding cause and to the effect that follows, and must thereby explain some of the bivariate association between the first cause and its ultimate result; the mediator explains how it happens. In our gun laws example, X3 might capture a key mediating variable such as the frequency of crimes involving handguns. Logically, if there are more guns in the population (X1), then whenever a crime occurs it may be more likely to involve a gun (X3); in turn, when guns are used in crimes, it is more likely that a fatal injury will occur (Y). Exogenous predictor variables are also sometimes referred to as "distal" causes, while mediating variables that immediately precede the outcome of interest are termed "proximal" causes (Greenland & Brumback, 2002). In the current example, an intervention aimed at a distal cause of firearm fatalities might focus on reducing the number of guns in the population, while an intervention targeting a more proximal cause might focus on reducing violent crime.

Finally, the box labeled X4 represents both a moderating variable and one that interacts with another causal factor in the system. As depicted, this variable exerts a direct effect on Y, but also modifies the pathway between X1 and Y (that is, is also a *moderator*); hence, the arrow leads to another arrow, rather than to a box. In our gun control example, X4 might stand for a variable measuring implementation of firearms laws, such as the extent to which states report disqualifying records to the National Instant Criminal Background Check System (NICS). The diagram would help us show that we expect NICS reporting to exert a direct effect in lowering risk of firearm fatalities (Y), but also to potentiate the effect of the law itself (X1)—interact with the law to produce a larger impact than the sum of each of these component causes' single effect. Another important way in which a moderating variable can operate is when a causal effect is stronger in one group than another, or when it works only in one group and not another. For example, Ludwig and Cook (2000) found that the

Brady Handgun Control Act significantly reduced suicides, but only in people over age fifty-five. Thus age was found to be a "moderator" of the law's effect.

It is important to recognize that building a CD is an iterative process; as an evolving model confronts new theoretical ideas or evidence, new mediators or moderators may be added, blocks may change position or be removed, and the direction of arrows may even reverse. The descriptive example here is just one way in which to create a CD. Ultimately, the CD should provide one-to-one correspondence between the theoretical constructs and a testable empirical model. CDs are helpful to evaluate how well constructs in the model are operationalized with available data. Next, we move on to review a range of different options for constructing CDs and note the strengths and weaknesses of each approach in relation to PHLR. However, all of these models proceed from the same basic idea of working through time with the inputs on the left and the outcomes on the right.

Variations on the Theme

Several different types of causal diagrams may be useful in PHLR. These serve distinct but complementary purposes, and some of them follow the conventions we have just described more closely than others. There is no one-size-fits-all approach, and it is important for the researcher to modify the CD according to the features and complexity of the specific study.

A Common Understanding

The first purpose of CDs is descriptive classification, addressing the need for a specific, common understanding of the thing to be studied. For example, suppose we wish to examine whether involuntary outpatient commitment laws improve population health and safety. As a general definition, outpatient commitment is a civil court order requiring that a person with mental illness meeting certain criteria participate in outpatient psychiatric treatment.

However, there are several types of legal outpatient commitment (Swartz, Swanson, Kim, & Petrila, 2006); without understanding these types and distinguishing them from each other, it would be difficult to proceed with an informative study of outpatient commitment. Figure 10.2 illustrates how a CD can be used to define and graphically describe the different types of outpatient commitment laws (OPCs), showing the pathways by which someone in a mental health crisis may qualify for each type.

A Process Blueprint

A variation on the descriptive purpose of CDs is process modeling for a specific legal intervention, policy, or program. The goal of process modeling in PHLR is

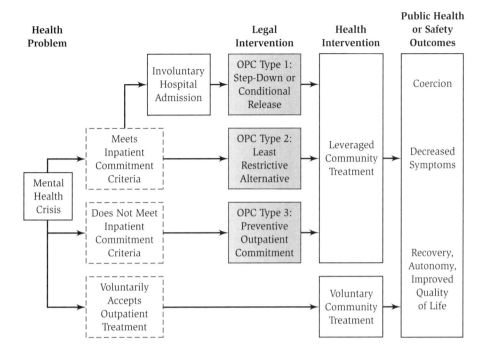

Figure 10.2. Types of Involuntary Outpatient Commitment.

to provide a detailed blueprint of a given legal intervention and how it is designed to function. By analogy, if a generic descriptive CD defines an automobile and distinguishes generally between cars and trucks and buses, a process model CD would "lift the hood" of a particular vehicle and show how the engine works.

Figure 10.3 illustrates such a diagram for a program of legal outpatient commitment, New York's Assisted Outpatient Treatment Program (AOT) (New York State Office of Mental Health, 2011). This type of model can also be used as an action map or decision guide for system actors who are involved with the AOT program. The CD moves from referral to investigation to assessment and service delivery, highlighting the range of potential mechanisms involving clinical and legal actors.

Sometimes the same information can be conveyed using different types of CDs to reach different audiences. While graphical boxes labeled with different types of actors and organizations may be useful for program administrators, these images may be meaningless to the general public or policy makers. As an alternative, Figure 10.4 presents a CD on the same New York AOT program, but directed toward a general lay audience (Pataki & Carpinello, 2005); this CD is centered on the perspective of an individual trying to navigate the system.

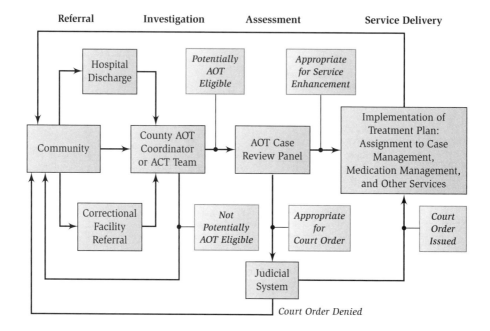

Figure 10.3. Schematic Representation of AOT Processes in Nine Areas of New York State.

Source: New York State Office of Mental Health, 2011.

Mapping Multiple Interventions

The CD can also be used to map the cumulative and interacting effects of a range of interventions that address a specific health topic. Figure 10.5 provides an example of a model depicting ways to curtail youth consumption of alcohol, such as reducing economic and physical access to alcohol, enforcing societal norms, and exercising other social control mechanisms. The model combines theoretical elements from several disciplines, including social and behavioral sciences and economics, and engages the issue of underage drinking from the perspectives of several key actors, including the minor who would consume alcohol, the retailer who would sell alcohol to minors, and the law enforcement officer who would detain the minor (Wagenaar & Perry, 1994). While this is a complex model, it represents an inherently complex set of interconnecting phenomena, and does so in a comprehensible way that provides an opportunity to consider multiple points of potential modification to existing laws and legal practices.

Theoretical Foundations

A fourth important purpose of CDs is theoretical explanation, or the articulation of a causal theory. Here the diagram identifies a particular phenomenon to be

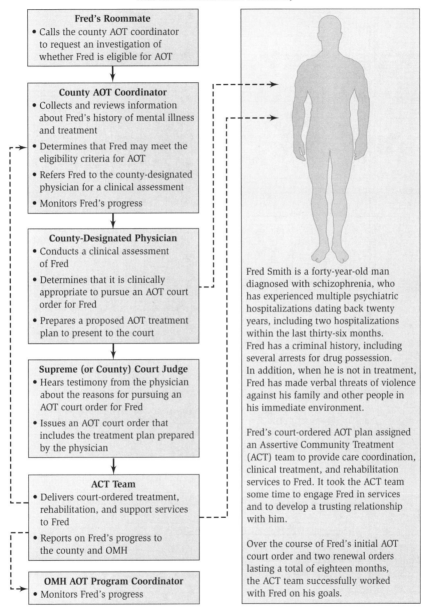

Fred Smith's Experience with AOT
(To prevent recognition, "Fred Smith" is a composite of several actual AOT cases with similar histories and outcomes.)

Fred's Roommate
- Calls the county AOT coordinator to request an investigation of whether Fred is eligible for AOT

County AOT Coordinator
- Collects and reviews information about Fred's history of mental illness and treatment
- Determines that Fred may meet the eligibility criteria for AOT
- Refers Fred to the county-designated physician for a clinical assessment
- Monitors Fred's progress

County-Designated Physician
- Conducts a clinical assessment of Fred
- Determines that it is clinically appropriate to pursue an AOT court order for Fred
- Prepares a proposed AOT treatment plan to present to the court

Supreme (or County) Court Judge
- Hears testimony from the physician about the reasons for pursuing an AOT court order for Fred
- Issues an AOT court order that includes the treatment plan prepared by the physician

ACT Team
- Delivers court-ordered treatment, rehabilitation, and support services to Fred
- Reports on Fred's progress to the county and OMH

OMH AOT Program Coordinator
- Monitors Fred's progress

Fred Smith is a forty-year-old man diagnosed with schizophrenia, who has experienced multiple psychiatric hospitalizations dating back twenty years, including two hospitalizations within the last thirty-six months. Fred has a criminal history, including several arrests for drug possession. In addition, when he is not in treatment, Fred has made verbal threats of violence against his family and other people in his immediate environment.

Fred's court-ordered AOT plan assigned an Assertive Community Treatment (ACT) team to provide care coordination, clinical treatment, and rehabilitation services to Fred. It took the ACT team some time to engage Fred in services and to develop a trusting relationship with him.

Over the course of Fred's initial AOT court order and two renewal orders lasting a total of eighteen months, the ACT team successfully worked with Fred on his goals.

Figure 10.4. New York State Office of Mental Health Diagram Explaining AOT to the Public.

Source: Pataki & Carpinello, 2005, p. 6.

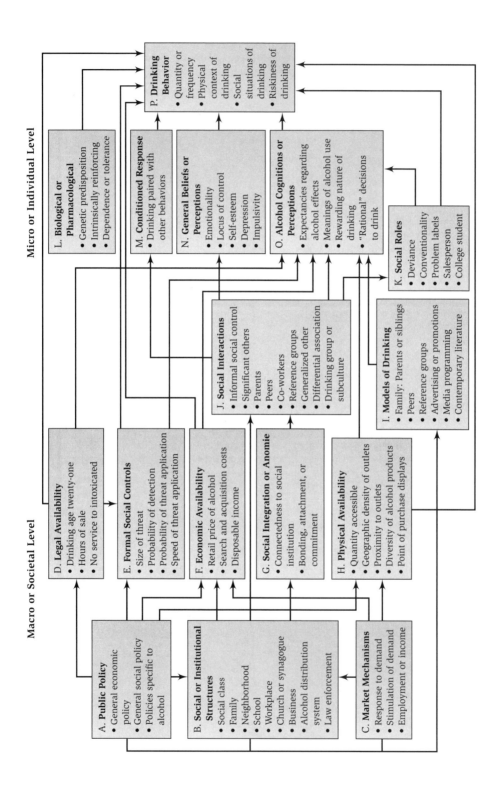

Figure 10.5. An Integrated Theory of Drinking Behavior.

Source: Wagenaar & Perry, 1994, p. 322.

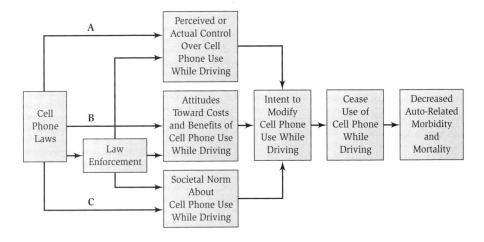

Figure 10.6. Use of Theory of Planned Behavior to Frame Distracted Driving Behaviors.

explained, sets forth a proposed cause or multiple component causes of the phenomenon, and specifies the pathways of association—patterns of common, sequential occurrence—that theoretically connect the causal factors to the effect of interest. Figure 10.6 draws from behavioral theory and applies the theory of planned behavior (TPB) to explain how a law restricting or prohibiting cell phone use while driving can result in a behavior change and improvements in health outcomes.

In this model, we offer three potential hypotheses for how TPB can be used to explain mechanisms for expected legal effects on population health and safety. The diagram clarifies theoretical mechanisms by which legally restricting cell phone use while driving can be expected to change driving practices, and potentially reduce mortality associated with distracted driving. This specific example demonstrates the integration of a classic behavioral sciences theory with classic legal theory on deterrence.

First, a "fear hypothesis" (path A in Figure 10.6) would posit that fear of being caught and punished—deterrence, in legal terms—inhibits the individual's independent action of using a cell phone while driving. A second option is the "guilt hypothesis" (path B), which posits that negative social sanctions attaching to the behavior of using cell phones while driving affects the actor's attitude toward these behaviors and persons who engage in them. Finally, the "shame hypothesis" (path C) posits that laws and law enforcement activities can induce in the actor a sense that others look down on the sanctioned behavior, in this case that fellow drivers will be annoyed and irritated by someone using a cell phone while driving. These attitudes determine the intention to use a cell phone while driving.

If the law is working, one or more of these mediating mechanisms will modify the subjects' intention and behavior, and eventually the risky practice of driving while using a cell phone will decrease across the population. Given valid measures and sufficient observations of data from a representative sample, such an effect would be detected as predicted by the model. We could also expand the model to include mediators and moderators of the relationship between the intent to modify the behavior of using a cell phone while driving and actually stopping the behavior. However, it is best to keep the CD focused on a few elements that are both theoretically relevant and empirically testable, rather than to include any number of extraneous variables that might possibly co-vary with the law and correlate with its outcome.

Moving from Pictures to Measures

A fifth purpose of CDs in public health law research is to guide tests of direct and indirect causal effects of laws on public health outcomes (Rothman & Greenland, 2005). To illustrate, Figure 10.7 articulates testable mechanisms by which various tobacco control policies could modify smoking behavior (Fong, Cummings, Borland, et al., 2006). Any policy's effect is likely to be moderated by individual characteristics—from sociodemographic descriptors to personality features and previous smoking behaviors—and mediated by psychosocial factors such as shared beliefs and attitudes, group norms, and perceptions of risk. The model allows us to think about the specific measures and sources of data that would be necessary to test alternative and complementary hypotheses. While the model was created mainly as a general framework for tobacco control policy efforts, it also provides a useful catalogue of mediating variables that specific policies might target, and which could be measured to test these policies' effects.

A final purpose of CDs in public health law research is to depict and guide the process of research or evaluation itself. An extensive literature exists that explains the use of "logic models" in public health program evaluation (W. K. Kellogg Foundation, 2004). The main distinguishing feature of these types of CDs is a depiction of programs' "theory of change," including "resources, inputs, activities, and outputs" in order to demonstrate and evaluate effectiveness. Beyond use for research or evaluation, CDs may also be deployed as a tool for policy making and analysis, particularly in cases when policy makers must make decisions without the benefit of strong evidence for the likely effectiveness or adverse consequences of a course of action. By graphically unpacking a policy's potential requirements, goals, and expected pathways of effect, the CD provides an opportunity to consider hidden assumptions, barriers, or unintended "side effects" that might not otherwise be debated.

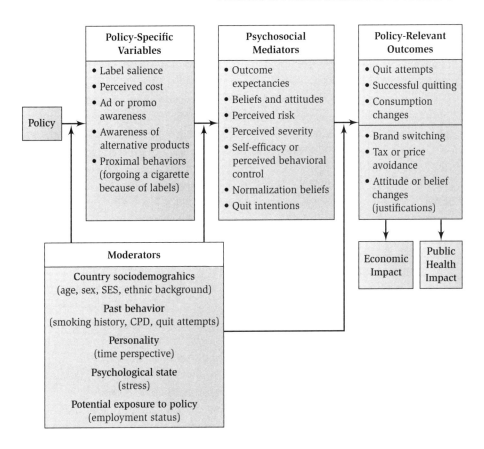

Figure 10.7. Conceptual Model of the Impact of Tobacco Control Policies Over Time.

Source: Fong, Cummings, Borland, et al., 2006, p. iii5.

What Makes a Good Causal Diagram?

Scholars have described several criteria to evaluate the adequacy of representational diagrams used in process modeling, particularly in the context of business and information sciences (Recker, Rosemann, Indulska, & Green, 2009). The ideas underlying several of these criteria can be adapted to evaluate CDs for public health law research and to identify specific problems that may arise with these models. We propose related criteria that can be summarized as the "Three C's": correspondence, comprehensiveness, and clarity.

Correspondence

The first criterion for evaluating CDs is *correspondence*, meaning that a given concept or construct in the model must correspond in a valid, specific way to the particular phenomena or set of observations that it purports to describe in the real world. Since the basic premise of the model is to explain real-world phenomena to facilitate research, it is important that each box has a clearly defined connection to some element directly or indirectly observed in reality.

To illustrate this criterion, consider a CD that is designed to illustrate a test of whether states' laws against driving while using a mobile communications device prevent motor vehicle crashes and injuries. Imagine that the CD depicted in Figure 10.6 had included separate boxes labeled "distracted driving laws" and "laws against texting and driving." The first problem with such a model would be *poor correspondence* between at least one of the constructs and the real-world phenomena of interest.

Specifically, the box labeled "distracted driving laws" would suffer from what Recker and colleagues (2009) call "construct overload." As they explain (in the context of business process modeling), construct overload occurs when a term "provides language constructs that appear to have multiple real-world meanings and, thus, can be used to describe various real-world phenomena. These cases are undesirable, as they require users to bring to bear knowledge external to the model in order to understand the capacity in which such a construct is used in a particular scenario" (p. 349). In short, "distracted driving laws" could refer to distractions such as eating, doing make-up, reading, and a whole host of other activities that individuals may do while driving, rather than the intended focus on the use of mobile communications devices while driving.

Second, the inclusion of two boxes labeled with slightly different definitions of the law, and with varying degrees of specificity, would also show poor correspondence. The logical deficit here could be called *concept redundancy*. A PHLR model containing constructs with overlapping meanings and real-world referents is difficult to understand, impossible to test, and hopeless to apply to policy making. As mentioned earlier, it is possible to create a CD that includes multiple legal interventions to address a particular public health issue, but it is imperative that each box has a mutually exclusive definition within that model, and that hypothesized interactions are depicted with appropriate precision.

Comprehensiveness

A useful CD should incorporate all necessary elements to achieve its specific purpose—whether description, classification, explanation, testing, or evaluation. Thus the model must include sufficient detail to adequately represent the hypothesized legal causes, hypothesized mediators, and health effects to be examined in a PHLR project; it should not omit relevant variables and pathways. At the same time, the model should not be made more complex than necessary in an attempt to "represent the whole world." Just as a figure that is too basic invites misinterpretation, a diagram that is too complicated may create

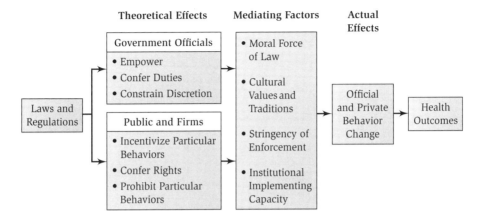

Figure 10.8. Conceptual Model of the Effect of Law on Public Health Outcomes.

confusion. The goal is to construct a model that strikes an appropriate balance between the bare bones and the byzantine.

Figure 10.8 is a CD designed to explain the ways in which laws and regulations influence the behaviors of the public and government and private entities, resulting in a change in health outcomes (Mello, Powlowski, Nañagas, & Bossert, 2006). The model provides an example of a CD that avoids the clutter of irrelevant details, yet does not oversimplify its relevant constructs and connections. The model is thus able to achieve its goal of visually representing, and therefore illuminating, the link between theoretical and actual effects of law on public health outcomes. Moreover, while the model provides an overall picture, it is possible to segment out one section of the model—for example, government actors only—and create a more granular version that elaborates on the mediating and moderating factors. The comprehensiveness criterion is also related to the term *parsimony* as used to evaluate theories in philosophy of science: all things considered, the simplest explanation is the best.

Clarity

The final CD criterion that we will mention here is clarity, which refers both to visual intelligibility and conceptual lucidity. Clarity means, in essence, that a CD's images and accompanying labels should be easy to read, and they should make the concepts they stand for easy to understand. While this is related to considerations of correspondence and comprehensiveness, the clarity criterion expresses the model's intuitive logical appeal, and the extent to which it conveys an intended message with sufficient detail in definition—the elements in sharp focus with a minimum of surrounding "fog." The diagram must also be visually appealing and easy to follow; the reader should spend time thinking

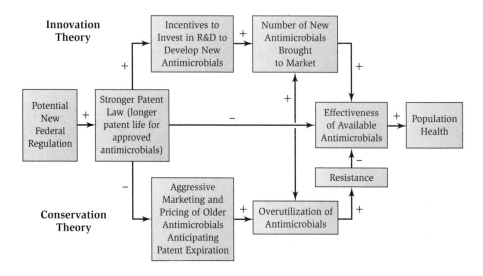

Figure 10.9. How Stronger Patent Laws Could Improve Antimicrobial Effectiveness.

about the ideas, not figuring out how to interpret the boxes and arrows. It is possible for a model to be relatively simple, even to have good correspondence between constructs and their real-world referents, and still not be clear. For example, consider a model designed to depict the population health effects of regulatory action on pharmaceutical companies' innovation in developing new antimicrobial medications. Imagine a series of boxes labeled "regulation," "innovation," "incentives," "overutilization," "resistance," "effectiveness," and "population health," with multiple arrows connecting the boxes. The main problem with such a model would be lack of clarity: What does it mean? How do these elements fit together according to some logical scheme?

Figure 10.9 presents a model of clarity using the same basic concepts, but lays out the logic for two different approaches to solving the public health problem of antibiotic resistance—innovation and conservation—and shows how strengthening patent law could plausibly work through both mechanisms simultaneously (adapted from Outterson, 2005). The picture is clear and it is easy to see potential research questions, hypotheses to be tested, and measures to represent each box. This is the ultimate goal of CDs.

How to Create an Effective Causal Diagram

An informative and effective CD begins with careful preparation. The creative activity of sketching boxes and arrows should follow from, not precede, a solid understanding of the substantive topic at hand. Thus the first step should be to selectively review current academic literature on several facets of the subject:

the basic dimensions of the public health problem at hand; its established or putative causes; contours of the law, policy, or regulatory scheme whose possible effects on health are the subject of inquiry; and what may already be known about the mechanisms of these laws' effect on health. This selective literature review should be carried out with the purpose of extracting key constructs, ideas, and causal relationships that recur in the literature across relevant fields of study, or that seem to bridge parallel understandings in diverse disciplines—from the health sciences to social sciences and the law.

The selective literature review should be driven by several basic theoretical questions that could also become research questions: What are the major causes of this public health problem? How could law, policy, or regulation conceivably affect the problem? What factors could modify or strengthen the law's effect on the health problem? Are there reasons to posit a fairly direct link between law and health in this instance? Or is it more likely that complex processes—environmental change, structural change, behavioral change, or all three—would intervene as foreseeable mechanisms of effect?

Armed with a basic understanding of key concepts and how they might fit together, there are many ways to actually draw a CD. Here is one: start by sketching a box that represents the health problem—the main outcome to be affected—on the right-hand side of a sheet of paper (or its computer-screen equivalent.) Next, sketch a box representing the legal intervention on the left of the drawing space. Connect the two boxes with a long arrow from left to right; keep in mind, the diagram "moves" chronologically from left to right. Next, stop and ponder: What other important variables could influence the health problem, and how might they be affected by the law as well? Add these variables to the diagram in the form of labeled boxes positioned above or below the central horizontal arrow, and suspended between the legal intervention on the left and the health outcome on the right. Connect these middle boxes with diagonal arrows coming from the law and proceeding to the health outcome.

The final step involves revising the diagram with an eye to the whole picture—repositioning boxes, adding or subtracting arrows—until the CD begins to form a clear, legible, and intelligible portrait of a health problem and its potential legal solution, along with any necessary "scaffolding" to make it work. While described here in few steps, in practice this is an iterative process. The final result should be a CD that is sufficiently detailed to convey all the information that is necessary to represent the theory or research problem at hand, but without extraneous conceptual or visual clutter.

Conclusion

Causal models have become increasingly common in the presentation of theory-driven research schemes across a variety of disciplines. However, there are few clear conventions in current practice of graphic representation of variables, associations, interactions, and time that allow such pictures to be understood across disciplines. In this chapter, we have described a set of simple conventions for using causal diagrams as heuristic models to visually represent key independent and dependent variables, hypothesized mediators, moderators, and direct and indirect pathways of effect. The use of these models in PHLR can yield powerful insights into the intended and unintended effects of laws on population health, as well as the social and institutional contexts in which they occur.

Causal diagrams can do important work in PHLR, insofar as they answer several kinds of questions. They can help to describe ("how things are now"), classify ("why things go together"), explain ("how things really work"), predict ("what will happen if"), and decide ("what you should do now"). As conceptual models, CDs not only map the steps by which law may impact health but also allow a researcher to more carefully consider the set of measures to be used in developing a methodologically rigorous study. Models that exhibit valid correspondence and are appropriately complex yet clear will help PHLR researchers plan and carry out their work. Images that accurately represent the topic at hand may also be useful for policy makers in understanding new evidence for the many ways that laws may improve population health.

Summary

Given the multidisciplinary perspectives of public health law research and the wide range of topics included in PHLR, the use of commonly understood pictures to illustrate the ways in which law and health interact can be invaluable (Burris, Wagenaar, Swanson, 2010). Ranging from laws that prohibit individual behaviors to laws that provide authority to act to laws that regulate organizational practices, PHLR seeks to understand the mechanisms by which laws can improve health; visualizing these mechanisms in diagrams is an important tool for achieving such an understanding. The purpose of this chapter is to review some basic conventions used to create visual models, evaluate relevant examples of models in published PHLR studies, and offer recommendations for constructing clear and informative models.

Causal diagrams can do important work in PHLR, insofar as they answer several kinds of questions. They can help to describe ("how things are now"), classify ("why things go together"), explain ("how things really work"), predict ("what will happen if"), and decide ("what you should do now") As conceptual models, CDs not only map the steps by which law may impact health but also allow a researcher to more carefully consider the set of measures to be used in developing a methodologically rigorous study. Models that exhibit valid correspondence and are appropriately complex yet clear will help PHLR researchers plan and carry out their work. Images that accurately represent the topic at hand may also be useful for policy makers in understanding new evidence for the many ways that laws may improve population health.

Further Reading

Coryn, C.L.S., & Scriven, M. (2008). The logic of research evaluation. In C.L.S. Coryn & M. M. Scriven (Eds.), *Reforming the evaluation of research* (*New Directions for Evaluation*, Vol. 118, pp. 89–105). San Francisco: Jossey-Bass and American Evaluation Association.

Dansereau, D. F., & Simpson, D. D. (2009). A picture is worth a thousand words: The case for graphic representations. *Professional Psychology: Research and Practice, 40*(1), 104–110.

Ellermann, C. R., Kataoka-Yahiro, M. R., & Wong, L. C. (2006). Logic models used to enhance critical thinking. *The Journal of Nursing Education, 45*(6), 220–227.

W. K. Kellogg Foundation. (2004). *Logic model development guide: Using logic models to bring together planning, evaluation*. Battle Creek, MI: W.K. Kellogg Foundation.

Chapter 11

Measuring Statutory Law and Regulations for Empirical Research

Evan D. Anderson   Charles Tremper   Sue Thomas

Alexander C. Wagenaar

Learning Objectives

- Describe the importance of selecting a legal framework at the beginning of a law measurement effort.
- List the steps in a systematic process for measuring law and creating a numeric legal dataset.
- Explain the importance of composite measures in coding statutory law.

Law affects health in many ways. Policy makers use law to reduce health risks and harms. The effects of law on health, however, extend far beyond deliberate uses of law by health-oriented policy makers. Few of our environments or behaviors remain untouched in some significant way by law. This chapter focuses on how to measure law to enable rigorous evaluation of its effects.

Measuring law as the term is used here is determining dimensions or components of an area of law relevant for a particular area of research, categorizing the legal elements of a policy, and using the resultant categorization schema to produce accurate representations of the law in terms of counts and numeric indicators. The process for measuring law relies on techniques that are common practice in both quantitative and qualitative research. While few of these techniques are conceptually challenging, their application to the law can be difficult.

The bulk of this chapter is devoted to providing a step-by-step guide for reflecting variation in laws across time, space, or both for purposes of evaluation research. To provide context and make clear the importance of these steps, the chapter begins with a short section explaining some of the basic principles underlying the process. A final section describes common challenges and offers suggestions for addressing them.

The Impetus Behind Measuring—or Mapping—Law

Supreme Court Justice Louis Brandeis famously remarked that "it is one of the happy incidents of our federal system that a single courageous state may, if its citizens choose, serve as a laboratory; and try novel social and economic experiments without risk to the rest of the country" (New State Ice Co. *v.* Liebman, 1932, p. 311). Innovation by states and other political units is vital to having an effective regulatory system. Policy experimentation by localities and states is frequently a necessary step on the way to identifying effective public health laws. Consider the problem of motor vehicle crashes for teenagers and graduated driver licensing (GDL) laws. In the mid-1990s, a few states began experimenting with laws that restrict when and under what circumstances teenage drivers could operate a motor vehicle. As these laws proliferated in number and type, researchers evaluated their effects, first in studies comparing crash rates in single states before and after the adoption of a GDL restriction, and then in studies comparing changes in crash rates in states adopting GDL laws of varying restrictiveness. As these studies accumulated, it became very clear that restrictive laws saved lives. Less than fifteen years later, almost every state has adopted similarly restrictive laws, though important variation in the law across states remains. Teen crash rates have declined continuously since, marking GDL laws as one of the great modern examples of how policy innovation, rigorous evaluation, and evidenced-based dissemination save lives (Preusser & Tison, 2007).

Two factors made GDL research possible. First, there was variation in both state laws and state motor vehicle crash rates. Second, there were methods for measuring that variation that enabled statistical comparisons. Measuring crash-related harms is accomplished by generating counts through police reports, hospitals, and other administrative data. But how does one measure and quantify something textual like the law? The answer turns out to be that it is not too difficult using one or more experienced legal researchers, careful consideration of a handful of persistent areas of error, and attention to the usual basic principles of science. As any qualitative researcher can attest, characteristics of texts can be observed and these observations can be easily converted into numeric indicators, or *coded* as it is often called. At its core, the task of a coding law is not altogether different from coding an open-ended interview transcript.

In each instance, researchers strive to measure the apparent features of the texts in ways that are consistent with scientific standards of validity and reliability.

There are two primary sources of difficulty in the process of measuring law. The first is typical of almost all research that involves analyzing the meaning or contents of texts. Law is, by its nature, an abstraction with at best an uncertain underlying empirical foundation. For this reason, measurements of law themselves cannot be directly validated against observable phenomena in the natural world (see Singer, 1984). The method for measuring law offered in this chapter is more similar in many ways to observation than traditional legal interpretation. But few observations can be made of laws that do not require some predicate legal decision making based on assumptions about the nature of the legal text being examined. The types of observations of laws that are defensible regardless of context or purpose—like the number of words in a statute or whether it includes a specific term—tend not to provide much value by themselves in public health law evaluations. The decisions that shape which laws are collected and how they are understood increase the importance of reporting how and, in some instances, why specific legal measures were adopted to represent a particular construct.

The second primary source of difficulty in measuring law is identifying the right legal texts to collect and examine. Unlike the qualitative researcher who creates a file of transcripts for coding by, for example, interviewing some defined group of people, the legal rules that regulate life in the United States are distributed over space, time, levels of government, and types of law. Determining the prevailing law governing the sale of sugar-sweetened beverages in a selection of cities, for example, might necessitate gathering laws from different sources (legislative, executive, judicial, electoral, and constitutional) and at different levels of government (federal, state, and local). In addition to difficulties finding the right provisions, researchers also have to consider how provisions interact within a broader legal framework. In most instances, lawyers are needed to help determine which laws are relevant, how to find them, and, in some instances, how they are to be interpreted—which means that for empirical researchers embarking on an evaluation of law, collaboration with legal colleagues is almost always necessary to avoid errors in coding laws.

While legal expertise is essential to measuring law it is not sufficient to generating valid data. The bulwark against error in legal measurement is a deliberate commitment to standard principles and practices of good science. The method described here provides steps for operationalizing those principles and practices in legal research. Some standard scientific practices—such as the creation of a detailed research protocol that enables replication and updating of data—might seem odd at first to legal colleagues who are accustomed to the more normative and interpretive world of traditional legal research in which the process for doing research is closely guarded as the lawyer's stock in trade.

But our experience is that legal researchers quickly internalize these rules and procedures; indeed, they often find them valuable in other areas of their work.

Projects that blend legal and empirical research fall into two primary categories. In the first, legal research measuring the features of law is driven by the goal of testing a specific hypothesis. A hypothesis-driven project might be, for example, investigating whether increasing the age at which individuals can drink will reduce fatalities from motor vehicle crashes (Wagenaar, 1983b). In such instances, decisions about measurement are guided by, and typically limited to, the question of interest. Suppose that state law bans use of cell phones by bus drivers and novice drivers. Researchers evaluating the effect of the law on novices normally will not include the bus-driver ban in their data. In the second category, what we refer to as *legal mapping studies*, the purpose is to survey the legal terrain in a policy domain capturing all major characteristics that vary in ways plausibly related to health. When conducted with appropriate rigor and transparency, legal mapping studies yield datasets that can be used in empirical evaluations examining many different hypotheses. This chapter focuses on measuring law for hypothesis testing, but the same principles and practices are, with some exceptions, required for legal mapping studies.

A few final words about terminology bear mentioning. Throughout this book, law is understood in its broadest terms to encompass both legal texts and the whole range of institutions, practices, and beliefs through which laws influence health and the determinants of health. This chapter is devoted exclusively to law as it is set out in constitutions, statutes, regulations, ordinances, and other legal texts. *Provisions"* are clauses or sections of laws. We use the term *policy* to represent the operation of two or more laws. So, for example, a state policy regulating the use of mobile communication devices by drivers might include a statute specifying a prohibition (for example, a ban on drivers under age nineteen from texting while driving), a statute specifying the fine for a violation, and a statute specifying the extent to which police officers can enforce the prohibition as a primary or secondary offense (Ibrahim, Anderson, Burris, & Wagenaar, 2011). This contrasts with definitions of policy that include a broader range of political outputs expressed as goals, preferences, long-range objectives, and the means by which ends are sought (Plano, Riggs, & Robin, 1982).

The Process for Measuring Law

As is the case in all scientific research, questions of interest and availability of data define measurement objectives. The types of legal data pertinent to evaluation research vary widely depending on, among other things, whether legal measures are to be used as independent or dependent variables, and the particular research design chosen for the study. Notwithstanding these differences, the process for measuring law depicted in Figure 11.1 is composed of steps that are

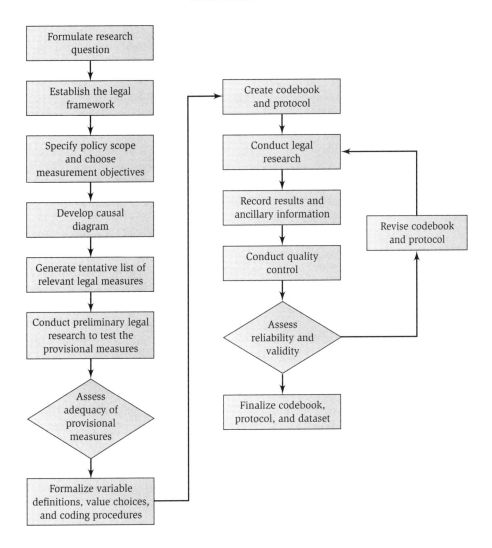

Figure 11.1. Process for Measuring Law.

essential in all legal measurement projects. The process is generally iterative, with one or more steps being repeated as discoveries at one stage expose inadequacies of constructs developed at a previous stage. The following sections describe each step in the figure except the first, which is addressed in other chapters.

Establish the Legal Framework

The first step in any legal measurement project is to identify the legal framework of interest. It is seldom practical or feasible to study every possible law related to a health issue. Consider the problem of distracted driving. It is clear that using a mobile communication device while operating a motor vehicle is a dangerous behavior. Many states and localities have responded by prohibiting activity with such devices for different groups of drivers. For empirical researchers interested in understanding the relationship between law and this high-risk behavior, these interventional laws have obvious importance. But they are not the only or even necessarily the best place to start. The tort system could exert an equal if not greater influence on drivers' tendencies to answer a call or send a text message. Or it could be that law regulating insurance or employer liability is a plausible factor affecting distracted driving. Decisions about the type of law to study depend on the purpose of the study and theorized relationships of interest.

Assume that a researcher decides to focus on state laws that specifically prohibit activity with mobile communication devices. These laws exist at the local and federal levels too (for example, those that apply to long-haul truckers). Choice of legal framework is in this way also a choice of at which level or levels of government law will be studied. Table 11.1 displays a familiar categorization of law by level of government and by source, with the most common type of law in each cell. Statutes enacted by Congress or state legislatures are generally the easiest source of law to measure because they are readily accessible and—compared to common law created by courts—relatively straightforward. The ordinances of cities, counties, and other units of government below the state level offer similar advantages, although they may require more effort to locate. Bills under consideration by a legislature may also be of interest. For example, Wagenaar and colleagues (2006) used measures of bill introductions as an

Table 11.1. Types of Law by Level and Source.

	Federal	*State*	*Local*
Legislative	Statutes	Statutes	Ordinances
Executive	Regulations Executive orders Administrative judgments	Regulations Executive orders Administrative judgments	Regulations Executive orders Administrative judgments
Judicial	Case law (common law)	Case law (common law)	Case law (common law)
Electoral	—	Initiatives Referenda	Initiatives Referenda
Basic Law	Constitutions	Constitutions	Home rule charter

Note: Dash indicates the absence of a law.

intermediate outcome in a national evaluation of statewide coalitions whose objective was to reduce the availability of alcohol to youth. In this study, bill introductions functioned as one indicator of policy attention to an issue. For some policy domains, law emanating from the executive branch (for example, regulations, executive orders) is equally as important to measure as statutes and ordinances.

All, none, or some other combination of these legal frameworks might yield levers for effectively reducing mobile communication device use by drivers. In choosing a legal framework, there is no right or wrong answer a priori. But the decision should be a mindful one supported by plausible theories—both legally and behaviorally or biologically, depending on the nature of the exposure—about how laws within the framework relate to a health outcome of interest.

Specify the Policy Scope and Choose Measurement Objectives

To conserve resources and ensure that the ultimate legal measures generate data capable of illuminating the hypothesis of interest, it is important to define measurement objectives at the start even if they change during legal research and preliminary coding. In a study of distracted driving, for example, one might begin with the objective to capture how state laws prohibiting driver activity with mobile communication devices have evolved over a ten-year period (chosen perhaps because of the availability of crash data) in regard to covered activity, devices, and classes of drivers. The preceding sentence is deliberately vague on one point: What is the right unit of analysis? Is it individual legal texts or state policy? The answer depends on the purpose of the measurement. An example of a study that focuses on counts of specific laws as the unit of analysis is the Wagenaar and colleagues (2006) study, mentioned earlier, which used measures of bill introductions as an intermediate outcome in a national evaluation of statewide coalitions whose objective was to reduce the availability of alcohol to youth.

In most evaluations, the ultimate unit of analysis is state policy and not specific legal provisions. That is, each record—or row in a two-dimensional table—represents all the characteristics of state policy—for example, the legal drinking age and its enforcement—whether determined by one legal provision or multiple provisions set out in numerous statutes. A dataset reflecting variation in law for all U.S. states and the District of Columbia would therefore have fifty-one rows excluding headings (and leaving aside for the moment the issue of data encompassing changes in the policy over time). The columns in the table would represent variables and the characteristics of state law those variables describe. While that is almost always the intended structure of the final dataset, seldom is it the easiest way for organizing and making sense of laws in the early stages of research. This is especially true in instances in which there are many related or similar provisions in a single state.

Periodic discussion and clarity regarding the unit of analysis ensures that different ways of organizing the search returns in early phases of the research do not muddle the purpose of the legal measurement and therefore its ability to inform the hypothesis of interest. Casual and somewhat inevitable short-hand descriptions of the legal research increase the chance of confusion; it is easy to describe the example in this section simply as a study of "distracted driving laws." A truer articulation of the project and the underlying measurement objective is to determine which activities with mobile communication devices are prohibited for specified drivers under state statutory law, how those prohibitions are enforced, and what the fines are for associated violations.

Develop a Causal Diagram

Having defined the scope of laws to be collected, the next question is simply which characteristics of the laws are to be measured. Causal diagrams—as described in more detail in Chapter 10—are valuable tools for this purpose. By forcing researchers to identify and clarify plausible links between law and health outcomes, causal diagrams help flush out the legal inputs relevant to the question of interest. In the distracted driving context, for example, researchers might suspect that the primary legal mechanism mediating reductions in device use is deterrence. In other words, laws that are easier to enforce and carry higher penalties result in the greater reductions in high-risk behavior. In that instance, provisions specifying whether police officers can enforce prohibitions as a primary offense—that is, without needing another pretext to make stops—have obvious importance. Also important in that scenario are provisions specifying fines or other penalties such as suspensions for drivers on learner's permits. A causal diagram based in part or entirely on different mechanisms might suggest measurement of different sets of legal inputs.

Generate a Tentative List of Relevant Legal Measures

In hypothesis-driven research, causal diagrams limit the laws that will be studied on the basis of theories about how those legal inputs relate to some other outcome. The legal inputs themselves are often until this point broadly understood as concepts such as manner of enforcement, scope, and severity of fine. To capture how these conceptual legal inputs vary, the important components of each must be identified. Then the task is to formulate simple schemes for describing that variation. Operationally speaking, this is the point in the process to start creating variables. They need not be dichotomous, which is, as noted further on, sometimes preferable for variables in the final dataset. For the case of distracted driving laws, a sufficient set of preliminary measures to describe the scope of the laws might be categorical variables reflecting activities prohibited (for example, only texting, only talking, talking and texting, other), classes of drivers covered (for example, all drivers, bus drivers, inexperienced drivers, other) and devices (for example, cell phones, personal digital assistants, laptop computers, other) subject to the law.

Conduct Preliminary Legal Research

Whether the tentative measures align with relevant variation in extant laws is an empirical question that should be tested on a sample of the jurisdictions to be studied. If little is known about the variation in the law across jurisdictions, a random sample of jurisdictions increases the value of preliminary review. If the structure or operation of law in the area of interest is known to vary systematically across jurisdictions in terms of a small number of major characteristics, purposely sampling jurisdictions across such strata is best. The size of the sample depends on the law being studied and the a priori knowledge that the research team possesses about legal variation in the area. In addition to examining a handful of jurisdictions, surveying literature that describes the policy environment, whether in legal journals or other social science research, sets the research on much firmer ground moving forward. Preliminary research illuminates relevant dimensions of the law and provides the research team with a basis for estimating the breadth and complexity of the law being studied and the resources needed to systematically collect and analyze it moving forward.

Assess the Adequacy of Provisional Measures

Pausing to test the adequacy of provisional measures reduces the likelihood of wholesale recoding that would be necessary were the coding scheme to be found later in the research process to be incapable of reliably and validly capturing relevant variation. At this stage in the process, insights about important dimensions of variation in the law and how to elicit that variation through coding questions should be crystallizing in the minds of the research team. For the distracted driving example, researchers might decide that the provisional measure describing classes of covered drivers is insufficiently specific. Rather than lumping all inexperienced drivers into one group, the variable could be refined to distinguish between laws that cover drivers by age (that is, at ages sixteen, seventeen, eighteen, nineteen, and above) and laws that apply to all new drivers regardless of age. It might also become apparent, at this point, that a handful of exceptions reduce the scope or enforceability of prohibitions, such as exceptions for hands-free use or exceptions in statutes banning texting that permit typing keys to start or end a call.

Formalize Variable Definitions and Coding Procedures

It is in coding that measurement of law differs most significantly from traditional legal research. Traditional legal research typically produces narrative descriptions of how one or more laws differ in both their text and their meaning; measurement of law for empirical research determines how laws vary on specific characteristics in specified units. From an operational perspective, this means first identifying all the relevant ways that laws vary and then finding numeric schemes (or preliminary textual ones such as "yes" and "no") to capture that variation. Although it is a bit counterintuitive and may strike coders as odd at first, coding questions, and the variables they define, should be precise and should minimize human judgment. Coding questions requiring interpretation undermine reliability because of innate differences between coders. Consider a coding question asking whether a law prohibiting communication on wireless telephones by drivers applies to talking over an Internet connection through a headset attached to a laptop. Different coders could reach entirely defensible but different conclusions depending on how they interpret the operative terms and ultimate meaning of the rule (that is, "a computer is not a wireless telephone" versus "anything that allows electronic transmission of oral communication is a telephone even if embedded in something that has other purposes").

Adding a "not sure" category to the coding choices for a variable provides a useful safety valve, especially in the early stages of coding. The "not sure" category gives coders an option for handling ambiguity and conflicts that may or may not be resolved by additional research or subsequent developments such as a court ruling during the course of the study. And, regular review of "not sure" cases by the entire research team often leads to revision of the coding protocol, increasing reliability, precision, and comprehensiveness. Sometimes a "not sure" or "unsettled" code will remain in the final dataset so that those records can be excluded from analyses or addressed separately in a substudy.

The use of dichotomous "law or no law" variables to code the presence or absence of a particular type of law is useful only for some limited types of research questions and study designs. Dichotomous variables can easily obscure a great deal of legal variability and hence limit the value of a dataset for analyzing, adopting, and evaluating policies. Consider an example from the Alcohol Policy Information System dataset (National Institute on Alcohol Abuse and Alcoholism, 2011b). A dichotomous law or no law variable initially might seem adequate for indicating whether a state prohibits people under age twenty-one from purchasing alcoholic beverages. Most states have such prohibitions, and almost all of the laws on the topic are clear and simple. Several states, though, permit purchases by youths in some situations, such as acting in conjunction with law enforcement. The laws in New York and Delaware are less straightforward. Although these two states do *not* prohibit underage purchase, they do prohibit obtaining alcohol in connection with making a false statement. Rather than trying to shoehorn these laws into a dichotomous law or no law variable, a polychotomous variable could be created, in this case with four codes to include an absolute prohibition, a prohibition with exceptions, a prohibition against purchase in connection with making a false statement, and no restrictions. Better still, the categorical variable could be separated into four dichotomous variables, each measuring one dimension, an approach adhering to the principle that a measure in general should concern a single distinct, unitary attribute.

One of the preliminary measures identified for distracted driving defined the possibilities for regulated activity as (1) only texting, (2) only talking, (3) talking and texting, and (4) other. A simpler approach is to create two dichotomous variables that respectively answer the questions "Does the law prohibit texting?" and "Does the law prohibit talking?" These unidimensional variables can easily be combined with each other to reflect instances when both activities are prohibited or combined with other variables defining the existence of exceptions (for example, Is there an exception for hands-free use?) to represent all major regulatory permutations.

For the coding of legal texts, classifying features of laws into categories—that is, using categorical variables—is the most common way to reflect variance. The categories—or attributes—of a categorical variable have no natural numeric ordering or quantitative relationship. In contrast, the attributes of ordinal variables have a natural ordering (for example, low, medium, high). Interval variables are a special type of ordinal variable in which the difference between attributes is meaningful and assumed to be equal across the distribution (for example, separation into first, second, third, and fourth quartiles). Some features of the law can be measured at ordinal or interval levels, thereby enabling dose-response analyses, possibly enhancing statistical power to detect the law's effects, or more closely matching the analytic model to theory. Penalty type, for example, can be coded as an ordinal variable, with civil infractions, misdemeanors, felonies, and capital crimes as values representing ascending severity as defined by the law.

Continuous variables, which can take any numeric value (for example, temperature in Celsius), provide even more analytic benefits than ordinal variables. Attributes such as length of jail terms, appropriation amounts, and legal thresholds (for example, alcohol-impaired driving defined as blood alcohol content over 0.08), are often measurable with continuous variables. Careful definitions and coding protocols can also produce continuous variables based on a policy's non-numerical features. This is distinguishable from a combination of multiple variables to create a composite measure of a larger characteristic of the law. For example, researchers might use length of jail sentence, magnitude of fine, and the availability of defenses to create a composite measure of "stringency." Composite measures are potentially powerful as analytic tools but can be difficult to validate. This synthetic approach—or second-level coding—is discussed as a special case in the final section.

Create a Codebook and Protocol

Creating a codebook and a well-defined, precise coding protocol to capture the decisions made during the design phase facilitates both the initial legal research process and any subsequent attempts to replicate or update the data. The codebook should reflect the standards of any good data-collection documentation as well as the special considerations described earlier for coding laws. Elements include a description of the study; scope of data collection; variable definitions; values (codes and their definitions); algorithms for constructing scales; technical information about files—tables, records, relationships, number of records for each case (some jurisdictions have multiple related laws); and details about the data (columns, text, numeric, Boolean).

A codebook alone is inadequate for any but the simplest study because potentially critical decisions about coding conventions and procedures for legal data are rarely apparent from examination of a codebook alone. A comprehensive protocol includes information about how the laws were collected (for example, exact legal text databases searched, exact search terms and syntax); inclusion and exclusion criteria for defining the body of legal texts to be coded; precise rules for coding the variables (which legal terms support classification into a specific category); conventions used regarding effective dates or other determinations about a law's operation; and standards for collecting legal citations.

For teams composed of empirical and legal researchers, up until this point, most of the activity should have been joint effort with a lot of dialogue. In the next phase, however, the distribution of labor shifts considerably. Collecting the relevant laws requires legal training. Especially if legal researchers have not been integrated into the earlier steps, but even if they have, this is an ideal time for training all of the coders. It is imperative that law students and other legal researchers understand not only what they are looking for but also why so that they can report on unanticipated nuances in the law. Legal researchers must follow good legal research practices such as reading provisions in context by carefully locating and considering the definition of all operative terms. Relevant provisions are often located by key word searches; without explicit instruction some legal researchers will not inspect other provisions in the same part of the statutory code. The use of statutory tables of contents is not always emphasized in training of law students but is indispensable for making sense of statutory schemes, especially across jurisdictions. Being observant for court decisions that substantially influence the legal meaning of status of the law is also essential. Key points of emphasis in discussions with attorney or law student coders include keeping records of any needed modifications in the research protocol, erring on the side of over-inclusion in the collection of law, and raising questions for discussion with supervisors. The training of legal researchers naturally coincides with collective review of the protocol and codebook. Whether the legal researchers are students or experienced lawyers, from this point forward, the protocol and codebook should provide a high degree of clarity to guide the location, organization, and eventual coding of legal texts.

Conduct Legal Research

Having tested and refined the coding scheme, a project team can then proceed to the task of systematically collecting and coding the relevant law. Available resources to perform original legal research include Westlaw and Lexis, both comprehensive proprietary online legal research services. HeinOnline is another proprietary source that provides access to state session laws going back in some instances to the 1840s. Alternatives to these tools that can suffice for some studies include the commercial service Loislaw and publicly available online sources such as the Library of Congress website at www.thomas.gov for federal material. The commercial service StateNet, www.statenet.com, offers access to recently enacted statutes and pending bills. An excellent resource for studying legislative activity is LexisNexis Advanced Legislative Service (ALS), which catalogues only bills that were eventually adopted. The returns from ALS provide a valuable picture of how law has evolved in a particular area and can be used for updating or checking established legal datasets. Conducting searches in these databases and making sense of returns requires legal training in almost all instances. For large projects, consulting with legal librarians and database vendors—which typically offer assistance free of charge for law students and many other legal researchers—can increase efficiency of research even for experienced lawyers.

Finding legal materials at the city and county levels is often difficult. There is currently no comprehensive or authoritative collection of local laws. Lexis, Westlaw, and FindLaw maintain partial collections of municipal ordinances, and some jurisdictions publish their own materials online. Growing repositories are also available at www.municode.com, www.amlegal.com, and www.statelocalgov.net. If the research goal is limited to one or a few local jurisdictions, finding the relevant ordinances is often feasible. As the number of jurisdictions expands, the task quickly becomes unwieldy and will require extensive investment of researcher time to search multiple databases and, in some occasions, query local governments directly.

Record Results and Ancillary Information

Well-designed data-collection systems for gathering legal source material are crucial for a smooth measurement process. An adequate data-collection system for coding the law stores much more than the final resulting data for each variable. The system needs to retain ancillary information that supports the coding, typically in the form of extended blocks of legal text. The system should allow for changes to variables and codes as the project progresses, knowledge is gained, and previous errors are corrected, as well as keep a record of such changes. At a minimum, all relevant statutory, regulatory, and case law citations should be collected and recorded. Because coding of a single variable may depend on a legal analysis based on several sources of law (for example, three regulations, two statutes, and a court case), a data field with no character limit is generally best for citations. Ideally, citations should be stored in records that have a many-to-one relationship with the coding record so that each citation can have its own field and be stored together with additional information.

Along with citations, collecting relevant text facilitates subsequent review of coding decisions. Microsoft Access, which permits up to sixty thousand characters of text in each data field, can be used for cataloguing small- or medium-sized laws. Custom-designed databases can also be purchased from commercial vendors for large legal measurement projects. Rigorous and consistent coding decisions are enhanced by recording rationales for coding in the data-collection system, especially in instances when there is latent ambiguity. In addition to storing legal information, retention of the coders' notes, comments, and questions offers a big advantage, not only to the entire present research team but also to potential future users of the dataset. Maintaining records of each coding decision helps immensely. Although coding decisions should, as noted, have a solid basis in the observable features of the legal text, there may also be instances when the text of a law is explicit but some important extrinsic information exists that changes the effect of the legal text—for example, a law enforcement agency choosing not to enforce a law through an organizational policy that is not included in the data. There may also be instances when the answer to a coding question is clear but some feature of the legal text is noteworthy. For example, consider a study measuring whether states include syringes within the definition of prohibited drug paraphernalia. Every state that defines a class of such objects refers to it as drug paraphernalia except Georgia, which uses a different term, *drug-related objects*. Noting this sort of nuance in terminology is another appropriate use of comment boxes and can greatly reduce inaccuracies and confusion during later analyses.

As with all tasks that require repeated actions and fine-tuned manual manipulations, random human error is an inevitable threat to data integrity. The traditional model of coding texts involved three objects: a codebook describing the coding question, a datasheet in which coding decisions were placed (typically an Excel file or other sheet with lots of rows and columns), and the text to be coded. Moving between the three materials provides coders with many opportunities to make mistakes. This sort of error can be greatly reduced through the use of coding platforms that integrate codebooks, datasheets, and the legal text being coded. Data entry forms designed in Microsoft Access or Filemaker Pro, for example, enable researchers to create templates in which the legal text to be coded is visible next to coding questions that drive data to an underlying data table.

Clear coding roles for each person and adherence to rigorous implementation procedures reduce both outright errors and subtle distinctions that might otherwise go unnoticed. Regardless of how many coders work on the project, each will need to scrupulously follow clearly defined protocols and adhere to all coding guidelines. This is true for all types of research, and no less so when measuring law. Coders not only must be thoroughly versed in conventions adopted at the design stage of the research project, they also must be empowered to alert the principal investigator to oddities that arise in the course of coding that may require modification of those conventions, or the use of caveats and elaborations in subsequent descriptions of the research.

Conduct Quality Control

Systematic quality control is essential to accurately measure law. Having at least two legal researchers concur on coding decisions is a minimal standard for achieving accurate codes. The two coders should work completely *independently* in coding each variable and recording results without reference to each other's work (that is, blinded double coding). In a significantly less rigorous protocol, one researcher codes the data initially and the other then checks the coding. This more streamlined option catches many errors but does little to find mistakes arising from laws that the first researcher missed.

A second important step in assessing accuracy of data gathering and coding is comparison to secondary sources or checking with government officials. In many instances, at least one legal survey exists that provides a good cross-reference. The value of these secondary sources is strengthened by the fact that many are created through different methods, such as surveys of informants in state agencies or professional organizations (although keep in mind they often contain errors).

Measures adopted to minimize error should be included in the research documentation. Not only might such protocols facilitate future corrections of errors in specific legal compilations, their use will more broadly advance the quality of the science and the state of knowledge. Future researchers can adapt, modify, and enhance the application of these protocols to improve understanding of the specific topic initially under study as well as a wide range of related policy issues.

Assess Reliability and Validity

Quality control measures are intended to test how well legal researchers have applied the protocol and coding scheme. Even perfectly executed protocols and codebooks can generate misleading data. Blinded redundant coding reduces the likelihood of random or careless error; comparing the two resulting datasets for inconsistencies points to possible areas of underspecified coding conventions. Double-coding also provides a direct assessment of reliability. Per standard scientific practice, all legal dataset collectors should report cross-coder reliabilities achieved. But sometimes even independent coders share similarities that bias their treatment of the law. Being systematically integrated into a research project can subtly influence how the coder collects or codes law; likewise, coders often share characteristics that predispose them to similar patterns of observation or analysis, which could bias resulting data. A final important step to address these concerns is to have a third legal researcher who is totally naive to the project recode a randomly selected portion of the records. If desired, the rate of divergence can be reported as a crude rate or as a rate that adjusts for the probability of randomly selecting the "right" answer. Cohen's Kappa provides a more conservative estimate of the reliability of a test than the crude rate of divergence by accounting for the fact that, for example, on a dichotomous variable independent coders picking randomly will get the same result half of the time simply by chance. The use of statistics such as Cohen's Kappa depends on the dataset's context and the scale. In general, however, simple divergence rates may be sufficient. And unlike with survey research, there are no clear thresholds for deciding when divergence rates are too high. Generally speaking, however, anything more than the occasional discordance (that is, divergence rates of greater than 1 or 2 percent) is cause for concern.

Revise Codebook and Protocol

After assessing reliability and validity, the codebook and protocol specifications typically are revised to improve coding of some of the measures. The research team then cycles back to conducting legal research with the newly revised protocols, repeating the quality control and assessing reliability and validity steps. After multiple rounds of revisions and testing each round of revision, when the highest practically achievable levels of reliability and validity are attained, the research team advances to the final step.

Finalize Codebook, Protocol, and Dataset

In the final phase of original legal research, the codebook and protocol should be reviewed to ensure that they reflect any changes in definitions, coding conventions, or other matters that occurred during the research process. The final codebook and protocol should be sufficiently specific to enable exact replication of the dataset if those procedures are implemented by a separate team. The codebook and protocol also greatly facilitate future updates and ensure comparability of the data collected at different times and by different teams.

Challenges and Next Steps

Challenges unique to measuring law for empirical research pervade a number of steps in the process and deserve additional discussion.

Comparing Law Across Jurisdictions

Jurisdictions have considerable authority to create law. This independence extends not only to the substantive features of law but also to the way in which policies are drafted as provisions and organized as statutory code. As a result, statutory regimes vary considerably across states. States can accomplish identical policy positions through a variety of legal strategies and mechanisms. In some states, for example, a single comprehensive statute specifies different options for mental health care directives (Swanson, McCrary, Swartz, Elbogen, & Van Dorn, 2006); other states have a legal arrangement that creates a functionally equivalent policy through provisions that are scattered across probate codes, health and safety codes, and civil practice and remedies codes. In the distracted driving example, some states define the regulated activity, the fine for violations, and the manner of enforcement in one statute; others specify these details in multiple statutes. Some laws are detailed; in others a broad mandate is filled in by executive agency regulations.

It is not just that the text of provisions varies across states. Even if texts are identical, laws operate within regulatory structures, and those structures differ, sometimes markedly, between jurisdictions. Failure to account for the broader legal context in which a law exists can produce misleading comparisons. Consider, for example, a researcher interested in determining whether states where syringe exchange programs are legal have lower incidence of HIV/AIDS. For that researcher, a reasonable way to start might be to collect all the laws that explicitly authorize syringe exchange programs. If the collection of law stopped there, however, the resulting findings would present an incomplete and inaccurate picture of the relevant state law. In some states, syringe exchange is legal under state law simply because no laws forbid it; categorizing such states as prohibiting syringe exchange because they have not explicitly authorized syringe exchange would be legally invalid. Accurately measuring how states vary with respect to the legality of syringes requires collecting not only public health laws that explicitly authorize syringe exchange but also criminal paraphernalia laws regulating possession and distribution of syringes, pharmacy statutes and regulations defining restrictions on the delivery of syringes, and criminal laws banning drug possession that could potentially apply to residue in used syringes that are possessed prior to exchange (Burris, Anderson, Craigg, Davis, & Case, 2010). These sorts of challenges highlight the need for project teams to incorporate legal expertise early at the stages of conceptualization and design of the study, as well as during implementation.

Tracking Change Over Time

The weakness of purely cross-sectional comparisons for inferring causal effects is well known. Studies of *changes* in law, best with longitudinal data over many years, are much stronger. This chapter takes as given the necessity of determining when a law was enacted or became effective and whether subsequent legislative or judicial action nullified it or modified it in ways relevant to the research—the question is which dates and how. In most states and at the federal level, except for emergency legislation, there is a lag between the date of enactment of legislation and the effective date. For evaluation research, the effective date of a law is usually the most appropriate measure for the law's onset, because many studies assume that a law cannot affect health outcomes until it legally takes effect and is therefore enforceable. For some studies, such as those examining correlates of policy choice in legislatures or those evaluating the relationship between legislation and social norms, the date of enactment may be more appropriate.

Effective dates are usually determined either by a specific clause in legislation or by the jurisdiction's legislative rules, which to the uninitiated can be quite obtuse and confusing. Identifying changes in the law over long periods can be time and labor intensive. Lexis, Westlaw, and a few specialized services such as HeinOnline compile archived statutes and other legislative materials, which can make coding and validation easier. However, these historical materials tend to have more anomalies and interjurisdictional variations (for example, differences in years of coverage for archived statutes across states) than collections of current law. To perform historical legal research, coders typically need additional training. Effective dates tend not to appear in the text of legislation or statutes and or refer to an extra-legal event, for example "60 days after the end of the legislative session" or similar referent. StateScape's free online fifty-state chart is invaluable (www.statescape.com/resources/Effective_dates/effective_dates.asp), although only for current, not historical, practices. Retrospective research may be impossible at the local level or for state regulations because of the inaccessibility of historical records.

Amendments or other changes that occur after a law has been enacted and takes effect also require attention. Subsequent legislation that either directly amends a statute or repeals it entirely is the most obvious example of a modification. A sunset clause in a bill that nullifies it after a period of time is another important source of possible change. The judiciary, too, can invalidate a statute either in whole or in part. Such legal changes must be carefully examined to determine relevance to the research topic. Very high accuracy in coded effective dates is essential for public health law evaluation research because errors in effective dates can invalidate studies.

Reliance on Secondary Sources

At the start of a public health law evaluation project, discovering that someone else has already produced a summary of applicable laws might seem like a windfall that obviates the need for painstaking legal research. Many advocacy and think-tank websites and publications offer authoritative-looking fifty-state lists and similar compendia of "the law" on various topics. These secondary sources can be very useful for getting an overview of the law at a particular time and for use in the quality assurance process, but they are rarely sufficient sources of legal data for research projects. With few exceptions, these lists have one or more serious flaws, including that they do not result from rigorous research and verification processes; lack effective dates or other indications of the period during which a law is in effect; provide data only for one point in time, which usually is not specified; lack documentation of the research process and coding conventions used to produce them (thereby preventing replication of the research); and often contain significant errors.

Another seemingly sensible shortcut is to use key informant interviews or surveys, perhaps targeting agency staff presumed to know the law they are charged with administering. Experience has repeatedly demonstrated, however, that agency staff members do not always have the right answers. Surveys or other instruments addressed to an appropriately knowledgeable official at an under-staffed agency may be completed by a subordinate and returned without review by the expert. A study by LaFond and colleagues (2000) comparing legal data compiled from key informant interviews; surveys of agency directors and staff; and rigorous, original legal research found that original legal research produced the most accurate results. Error rates for some data collected by surveying agency personnel exceeded 50 percent.

There are few high-quality sources of legal data available. One of these, the Alcohol Policy Information System (APIS, alcoholpolicy.niaaa.nih.gov), developed by the National Institute on Alcohol Abuse and Alcoholism, relies on research attorneys to classify legal data on alcohol policy topics for all fifty states, the federal government, and the District of Columbia. Another example is the State Cancer Legislative Database Program (www.scld-nci.net), developed by the National Cancer Institute, which features a compendium of state statutes and resolutions on cancer-related policies. Notwithstanding APIS and a few other examples, obtaining legal data for an evaluation research project almost always entails conducting original legal research, which requires specialized legal and conceptual expertise beyond simple familiarity with a particular policy. Especially for multistate studies, anyone conducting research without considerable legal training and experience will be unlikely to produce reliable and accurate datasets.

Creating Composite Measures

The development of indices and scales can substantially increase the value of empirical legal datasets. For some studies, collapsing multiple variables into summary measures is required for analytic purposes. The dataset for distracted driving laws (www.phlr.org/datasets) includes well over a hundred variables. Statistical analyses are difficult if dozens or hundreds of variables are simultaneously included. Granular coding of legal features into many specific variables provides the basis for classifying a jurisdiction's laws, and starting with granular coding allows much more diverse sets of analyses later. Various composite measures use the detailed codes to represent broader constructs such as stringency, severity, or comprehensiveness of the law.

Developing good scales for legal measures remains particularly difficult, and few flawless examples exist. Among the best are rating systems such as the "Tobacco Policy Rating" based on data in the National Cancer Institute's State Cancer Legislative Database (www.scld-nci.net). Development of this scale bears several hallmarks that distinguish well-developed complex measures. First, the scale is firmly grounded in a causal diagram that links its components with tobacco use outcomes. Second, both legal and social science experts collaborate in constructing the scale. Third, a Delphi panel or other structured process is used for proposing, testing, and revising the scales. Because scales are by nature synthetic measures that encode assumptions along with observations, clarity and transparency regarding exactly how scales are constructed are essential to a study's integrity. All coding conventions and scaling procedures must be documented and reported. If data for the scale are to be analyzed using statistical techniques that require interval-level data, it is important to specify how increments between values are equalized as well as the scale's limitations (Chriqui and colleagues [2002] provide an excellent example of a description).

Creating simple scales based on the number of statutes in a jurisdiction or otherwise treating all laws as equally important produces a simple indicator that may be useful for certain purposes, but simple counts may be misleading because of omnibus legislation and interjurisdictional variations in codifying bills (for example, three statutes in one state may be equivalent to one statute in another or equal to a combination of statutes and regulations in a third).

In addition, some laws are likely to have much more effect than others. For example, a researcher might identify a dozen different state policies pertaining to child safety and use them in a study of childhood injuries. This design may mask the reality that a single law or combination of very few laws accounts for all of the influence of law on injuries; moreover, some of the specific laws in the scale may be inversely correlated with the outcome measure. How a scale is constructed is necessarily shaped by the underlying theoretical model, and a scale that is appropriate and useful for one purpose may be quite inappropriate for a different purpose.

Making Sense of Preemption and Federalism

The interplay among laws at the federal, state, and local levels adds another dimension of complexity to determining what the law "is" in any particular place. Sometimes the law being studied—say, state law aimed at regulating sugar-sweetened beverages—is contingent on law at other levels of government. At least two federal laws (the Child Nutrition Act of 1970 and the Child Nutrition and WIC Reauthorization Act of 2004) address this issue, as do statutes or regulations in at least thirty-four states (Mello, Pomeranz, & Moran, 2008). Moreover, some municipalities have their own ordinances, and many school districts have adopted policies as well. Evaluations of state limitations on sales of sugar-sweetened beverages in schools may be influenced by federal law and may show different results depending on whether local law is included or ignored.

Conflicts among laws at different levels of government generally are resolved by their hierarchy, with federal law being supreme and state law trumping anything at the local level. This seemingly straightforward arrangement is more complex than it initially appears, however. In some situations, federal law and conflicting state law may both be applied in the same jurisdiction, and state authorities may decline to enforce federal law. For example, since California decriminalized medical marijuana in 1996, state authorities have not enforced federal drug laws against dispensers or users of medical marijuana. Federal officers in California continue to apply U.S. drug laws. The varieties of preemption—a term that encompasses different arrangements of authority between levels of government—present some of the most interesting and complex legal questions. Here again, the need for guidance from a legal expert typically is required.

Research Design, Assumptions, and Inferences

Although this chapter is devoted to measurement, a few comments about inference and analysis bear mentioning. For empirical law evaluation studies there is an analog to the "If a tree falls in the woods" question: What if a law exists but no one follows it? Absence of compliance by relevant populations, varying enforcement by police or administrative personnel, unwillingness of prosecutors to bring charges, differing interpretations across jurisdictions, and inadequate funding for implementation or enforcement can create misleading evidence about the relationship between a law "on the books" and health outcomes "on the street." While the existence of a law supports an inference that it is being enforced, the possibility of non-enforcement or inconsistent enforcement can make a critical difference to compliance and measures of a policy's effect (see Wagenaar & Wolfson, 1994). Laws often have both deterrent and norms-shaping effects, and the latter can occur independently of enforcement. Research designs that include measures of enforcement and compliance better isolate the relative effects of different policies as written.

Even when a mandate is clearly stated, implementation may not necessarily follow. Particularly in studies of policies that require monetary appropriations for implementation, such as laws that create systems for providing treatment or give citizens a right to receive governmental services, another factor looms: whether adequate funds are available. Legislatures are more apt to pass authorizing legislation for a program than to pass appropriations to fund it. Executive agencies— which are charged primarily with enforcing laws—may divert or delay funds with little recourse for policy makers.

Legal texts are measured to determine government-sanctioned policy. This information is seldom sufficient by itself to sustain inferences about the effectiveness or harm of specific laws. This chapter demonstrates that law is measurable for scientific study like other phenomena. If you are reading this, you likely take it as a given that law is important to health. Collecting and coding legal texts, however, is only the start. One also needs to measure a range of implementation factors and other features of jurisdictions to understand how law and health relate.

Conclusion

This chapter describes methods for measuring law and creating datasets for use in public health law evaluations. The aim is to generate scientifically defensible data that reflect in quantitative forms how laws vary over space and time. In addition to adding rigor to the study of legal texts, it provides a method for increasing the efficiency of studying legal change over time, a key requirement for evaluation research. While these methods are still developing and specific uniform standards and best practices are evolving, measurement and coding issues are an essential if underappreciated element of public health law research. Implementing the suggestions and procedures offered in this chapter helps advance the field of evaluation research by increasing the utility and accuracy of research that uses legal data, ultimately improving public policy and its effectiveness in achieving important goals in advancing population health and well-being. By blending the knowledge and skills of social and health scientists with those of legal experts, scholars can produce more accurate and more useful policy evaluations. As the field continues to advance, adopting minimum measurement standards along the lines suggested here will elevate the threshold of acceptable quality for designing, funding, and conducting evaluations of public policies embodied in law.

Summary

Effectively studying the relationship between law and population health requires variation in both the law and health outcomes being studied, over space as well as time, and valid and reliable methods for capturing variation and representing it in forms that allow comparison and analyses. A rigorous method for measuring law generates numeric data representing variation in law. The key feature of the method—and that which distinguishes it most from traditional legal research—is that it relies on observation of the apparent features of legal texts. By eschewing deep legal interpretation, this restrained observational approach produces data that is replicable through a process that is transparent. Transparency and replicability are essential attributes of scientifically defensible data.

There are many challenges in measuring law. Relevant legal texts can be hard to find and when found can be rife with ambiguous and conflicting meanings. Formulating reliable and valid ways of reducing complex bodies of law into numeric data can be difficult. There are also cultural and logistical challenges to blending legal and empirical expertise. These challenges can be overcome by a methodical process of design, data collection, and analysis that adheres to scientific standards. Steps include the careful delineation of the legal questions to be addressed and the scope of the research; the iterative development and refinement of a coding scheme; quality control; and the production of a transparent research protocol and codebook to accompany the resulting legal dataset.

Further Reading

Ibrahim, J. K., Anderson, E. D., Burris, S. C., & Wagenaar, A. C. (2011). State laws restricting driver use of mobile communications devices: "Distracted-driving" provisions, 1992–2010. *American Journal of Preventive Medicine, 40*(6), 659–665.

Public Health Law Research. (2012). *LawAtlas*. Accessed September 26, 2012, from http://www.lawatlas.org.

Singer, J. W. (1984). The player and the cards: Nihilism and legal theory. *Yale Law Journal, 94*(1), 1–70.

Chapter 12

Coding Case Law for Public Health Law Evaluation

Mark Hall

Learning Objectives

- Describe strengths and limitations of content analysis in public health law research.
- Identify steps in the systematic identification and coding of case law.
- Design an analysis plan for coded case law.

This chapter explains how the research method of content analysis can be applied to study legal decisions. Content analysis is a method for systematically reading and analyzing "texts" of any kind. Developed by sociologists and political scientists, the method is also used widely in the communications field (Krippendorff, 1980; Neuendorf, 2002). It can be applied not only to conventional written material but also to images or audio content. Written texts abound, of course, in the legal sphere, including statutes, regulations, hearing transcripts, and court filings. But our sole focus here is one especially important legal text: judicial opinions.

The content of judicial opinions merits careful study not simply because opinions reflect or respond to the law, but because they *are* the law. Legal researchers are correct to recognize that it "is almost impossible to study law in a meaningful way without some attention to the [content of] opinions that contain these justifications" (Friedman, 2006, p. 266). For instance, a researcher wanting to know what effect the First Amendment's protection of speech, religion, and association might have on enforcement of various public health laws would need to analyze Supreme Court opinions as a primary source of law.

But more than this, judicial opinions are detailed repositories that show what kinds of disputes come before courts, how the parties frame their disputes, and how judges reason to their conclusions. For example, Haar and colleagues (1977) coded for the presence or absence of 167 different factors in each of seventy-nine zoning dispute cases decided by one state's Supreme Court over a twenty-five-year period, to determine which factors appear to influence the outcome of these cases. It is this factual and analytical richness of judicial opinions that establish both their substantive legal importance and their utility as instruments for public health research of various designs.

On the surface, content analysis appears simple, even trivial, to some. It boils down to three steps: (1) selecting cases, (2) coding cases, and (3) analyzing (often through statistics) the case coding. The method comes naturally to legal scholars because it resembles the classic scholarly routine of reading a collection of cases, finding common threads that link the opinions, and commenting on their significance (Hall & Wright, 2008). But content analysis is much more than a better way to read cases. It brings scientific rigor to the collection and analyses of case law, which could create a distinctively legal form of scientific empiricism. This approach to reading cases can be used profitably in three distinct types of studies: those that identify determinants of judicial decision making, those that measure consequences of judicial decisions, or those that document how the judicial system operates.

What Content Analysis Can and Cannot Tell Us

Content analysis is not a panacea. It has certain advantages, along with substantial limitations, compared with conventional legal analysis. At best, the method generates objective, falsifiable, and reproducible knowledge about what selected courts do and how and why they do it. But this method does not lead to the Holy Grail of a true legal science. It works best when each of the judicial opinions in a collection holds essentially equal value, but not when what is needed is a deeply reflective understanding of a single pivotal case. Content analysis therefore does not displace traditional interpretive legal scholarship. Nor does it reveal how all aspects of a legal system function (Hoffman, Izenman, & Lidicker, 2007). Instead, it offers distinctive insights that complement the types of understanding that traditional legal analysis can generate, or that could be obtained by more direct observation of legal systems.

Conventional Legal Analysis

Traditional legal scholarship relies, like the interpretation of literature, on the interpreter's authoritative expertise to select important cases and to draw out noteworthy themes and identify potential social effects that might flow from decisions. Audiences depend on the author's judgment about which cases are worth reading, which are the "leading cases" that best illustrate the historical moment in question. Interpretive legal scholars read opinions closely, looking for common themes running through several opinions. They ponder the meaning of a decision for future cases by asking how the outcome in the current case relates to its facts, procedural posture, and the court's reasoning.

Although legal writing in this mode may contain many assertions about how judges think or act, it is not a scientific form of empiricism. These legal analysts report what they see in key cases and how they interpret these observations, not unlike how a literary critic might interpret poetry. Establishing some plausible basis for the minimally empirical claims in such work is usually done simply by citing relevant sources that readers can verify if they wish.

Although content analysis has different epistemological aims, it can be seen as a logical extension of the school of jurisprudence known as Legal Realism. Over a century ago, Justice Oliver Wendell Holmes Jr. famously proclaimed that "prophecies of what the courts will do in fact, and nothing more pretentious, are what I mean by the law." This credo, once revolutionary, is now so widely accepted that it is sometimes said in the legal academy that "we are all legal realists." All that content analysis seeks to do is to use accepted scientific methods to support the verifiable claims that legal researchers frequently make about what judges do and say.

Content analysis can augment conventional analysis by identifying previously unnoticed patterns that warrant deeper study, or sometimes correcting misimpressions based on ad hoc surveys of atypical cases. Once detected, these previously unnoticed and unexpected features of the law, observed only on the surface, can be explored more deeply through other, richer methods. Scientists speak in terms of "triangulating" different methods—that is, exploring whether different approaches offer similar conclusions, each approach rigorous in its own way, but each illuminating different dimensions and potentially overcoming their respective shortcomings. Quantitative description can tell us the *what* of case law; other methods may be better suited to understanding the *why* and *wherefore*.

Neither type of scholarship standing alone is as strong as the different types combined. Content analysis reaches a thinner understanding of the law than that gained through more subjective interpretive methods. The coding of case content does not fully capture the strength of a particular judge's rhetoric, the level of generality used to describe the issue, and many other subtle clues about the precedential value of the opinion. Or, as an example to put the point more bluntly, the "legal and cultural salience of Roe *v.* Wade far outruns its statistical significance" (Goldsmith & Vermeule, 2002).

Inevitably, then, content analysis trades depth for breadth. Content analysis is valid if it accurately and reliably measures the particular components of the decision that the researcher wants to study. Using systematic defined coding protocols improves measurement by removing elements of researcher bias, enhancing thoroughness, precision, and accuracy. However, to the extent that content analysis cannot reach important aspects of legal interpretation that are impossible to code objectively (such as nuance related to infrequent or highly complex factual and procedural patterns), plain content analysis loses relevance. When uniform coding cannot capture important details about idiosyncratic decisions, content analysis alone is not capable of measuring what lawyers or scholars would consider to be a full and accurate statement of the law.

Still, content analysis holds value not only for conventional doctrinal analysis but also for more theoretically influenced work in major branches of jurisprudence, such as economic analysis or critical theory. Writers in each of these scholarly camps frequently claim that judges and law respond predictably to various social, political, and market conditions—empirical claims that can be tested systematically. Some schools of jurisprudence emphasize the bare outcomes of cases in relation to their raw facts, while others emphasize the importance of how judges explain their decisions. Although these fundamental differences hugely affect how content analysis might be employed, the method itself is adaptable to any branch of legal theory that systematically studies judicial opinions. Moreover, the method is a key component of empirical studies evaluating effects of case law on the public's health. Such evaluative studies require transparent and reproducible numeric indices of law and how it varies across time and across jurisdictions, to examine how such variations affect population-level health-relevant exposures, behaviors, and outcomes.

Counting Case Outcomes

One basic use of content analysis is simply to document the bare outcomes of cases. Measuring who won and who lost differs fundamentally from measuring the law of a case. Case outcomes are much narrower and more objective questions, requiring much less legal judgment, than what legal principle a case embodies. One might, for instance, want to simply tote up the number of cases in which the authority of local public health laws was challenged, and who won and lost, either in one jurisdiction or many, over a period of time.

Counting case outcomes in this fashion is best done when each decision should receive equal weight, that is, when it is appropriate to regard the content of opinions as generic data. Coding and counting cases usually assumes that the information from one opinion is potentially as relevant as that from any other opinion. Because content analysis tends to regard all cases, judges, courts, and jurisdictions in the same way, it should be used only with great caution when any of these have a great deal more status or influence than the others, for the question addressed. Differential influence is often true in legal analysis because precedent and persuasiveness depend on various qualitative judgments about the reasons given or the source of the decision.

Taking this limitation into account, scholars have found that it is especially useful to code and count cases to document the *absence* of some element that is thought to be present in case law. "Proving a negative" is much harder than simply pointing to what is present in case law because the nay-saying researcher needs to demonstrate that he or she has looked exhaustively for all likely instances of the missing element.

Counting cases can also be useful in studying a wide range of social and economic phenomena that might affect judge-made law. Treating case outcomes as the dependent variable, the range of potential influences on judicial behavior that might be studied statistically is limited only by the bounds of a researcher's imagination. One study, for instance, explored whether the political makeup of Congress or changes in the presidential party in power affected the outcome of federal appellate cases in which health and safety regulations were challenged, over a twenty-five-year period (Revesz, 1997, 2001).

Case law can also be used as an independent variable, by asking how it influences various social and economic conditions. Law's effect on society is obviously a rich field of inquiry, but most such studies trace the effects only of statutory or regulatory law. Researchers have neglected the possible effects of judge-made law, including statutory interpretation. For instance, social host and bar owner liability for alcohol-related injuries is determined by both judicial decisions and statutory enactments, which vary widely by state and over time. These differences might contribute to a variety of public health effects of interest. With its diverse "laboratory of states," the United States offers boundless opportunities to learn from the "natural experiments" created by the inevitable differences in case law among jurisdictions and over time.

Evaluating Legal Doctrine

Opinion coding is not suited, however, to evaluating the legal correctness of judicial opinions. Certainly, many content analysts draw normative implications from what they observe, but their coding of cases aims only to document what judges do rather than to evaluate in a formal empirical manner how well they perform. Without an independent "gold standard" for what the law should be in any particular case or jurisdiction, who is to say its judges are legally wrong, in an empirical sense? After all, what judges say is the law. Therefore normative evaluation of legal doctrine ordinarily can be done convincingly only through some form of traditional legal analysis.

But beyond documenting merely the bare outcomes of legal disputes, content analysis might be used to study the legal principles one can extrapolate from those outcomes and the facts and reasons that contribute to those outcomes and principles. Such analyses raise important epistemological and jurisprudential issues.

"JURIMETRICS"

The most ambitious use of content analysis is to study the legal factors that determine the outcomes of cases, using sophisticated statistical methods to model or predict the behavior of judges. This general approach at one time was called "jurimetrics" (Loevinger, 1961). This kind of study might attempt to predict the likely result in a case when the parties present the judge with a particular combination of legally relevant factors. Often the stated purpose is to help practicing lawyers make better-informed decisions about handling particular cases. Other times, the purpose is more scholarly—to test various claims on the basis of legal theory.

An especially interesting subgenre uses content analysis to find some order and logic in a body of case law that, by conventional analysis, appears chaotic or haphazard. As Fred McChesney (1993) notes, "the academic history of American law generally is replete with instances in which scholars have proclaimed traditional common-law modes of distilling 'the law' from cases unworkable." These conventional legal analysts, throwing up their hands, conclude that the law on the topic is hopelessly confused and inconsistent, or, less pejoratively, dependent on individual facts. Nuisance law might be one relevant example. Are public nuisances solely "in the eye of the beholder," or are there patterns of factors that are associated with the likelihood of finding or not finding legally actionable public nuisance? Content analysis is well suited to answering this question in a body of case law that otherwise might appear unfathomable.

THE CIRCULARITY OF FACTS IN JUDICIAL OPINIONS

Naturally, correlation does not equate with causation. This is especially so in analyzing the content of judicial reasoning, considering a serious circularity problem. Judges marshal the facts and reasons that support the outcome of the case. Therefore, their opinions might not fully or accurately describe the real-world facts or the true nature of the judge's decision process. Indeed, there is every reason to think just the opposite.

This limitation entails two distinct problems: factual incompleteness and factual distortion. Incompleteness results because judges' presentations are meant only to explain as much of the facts as are necessary to justify the outcome. This judicial parsimony can severely distort analysts' measurement of facts that might be important across a range of cases. An apt example is the study of racial factors. Whites might be identified in only a fraction of cases in which race is mentioned, but most likely this is because courts usually do not consider it appropriate to mention race unless they think this might be legally relevant in a particular case.

The second problem is the possibility that judges distort the facts they report to justify the results they reach. This is a highly contentious charge, but distortion does not have to amount to outright misrepresentation. Instead, distortion arises simply from the inevitability that courts select and filter the facts as relevant to the explanation of their decision, but doing only that creates a serious methodologic challenge, since it is circular to predict judicial outcomes from facts that reflect rather than generate the result.

Answering the Skeptics

There are four possible responses to judicial skeptics. First, scientific data aim only to be a reasonable approximation of underlying reality. As a probabilistic endeavor, they can tolerate a degree of imprecision, especially when such imprecision is randomly distributed, not reflecting biased measurement (for example, when the measurement of a particular dimension of law systematically underestimates or overestimates). Similarly, for facts reported by judges, even though they may not be a full account of the "real facts," they may be as close an approximation as is reasonably available to study a particular question. This assumption is not heroic. Lawyers and law professors who stake their life's work on believing (by and large) judges' renditions of facts are, on the whole, hardly naive idealists.

Second, researchers specifically can examine the fidelity of reported facts, looking for indications of distortion or incompleteness, to determine if the facts are close enough to reality for use in statistical analysis. One such technique is to compare facts reported in an appellate opinion with those reported in either the trial court's opinion or a dissenting opinion.

Third, the "bias" created by courts' justifying their decisions may be precisely what a researcher wishes to study. After all, the facts and reasons the judge selects are the substance of the opinion that creates law and binding precedent, so they merit careful study for this very reason. This justification calls, however, for precision in setting the goals of study. Instead of predicting outcomes, content analysis can aim simply at studying judicial reasoning itself, retrospectively.

Finally, the fact that content analysis may not provide definite answers to factors affecting judicial decisions does not mean the method lacks all value. Even if doubts remain about cause-and-effect relationships with judicial decisions, identifying apparent or possible associations of interest can merit further study using additional, and perhaps more experimental, methods.

Exploring the Landscape of Case Law

Rather than trying to predict or explain case outcomes, content analysts can take advantage of the factual, rhetorical, and legal details in judicial opinions simply to describe or explore a body of case law. Observing and documenting what can be found in case law is more akin to mapping than to testing. Like a naturalist exploring new (or familiar) terrain, researchers can code cases to document trends in the case law and factors that appear important to case outcomes, such as the apparent effect of a new precedent, statute, or legal doctrine.

Wright and Huck (2002), for instance, code and analyze 440 decisions regarding milk production and purity standards during the eighty-year period starting in 1860, exploring the historical question of whether courts were hostile or receptive to state legislatures' progressive public health agendas. They conclude that judicial hostility was greater than legal and social historians frequently recognize.

The primary criticism of some descriptive or exploratory studies is that they can draw conclusions about features of the legal landscape that cannot be observed fully from judicial opinions. As discussed more further on, win-loss records from published opinions do not necessarily tell us about legal disputes that were never filed in court, or those that the parties settled, or those that judges resolved without written or published opinions. Nevertheless, even if judicial opinions offer a skewed view of what occurs elsewhere in the legal system, they are a highly valuable source for systematic study because they reveal the portion of the legal world that in many ways is most important. It is published opinions that set legal precedent and that guide lawyers.

Published opinions are especially probative of questions about the spread of ideas within the legal system or the types of information that judges appear to rely on. A number of studies analyze courts' reliance on different types of social science evidence (Hall & Wright, 2008). Naturally, caution is warranted in concluding that a mention of a source in an opinion indicates actual importance judges place on this type of evidence and argument. Still, with appropriate caveats on the claims being made, systematic study of how judges reason in their written decisions is perhaps the most compelling application of case content analysis because it best fits the method with the type of question that researchers are asking.

Finally, because published opinions represent "law," the amount, nature, and legal influence of particular dimensions of such law may well affect a diverse set of public health outcomes. To advance empirical study of the public health effects of law, we need counts, weights, scales, and other numeric indices of such law. Precise and specified procedures, and consistent implementation of such protocols, are required to meet scientific standards for reliable measurement.

Guidelines for Identifying and Coding Case Law

Assuming the decision has been made to conduct content analyses of case law (in contrast to traditional legal analysis), we next consider how best to design and implement such a content analysis. In brief, a content analyst selects a set of opinions on a particular subject via a predefined set of search-and-inclusion criteria; reads the documents systematically, recording features of each one in a consistent and reliable manner; and then draws inferences about the use and meaning of those documents.

Selecting Cases

The first decision in any case-coding project is which cases to select. There are two components to consider: sampling frame and selection method. The sampling frame is the theoretical universe of all relevant cases, and the selection method determines which cases will actually be sampled and studied. For both dimensions, researchers should specify exactly the protocol used (databases, search terms, repeated review and correction cycles, and so on) so that it is fully understood and reproducible by others.

SAMPLING FRAME AND BIASES

Frequently in empirical studies, it is not feasible to observe all or most members of a relevant population. Therefore the potential biases introduced by sampling method ordinarily are a topic of considerable methodological attention, so that a study sample accurately represents the true population of interest. Fortunately, most studies of legal decisions can avoid this concern because the sampling frame contains a small enough number of cases that *universal* sampling of *all* relevant cases is often feasible.

When the total population is too large to be manageable, however, sampling techniques might include true random sampling (best done by computer-generated list of random numbers); systematic sampling, such as every fifth case; quota sampling, such as all cases up to two hundred, per jurisdiction per year; or purposive sampling, such as cases that are cited by leading treatises and casebooks or cited by other cases.

The more troubling question is the relevant sampling *frame*. What are the boundaries of the subject matter in question? Obviously, this depends critically on the study's central questions and purposes. Study questions can be narrowed to fit the sample frame that is available, or a theoretical sample frame can be imagined that is unrealistically broad but that fits a more interesting or important set of questions the analyst wishes to pursue. Political scientists, for instance, often study political and institutional influences on judicial decision making by looking not at *all* Supreme Court cases or a random selection, but instead at a particularly controversial or value-laden set of decisions, such as those involving freedom of speech or unreasonable searches and seizures.

Whenever the actual cases selected do not fully match the sampling frame that theoretically applies to the questions posed or studied, an issue of sampling bias exists. For example, studies that sample cases until a certain date cannot, necessarily, claim with confidence that their findings reflect what happened after that date. (This is true as well for studies that sample from certain jurisdictions.) Researchers should at least reflect on these potential distortions or limitations, and mention in their reports those that merit explanation.

One scholar, for instance (who happens to be the author of this chapter), chose to explore how courts determine effectiveness of medical treatment in health insurance disputes by studying all *published* judicial opinions resolving such disputes (Hall, Rust Smith, Naughton, & Ebbers, 1996). That universe of observations might be relevant for a narrower question, such as how appellate courts reason their decisions on such issues, but the sample frame of all published opinions does not fully reflect what all courts do or how state trial courts actually make their decisions.

There is potential selection bias at each of many points in the litigation process. Only some human interactions produce disputes, only some disputes result in legal claims, many claims are settled, and many trial decisions are not appealed. Appellate courts regularly dispose of cases without opinions or decide not to publish some opinions, and computer databases inconsistently include cases that are not officially published. At each of these junctures, there are a variety of factors that potentially distort what one stage can reveal about the other. These biases can fundamentally threaten the validity or generalizability of a study's findings. In these situations, careful consideration of selection biases may lead to major redesign of a study as originally conceived.

Sometimes, however, agonized handwringing can be minimized or avoided. No concern arises if the researcher defines the research question in terms that match the population of cases actually sampled. For instance, if it is precedential law that one wants to study, rather than simply the generalized behavior or attitudes of judges, then unpublished opinions are irrelevant and so excluding them requires no justification. In other situations, when excluded cases are theoretically relevant, the exclusion can easily be justified if the likely direction of bias or distortion is considered. When the bias runs in the same general direction as the study's findings (that is, the excluded cases are even more likely to exhibit the observed pattern), then including the additional cases would likely only strengthen the findings. The only major harm from excluding them is potentially to have missed some additional findings of interest or to have produced a false observation of no effect.

In other situations, likely differences between studied cases and omitted cases are sufficiently inconsequential that the omission should create no more a concern than other limitations obvious and inherent in the sample frame itself, such as one date range rather than another. All empirical studies are imperfect—observational (non-experimental) studies especially. The realistic standard for selecting cases is not a perfect match between sample frame and research objectives, but only a strong connection between the two.

SELECTION TECHNIQUES AND REPLICABILITY

An essential attribute of scientific objectivity is the ability, at least in theory, to reproduce a project's findings using the same methods. Replicability is the overriding reason for using systematic content analysis, and transparency via reporting exact protocols used is a prerequisite for replicability. This is what confers scientific status on the findings and conclusions.

One component of replication is the method of selecting cases for study. Usually, this consists simply of specifying the particular structured search terms used to locate candidate cases in the Westlaw or LEXIS databases. However, mechanized searches are rarely refined enough to narrow the sample to only or mostly relevant cases. Cases that mention a topic of interest often do so only in passing. Those that decide an issue sometimes do so on technical or procedural grounds that are not relevant to a particular study. Therefore, further narrowing is usually needed in order to reduce an initial selection of candidate cases to those that are directly relevant to the research question.

Most legal researchers do so using somewhat subjective criteria of relevance that cannot be fully replicated. Another option, however, is to refine the initial mechanical search strategy. Useful strategies include searching case digests or headnotes rather than the full case itself, or searching a sample of cases selected initially because they cited particular statutes, or because they appear in a subject matter classification drawn by someone else, such as West's key numbering system or the publisher of a subject-matter-specific reporter. In effect, such researchers are relying on case selection criteria employed by someone else to establish probable relevance of cases.

Verifying the replicability of case selection is essential for a rigorous study, eliminating the possibility that a researcher subconsciously chose cases according to whether he or she appeared to support the researcher's preliminary hunches. Either formal reliability testing or case selection by someone who is otherwise uninvolved in the study is a way to guard against this potential bias.

Coding Cases

Once cases are selected, a defined coding scheme focuses attention systematically on various elements of cases, and mainly is a check against looking, either consciously or not, for confirmation of predetermined positions. This effort to articulate beforehand the features of a case worth studying also allows researchers to delegate some or all of the reading to assistants. More important, coding cases, even for just qualitative description and analysis, strengthens the objectivity and reproducibility of case law interpretation. Experts in content analysis outline four basic steps that should be followed in coding any material (Krippendorff, 2004; Neuendorf, 2007):

1. On the basis of questions most germane to the study, create a tentative set of coding categories a priori. After thorough evaluation, including feedback from colleagues, study team members or expert consultants refine these categories.

2. Write a coding sheet and set of coding instructions (called a "code-book"), and train coders to apply these to a sample of the material to be coded. Pilot test the reliability (consistency) among coders by having multiple people independently code some of the material, and calculate the correlation across coders (that is, inter-rater reliability).

3. Add, delete, or revise coding categories according to this pilot experience, and repeat reliability testing and coder training as required.

4. When the codebook is finalized, apply it to all the material. Then, or during that process, conduct a final, formal reliability test. This section elaborates on each of these steps.

CODING CATEGORIES AND INSTRUCTIONS

Categories used to code content of judicial decisions are tremendously diverse, owing to the wide range of questions that researchers pursue. Commonly used factors might be sorted into four general groups: parties' identities and attributes, types of legal issues raised and in what circumstances, basic outcome of the case or issue, and bases for decision. Coders often do not distinguish the "facts" of a case from various arguments that are made. Instead, they usually code simply for whether a variety of factual or legal factors are present in the case in some fashion. Coders should consider whether it suffices if these factors are merely alleged, realizing that the allegations may be sharply contested. If mere allegations are not sufficient, what is? Obviously, the procedural posture of a case (summary judgment versus post-trial) can complicate this evaluation.

Regarding the bases for decision, coders frequently distinguish between procedural and substantive rulings, and they record the various types of authorities that courts cite or rely upon. Some researchers also code for the degree of importance that various factual or legal factors have in the court's analysis or holding. A common focus of coding is also the court's style of analysis or approach to statutory or constitutional interpretation, categorized in various ways.

Coding is not restricted to manifest variables that are explicit in the text; it has been shown to work well also for some "latent" variables that require inference or evaluative judgment. For instance, Johnson (1987) demonstrates the ability of law students to code cases with some degree of reliability for the clarity, complexity, and completeness of their discussion of facts, issues, holding, reasoning, and the law.

Coding experts advise researchers to create more coding categories, and to make coding more fine-grained, than the categories they may ultimately use. Even though this produces more information than the project will eventually require, the advantage is allowing the researcher to test different categorization schemes to learn through trial and error which work best. Ultimately, the goal is to maximize the exhaustiveness of coding while keeping mutually exclusive categories—in other words, to capture all the relevant information, but to avoid having categories that duplicate or overlap each other. This does not mean, however, that a coding category must be devised for each possible nuance of relevance. Instead, categories should be used only if they occur with some frequency, or if the objective is to document their absence. Rare or unusual features can be coded simply with a miscellaneous "other" option.

A good example of exhaustive and mutually exclusive coding is categorizing case outcomes. It is usually not a simple matter to define what counts as a win or loss across a range of cases. Appellate cases arise in a variety of procedural postures, they usually involve multiple issues, and each issue can be resolved in several different ways. Case coding projects often have to devise complex categories to capture all the relevant detail. The United States Court of Appeals Database (http://www.wmich.edu/nsf-coa/), for instance, defines all possible case outcomes using nine categories. This illustrates that it is a better practice to be over-inclusive at the coding stage, waiting until the analysis stage to collapse the various categories into discrete win-loss columns.

When categories are finalized, it is essential to good coding practice to record their description and specific instructions for their application. Obviously, this is necessary if coding is done by someone other than the researcher, such as student assistants. Even if authors do their own coding, the scientific standard of replicability requires a clear written record of how categories were defined and applied, permitting other research teams to correctly replicate the procedure in future studies.

Experienced coders advise that errors will be reduced if coding forms are designed to minimize writing. For instance, a form might provide a checklist of factors to indicate presence or absence by ticking boxes rather than having to write in a number or letter. Also, while the objective is to reduce the need for coder judgment, detailed instructions can be conveyed either through the coding form itself, or in a supplemental manual. A balance should be struck between a form that is so spare it offers almost no on-the-spot instructional information for coders, forcing them to refer frequently to the detailed coding manual, and a coding form that is overlong because each form contains a full set of instructions. Thus it typically does not help to extensively revise succinct, well-written coding categories simply to satisfy the whim of each coder who might ask for more detailed instructions. It is inevitable that some measure of ambiguity will remain in how coding categories apply to atypical cases, and a residual notes file should be included to record unusual situations.

CHOOSING AND TRAINING CODERS

A major dilemma in coding cases is whether principal investigators should do this work themselves, or supervise students (or others). In theory, the most scientifically rigorous method is for researchers to train others to do the coding and for coders to work completely independently once they are trained. Using generic coders helps ensure that the researchers' preliminary hypotheses and personal views do not bias the coding. Also, this can save researchers considerable time and effort in large coding projects. Moreover, the imposed discipline of training and supervising coders ensures that coding instructions are written in a way that others can follow. Training and using multiple coders promotes the reproducibility that is essential for good science. Coding by law students is appropriate when some general legal knowledge is required but it is not necessary to be an expert in the field of study. Still, coding reliability improves the more that coders are trained. Researchers should describe how training was done in sufficient detail that others can replicate all of the steps.

Other considerations might counsel doing one's own coding, however. Training coders to achieve accurate and reliable results can be a difficult and time-consuming undertaking, one that may require considerably more resources and effort than would researchers simply doing their own coding, especially in smaller projects. A relevant selection of cases is often sufficiently small that a single reader can handle the coding alone. Also, even trained coders can make a surprising number of mistakes, even on seemingly simple and objective criteria such as dates. Although delegating coding may promote reliability, this can threaten the validity of results if the information that coders record is not accurate or is too "dumbed down" to be meaningful. It may be that student coders lack the level of expertise needed to code reliably the more complex or subtle, yet more meaningful, aspects of judicial opinions. If so, researchers will be sorely tempted to do their own coding. When this is done, however, it is especially important to conduct reliability tests by recruiting a colleague with similar expertise to independently double code at least a subset of cases. Resulting reliability estimates should always be recorded and published along with the substantive findings.

TESTING RELIABILITY

Demonstrating the reliability of coding is an essential aspect of good content analysis. If coding categories are so objective and straightforward that it is obvious they can be applied consistently, then perhaps this step is not necessary, though that is rarely the case. If there are significant elements of subjectivity or uncertainty in applying coding categories to legal decisions, scientific rigor requires evaluation of whether different people would code the documents consistently. This is essential because the theory of coding—the reason systematic content analysis is done at all—is the implicit claim of reproducibility, that other researchers using the same methods will achieve approximately the same results. This claim is undermined if coding reflects primarily the subjective, idiosyncratic interpretation of the particular individuals who read the cases, or if coding has large elements of error or arbitrariness.

It is true that even without any reliability testing it is perfectly possible that a coding scheme in fact is reliable. But this cannot be ensured unless investigators test coding reliability in some fashion. The best method is to conduct formal reliability tests during (at least) two stages in the process: initially, while piloting the draft coding process, and later, once coding categories and instructions are optimized. Formal testing calls for at least two coders independently to code a sample of cases and to compare their results statistically.

The most common statistic is simple percentage of agreement. However, a simple percentage does not account for the level of agreement that would be expected purely by chance. Because chance agreement varies according to the type of coding scheme (that is, a variable with two possible answers will naturally produce more agreement than a variable with eight possible answers), the best practice is to report one of several coefficients that reflect the extent of agreement beyond what is expected by chance. There are several such statistical tests, the most common of which is known as "Cohen's Kappa" (after its inventor) or simply the Kappa statistic. Ranging from 0 to 1, Kappa indicates the proportion of observed agreement that exceeds what would be expected by chance alone, with 0 indicating agreement entirely by chance and 1 indicating perfect agreement.

If statistics such as these are used, they must be employed correctly. One mistake is to test the overall reliability of all variables combined. The correct method is to test and report each variable's reliability because reliability can vary widely across items and aggregate statistics can mask serious problems with key variables. Also, when the response pattern for a variable is highly skewed (one of several available responses occurs much more frequently than the others), this should be noted or taken into account in the statistical measure used. Otherwise, the nominal level of agreement can be deceptive. If one were to code for the presence or absence of one hundred factors in each case, most likely only a dozen or so will appear in any one case. Testing for coding reliability may find a very high percentage of agreement then, but only because most factors are not present in most cases. The key question, though, is whether coders agree when they indicate a factor is present.

When reliability testing reveals discrepancies, as it almost always will, this will usually point to unresolved questions in the coding instructions, problems that can be corrected if the error appears after the pilot phase rather than after the completed coding. Also, poor reliability in the pilot round of coding often reveals conceptual ambiguity that can be clarified to more accurately measure the dimensions or their components that are actually most relevant to the particular research question.

After final coding, compulsive researchers might try to get to the bottom of remaining disagreements and resolve all discrepancies, both in the reliability testing sample and across the entire selection. When there are large numbers of cases being coded, resolving every discrepancy may be unnecessary and impractical. Disagreements sometimes arise from overt errors, but often they result simply from judgment calls or inevitable ambiguities that may be virtually impossible to eliminate without compromising the independence of individual coders. Perfect reliability is the goal, but rarely fully achieved. A key requirement of science is transparency—reporting the exact levels of reliability of the resulting data.

Refining coding rules to eliminate all elements of ambiguity is usually not possible, no matter how prescriptive the rules. Plus, each time the rules are rewritten, the best practice would be to retest the refined rules for reliability, producing a never-ending cycle in search of elusive perfection. Therefore coders should learn to live with a certain degree of imperfection once coding is found to be reasonably reliable, and draw appropriately modest conclusions when relying on variables with weaker levels of inter-coder reliability. Although there is broad agreement on the desirability of testing for reliability, and some agreement on the methods for doing so, there is not firm agreement on what *level* of reliability is the minimum that is acceptable. The goal is aspirational—to achieve high levels of agreement—rather than merely to rise somewhat above purely random agreement. One suggested rule of thumb is that a reliability coefficient of .8 (that is, data agree 80 percent more than mere chance agreement) is good, with indices from .67–.8 being sufficient for "tentative conclusions" (Krippendorff, 1980). Others claim that this is too demanding, especially for coding categories that produce highly skewed responses, since even small levels of disagreement can cause the statistical index to drop rapidly. Therefore, other methodologists provide a more lenient classification for the Kappa statistic (Lombard, Snyder-Duch, & Campanella Bracken, 2005): ≤ 0.00 is poor; 0.01–0.20 is "slight" agreement; 0.21–0.40 is fair; 0.41–0.60 is "moderate"; 0.61–0.80 is "substantial"; and 0.81–1.00 is "almost perfect." Keep in mind that these recommendations are for agreement levels beyond what is expected by chance. For a raw, unadjusted percentage, agreement levels below 70 to 80 percent are usually not considered to be good.

If coder agreement is not acceptable, researchers must either retrain coders, revise their coding categories, decide not to use the data, or use the data but with appropriate caveats. Following best practices, the first two options call for retesting of reliability. One convenient remedy is to combine marginally reliable detailed coding into a more aggregated category that has better reliability.

ALTERNATIVE CODING TECHNIQUES

Researchers might consider alternatives to independent coding by assistants. One is to have a group of assistants code each case and then assign the value that is coded by the majority. Group coding creates the impression of greater objectivity, and may in fact improve reliability, but this is not necessarily the case. Resolving split votes with whatever the third person thinks might be as arbitrary as using a single coder. The only way to find out for sure is to test the reliability of panel coding by coding a sample of cases independently with a different panel.

Similarly, some researchers have coders confer when they disagree in order to seek consensus, or the researcher uses her or his own expertise to resolve disagreements. Again, this may or may not improve reliability, but it does not *establish* reliability. The process of reaching consensus might be arbitrary, or the lead investigator's expert view might not be objectively reproducible.

A variation of these techniques is expert panel consensus. Developed for evaluating medical judgments, this has not been used so far for legal judgments but it is worth exploring. Following what is known as the Delphi technique, each expert first rates a case independently, then learns how peer experts have rated it, and then, following discussion, each expert gives an independent final rating, with the majority controlling when there is not unanimity (Shekelle, Kahan, Bernstein, et al., 1998). This has been shown to be a fairly reliable method for rating highly complex and judgmental aspects of medical decision making (Park, Fink, Brook, et al., 1986). It combines elements of "gold standard" expertise with consensus building and majority rule.

Finally, there is an innovative technique that avoids altogether the vagaries of training coders and demonstrating reliability: using completely mechanical forms of content analysis that can be done by computer or simple computation. For instance, some studies count the number of words or paragraphs devoted to discussing particular factors as an indication of the factors' relative importance. Also interesting is research that analyzes judicial texts entirely by computer, looking for revealing patterns in syntax or semantics (McGuire, Vanberg, Smith, & Caldeira, 2009; Wahlbeck, Spriggs, & Sigelman, 2002).

Analyzing Cases

A credible content analyst does not necessarily need to use complex or sophisticated statistics—or, indeed, any statistics at all. Often, researchers simply report counts and frequencies to show how commonly a given feature appears in the cases. Quantitative descriptive analyses may be sufficient to document trends in the case law, to challenge conventional wisdom, or to raise provocative questions meriting further study. Because many case-counting studies code the entire universe of relevant cases, statistics are not essential for analyzing the probability that the sample cases reflect the reality in a larger population.

Moreover, content analysis need not involve numbers at all. Instead, it can employ rigorous methods of purely qualitative analysis that focus on themes and patterns that are best understood through conceptual description and narrative illustrations rather than numbers. Empirically evaluating public health effects of case law, however, requires the use of counts and numeric indices and scales, and so statistical analyses are often essential.

One danger in using statistical testing in exploratory studies is that, without a tightly controlled analytical focus, such as a predefined set of theory-based hypotheses that are being tested, it becomes too easy to find associations and patterns of apparent significance entirely by chance. If enough variables are examined and enough comparisons are made, odds are that statistically significant findings will emerge, but some or all of these apparent findings could be due entirely to chance without additional statistical adjustments for the number of possibilities that were explored.

Potentially more revealing is multiple regression analysis, which can uncover hidden relationships among multiple factors, both internally within court decisions or between decisions and external factors. In attempting to explain the legal outcomes or health-related effects of a set of cases, for example, several factors may each appear significant by themselves, but when each is held constant, only one or two factors may emerge as the most important predictors of decisions. Sometimes, factors that legal analysts thought were dominant or important turn out to be red herrings. Alternatively, factors that, standing alone, may not appear significant might emerge as such once the influence of other factors is controlled statistically. It is advisable, however, to use regression analysis only for cases that are relatively homogenous, focusing on a single or narrow set of legal issues. Otherwise it may become too difficult to measure and control for all the relevant variables.

Another aspect of statistical analysis worth considering in broad perspective is whether each case (or part of a case) should be given equal weight. It is possible to weight each case according to an objective measure of its significance, such as how often it has been cited or followed, or where it stands in a line of precedent. The difficulty with this approach, however, is deciding how much weight to assign. Nascent efforts to apply network analysis to the citation patterns among cases may eventually prove fruitful in assigning appropriate weights to different cases (Smith, 2005). But, absent any objective means to assign different quantitative weights, the best option is to classify cases qualitatively into different categories and analyze each separately—such as major versus minor decisions, or leading versus following decisions.

A final concern is the appropriate unit of analysis. Rather than each case counting the same, case law can be grouped by separate jurisdiction to assign a legal rule to each location. Doing that enables exploration of how the adoption of particular rules of law relate to other occurrences, including health outcomes.

Conclusion

Content analysis is a valuable research tool for documenting what courts do and what they say. The insights gained from uniform content analysis of large numbers of opinions supplement the deeper understanding of individual opinions that comes from traditional interpretive techniques. The content of judicial opinions can be important in the study of the broader social, economic, and political systems that interact with judicial precedent, but cases are also well worth scientific study in their own right.

The major limitation of content analysis (a limit that applies equally to traditional interpretive methods) is that facts and reasons given in opinions cannot be treated as accurate and complete. Therefore, researchers should be cautious about the meanings they attach to observations made through content analysis. Within these bounds, content analysis is well suited to studying connections between judicial opinions and other parts of the social, political, or economic landscape.

Scientific methods complement conventional legal research methods in three key ways. Content analysis can verify or refute descriptions of case law that are based on more anecdotal or subjective study. Second, content analysis can identify surface patterns (which are sometimes hidden from the naked eye), to be explored more deeply through interpretive, theoretical, or normative legal analysis. Third, systematic numeric content coding of case law opens up major new avenues of research to better understand the many ways in which law affects population health.

Summary

This chapter explored the special considerations in coding text when the relevant legal materials are judicial decisions. The content of case law merits careful study not simply because judicial opinions reflect or respond to the law, but because they *are* the law. But more than this, judicial opinions are detailed repositories that show what kinds of disputes come before courts, how the parties frame their disputes, and how judges reason to their conclusions.

Content analysis of case law boils down to three steps: (1) selecting cases, (2) coding cases, and (3) analyzing (often through statistics) the case coding.

Insights gained from content analysis of large numbers of opinions supplement the deeper understanding of individual opinions that comes from traditional interpretive legal research techniques. The content of judicial opinions can be important in the study of the broader social, economic, and political systems that interact with judicial precedent, but cases are also well worth scientific study in their own right. For instance, content analysis can identify previously unnoticed patterns that warrant deeper study, or sometimes correct mis-impressions based on ad hoc surveys of atypical cases.

The major limitation of content analysis is that facts and reasons recorded in judicial opinions cannot be treated as accurate and complete. Therefore, researchers should be cautious about the meanings they attach to observations made through content analysis. With this caveat in mind, this chapter described a range of acceptable and best practices for systematically selecting relevant cases, forming coding categories, training coders, and testing for coding reliability.

Further Reading

Friedman, B. (2006). Taking law seriously. *Perspectives on Politics, 4*(2), 261–276.

Hall, M. A. (2003). The scope and limits of public health law. *Perspectives in Biology & Medicine, 46*(Suppl. 3), S199–S209.

Krippendorff, K. (2004). *Content analysis: An introduction to its methodology* (2nd ed.). Thousand Oaks, CA: Sage.

Part Four

Designing Public Health Law Evaluations

The most important determinant of the quality of a public health law evaluation is the research design. The fundamental objective of PHLR is to improve both knowledge on whether a particular law or regulation *causes* a change in population health and knowledge on the mechanisms of that effect (that is, how the effect was achieved). The level of confidence in a causal interpretation of an observed relationship between law and health is fundamentally related to the quality of the research design. Gerber, Green, and Carnegie begin the section by describing what is typically deemed the gold standard for research—the randomized experimental trial. To date, randomized trials have been rare in PHLR, since the researchers cannot control the passage and implementation of laws and thus cannot randomly assign some persons to get a law and others not. However, the scientific advantages of randomization are huge, and PHLR as a field could do much more to advocate for randomized experiments with new legal and regulatory approaches. With the creative cooperation of public health authorities and scientists, many more opportunities are possible for randomly timing new legal interventions and randomly rolling out new interventions across persons, organizations, or jurisdictions.

Wagenaar and Komro address the common situation in which laws and regulations are implemented by governments without researcher input—"natural experiments"—and random assignment to treatment or control groups is therefore not possible. The chapter presents many feasible design elements that enhance the plausibility of causal interpretations of observed effects, and emphasizes that any particular study should not simply select a workable research design but should creatively incorporate as many of the design elements as possible to maximize the validity of conclusions that a law caused changes in population health.

Two additional chapters follow on other useful approaches to public health law evaluation. Wood describes qualitative research strategies, which enhance quantitative approaches by providing more in-depth or nuanced information on how laws are designed or implemented and how available health outcome measures might not fully encompass the whole of legal effects. Results from such qualitative studies then often feed back into improved measurement and design of quantitative studies, more formally testing the effects suggested in qualitative research.

Public health officials and policy makers considering alternative laws and regulations not only want to know how many disease or injury cases are averted, but also want to know whether it is worth it in terms of costs involved. Miller and Hendrie describe how to conduct cost-effectiveness and cost-benefit studies, attending to the special considerations when estimating the costs and benefits of a law, rather than typical cost-benefit studies involving intervention programs that treat specific individuals.

We conclude the book with a chapter that points to the future of PHLR as an identifiable field of study, highlighting the importance of continual improvement in scientific methods and tighter integration of lawyers, sociolegal scholars, social scientists, and health scientists in PHLR.

Chapter 13

Evaluating Public Health Law Using Randomized Experiments

Alan S. Gerber   Donald P. Green   Allison J. Carnegie

Learning Objectives

- List the assumptions underlying experimental design and interpretation.
- Describe how randomized trials can be used to evaluate broader issues related to public health laws and policies.
- Explain the differences between a randomized controlled trial found in medical research and one designed for public health law research.

Estimation of treatment effects boils down to comparing outcomes of units that get an intervention to outcomes of those that do not. The key difficulty in measuring the effect of an intervention is to separate the treatment effect from other sources of difference across the treated and untreated subjects. In cases when the intervention is not randomly assigned, those who receive the treatment may be systematically different from those who do not, for many reasons. This problem is referred to as "selection bias." In many cases the researcher is interested in situations in which people or organizations get to choose among different "treatments." These choices reflect a subject's resources and preferences, and whether a given treatment is desirable to the individual or organization is often determined, in part, by the same outcome variable that interests the researcher. For instance, people who like to exercise and place a priority on fitness may also join gyms. The observed average difference in fitness among those who belong to a gym and those who do not would not measure the effect of gym membership and would not serve as a reasonable forecast of a policy that provides free gym memberships.

Random assignment overcomes the selection problem. In this chapter, we formalize the problem of estimating the treatment effect to demonstrate what is gained by random assignment and to describe the important additional assumptions that are necessary for an experiment to produce unbiased estimates of the treatment effect of interest to the researcher. We also discuss related issues of generalization beyond the experiment: Do the results of the experiment generalize to other groups beyond the experimental subjects, and can the experiment be generalized to interventions that are similar to the experiment but not identical to it? Do the experimental results apply to larger-scale versions of the experimental intervention?

A Potential Outcomes Model of Causal Effects

Suppose the researcher wants to measure the effect of a program or policy. For concreteness, suppose the researcher is interested in measuring the effect of health insurance coverage on health care utilization. For each unit of observation, which we will call a "subject" even if it happens to be an organization, city, or other entity, we measure whether the subject is "treated" or not. To be clear, although this chapter will focus on experimental work, the terminology of "treatments" and "outcomes" applies equally to experimental research and observational data. We denote the treatment status of subject i by D_i, and $D_i = 1$ if i is treated and 0 if untreated, regardless of whether treatments are assigned randomly. In our example, let $D_i = 1$ if unit i has good health insurance, and 0 if subject i has poor coverage or no insurance. The outcome of interest, in this example, is health care utilization, and we denote the outcome for subject i by Y_i. Datasets will often contain covariates, measuring other things about the subject beyond treatment status and the outcome. We ignore the other measured (pre-treatment) traits of the subjects for now; the discussion can be thought of as describing analysis within blocks formed by grouping subjects with similar background characteristics.

For each subject we define a pair of "potential outcomes," $Y_i(D_i)$, which are the values of the outcome variable Y that would be observed in two circumstances: when the subject is treated, $Y_i(D_i = 1)$, and when the subject is untreated, $Y_i(D_i = 0)$. Although both of these potential outcomes are real quantities that could in principle be measured, we will actually observe only one of these potential outcomes, depending on whether the subject is treated or not. The treatment effect for an individual, in our example the difference in health care usage with and without good insurance, is defined as $Y_i(1) - Y_i(0)$.

The average treatment effect for the collection of subjects, the sample average treatment effect (SATE), is $E(Y_i(1) - Y_i(0))$.

Random Assignment and Selection Bias

From the data available for our collection of subjects, we can calculate the difference in the average values of Y for the treated (those with good insurance) and the untreated (those without good insurance):

$$E(Y_i(1)|D_i = 1) - E(Y_i(0)|D_i = 0), \qquad (13.1)$$

where the notation $E(A_i|D_i = B)$ means the expected (that is, average) value of A_i among those subjects for which the condition $D_i = B$ holds.

In our example, this quantity is the difference in average health care use by the well insured versus use by those with poor or no insurance. Unfortunately, this is not equal to the average treatment effect from having "good versus bad" insurance. Rather, we learn the outcome for the treated subjects in their treated state (average health care usage for the insured) and the outcomes of the untreated subjects in their untreated state (average health care usage for the poorly insured). To see how this is different from the treatment effect (SATE), the expression (equation 1) can be rewritten as

$$E((Y_i(1) - Y_i(0))|D_i = 1) + [E(Y_i(0)|D_i = 1) - E(Y_i(0)|D_i = 0)]. \qquad (13.2)$$

The difference in the average outcome of the treated and untreated can be deconstructed into the sum of two quantities: the average treatment effect for a subset of the subjects (the treated) and a selection bias term. The selection bias term is the difference in what the outcome (Y) would have been for those who are treated had they been untreated and the value of Y observed among those who were not treated. This second term is an extra part of the difference in observed outcomes for the treated and untreated that is not the treatment effect. In the case of health insurance, among those with similar observables (for example age, class, race, and so on), standard economics arguments about adverse selection suggest that if future claims are, in part, anticipated by the individual but unobservable to the insurer, then those with higher expected claims will be more likely to buy insurance. That is, even if they did not have insurance, the insured might use more medical care than the uninsured. In the case that a selection bias term is positive, the observed difference in health care usage among the insured versus the uninsured will overestimate the treatment effect. More generally, however, it is difficult to know the magnitude of selection bias, and sometimes even the sign of the bias is unclear.

The selection problem is a solid obstacle to estimating causal effects from standard observational comparisons. Random assignment removes this obstacle. Intuitively, the difference in observed means across the treated and untreated is not equal to the average treatment effect because the quantities we measure are not the quantities we ideally want to measure. We observe group outcome averages among subjects who select into each group (treated or not) while wanting to obtain an average of a representative sample of the subjects in their treated states and untreated states. This is what random assignment provides. When random assignment is used to determine which group a subject is placed into, we know the process determining whether a unit is assigned to the treatment or not and we know (crucially) that the assignment is, by design, independent of the subject's potential outcomes. As a consequence, those randomly selected from the sample to form the treatment group are, except for the play of chance, representative selections from the group as a whole. This implies that, on average, they are expected to have the same treated potential outcomes as those randomly assigned to remain untreated (control group):

$$E(Y(1)|D=1) = E(Y(1)|D=0) = E(Y(1)). \tag{13.3}$$

By the same reasoning, those randomly assigned to the control group (to remain untreated) have, on average, the same outcomes in the untreated state as those assigned to the treatment group:

$$E(Y(0)|D=0) = E(Y(0)|D=1) = E(Y(0)). \tag{13.4}$$

There are two critical implications of random assignment. An implication of these equations is that when subjects are assigned using random assignment, the selection bias term vanishes and the difference of treatment and control group means measures the SATE. This can be shown by substituting equations (3) and (4) into equation (1):

$$[E(Y_i(1)|D_i=1) - E(Y_i(0)|D_i=1)] + [E(Y_i(0)|D_i=1) - E(Y_i(0)|D_i=0)] =$$
$$[E(Y_i(1)|D_i=1) - E(Y_i(0)|D_i=1)] = \tag{13.5}$$
$$E(Y(1)) - E(Y(0)) = E(Y(1) - Y(0)).$$

Random assignment solves the selection problem, which is why it is such an attractive research method. However, random assignment must be supplemented by two additional assumptions if we are to draw meaningful causal inferences. We next discuss these two important assumptions.

Key Assumptions for Measuring the Effect of the Intended Treatment

Two essential assumptions underlie the process of measuring the effect of the intended treatment—exclusion restriction and non-interference.

Exclusion Restriction

First, the effect of a subject being assigned to the treatment group (or the control group) must be produced by the treatment itself rather than through some other channel that accompanies a subject's group assignment. To discuss this issue precisely, we need to introduce additional notation. Let $Z_i = 1$ if a subject is assigned to the treatment group, and $Z_i = 0$ if the subject is assigned to the control group. The exclusion restriction assumption is satisfied when

$$Y_i(D_i, Z_i) = Y_i(D_i) \text{ all } D_i, Z_i, \tag{13.6}$$

where $D_i = 1$ if the subject is treated and 0 otherwise.

In the simplest experiments, all of those assigned to the treatment group $(Z_i = 1)$ also receive the treatment $(D_i = 1)$ and all those assigned to the control group $(Z_i = 0)$ do not receive the treatment $(D_i = 0)$. This suggests that the exclusion restriction is an assumption and not something that can be empirically investigated.

There are two main ways that the exclusion restriction is violated. First, the treatment designed by the researcher may combine the channel of interest, D, with some other "active" ingredient. If so, the experiment provides an unbiased estimate of the treatment combination, but it does not estimate the separate effect of the portion of the treatment that embodies the principle motivating the experiment. The Hawthorne effect, whereby people act differently when being observed by others, may be thought of as an exclusion restriction violation, if the researcher is interested in the posited effect of the program rather than the incidental effect of being observed. Placebo effects can be considered exclusion restriction violations as well, if the control group gets no treatment rather than a placebo treatment. As an example of compound treatments, consider an experiment in which applicants are selected by lottery to receive health insurance. Let Z_i equal 1 if the subject wins the lottery, 0 otherwise. Suppose that the researcher wishes to interpret the treatment effect as the effect of providing insurance, but the actual treatment that is implemented combines health insurance with other forms of support and assistance, such as health counseling and information about other government health programs that might be of interest to the lottery winners. Let $D_i = 1$ if a subject gets health insurance, 0 otherwise. Note that assignment to the treatment group involves much more than just the health insurance, which is just part of the collection of things that follow the lottery win. In this example, the difference of treatment group and control group means is not an unbiased estimate of the treatment effect of the insurance alone. To link this to the formal statement of the exclusion restriction, $Y(0,1)$ is the (theoretical) health care usage when the subject does not get health insurance but gets everything else a lottery winner gets, and $Y(0,0)$ is usage when the subject does not get health insurance and is a lottery loser. $Y(0,1)$ does not equal $Y(0,0)$ if the health counseling and information about other programs has an effect on the outcome, Y. If the researcher is interested in measuring the effect of the "full package" rather than a component of it (the insurance alone), then there is no violation of the exclusion restriction.

More subtly, any aspect of the experimental design that disturbs symmetric handling of the treatment group and the control group threatens to cause biases. In contrast to combination treatments, symmetry violations are typically inadvertent. Asymmetric measurement, for instance, may produce biased results. For example, suppose that all subjects in a health insurance experiment are called every month and asked about their health care usage. In addition, for those in the treatment group, the survey reports are augmented by the records generated whenever a subject uses his or her insurance card. This asymmetry will create bias, since measurement error will differ across treatment groups and control groups. The basic injunction in both design and measurement is to avoid *anything* that creates a difference in the treatment group and control group outcomes through some channel other than the intended treatment.

The exclusion restriction may be especially important in cases in which a substantial portion of those assigned to the treatment group do not actually get treated. When subjects assigned to a group do not receive what is intended, we say there is non-compliance (that is, $Z_i = 1$ but $D_i = 0$, or $Z_i = 0$ but $D_i = 1$). Non-compliance is common in field experiments. For many experimental designs, especially those involving government programs, subjects randomly assigned to the treatment group (that is, for whom $Z_i = 1$) have won a lottery granting eligibility for a benefit, such as a private school voucher or an insurance program. Of those who win eligibility, only a fraction exercise their option to enroll in the program, and therefore many in the treatment group remain untreated (they do not receive a private school education or the insurance program). In the simplest case of non-compliance, such as the example just provided, the non-compliance is "one-sided," which means that some of those assigned to the treatment group fail to be treated, while all of those assigned to the control group remain untreated. In such cases, the average treatment effect from the program among those who take the treatment if assigned is calculated by dividing the difference between the average treatment group outcome (the entire treatment group, including those who were not treated) and the average control group outcome by the proportion of the treatment group actually treated. The observed difference between the treatment and control group averages is inflated by dividing the difference in group averages by the fraction actually treated. For example, if one-third of those who are randomly granted eligibility for insurance actually receive the insurance, then the observed difference between the average outcome for the entire treatment and control is multiplied by three in order to estimate the effect of the treatment on those assigned for treatment.

To see how a violation of the exclusion restriction might affect treatment effect estimates when there is substantial non-compliance, suppose that winners of an insurance eligibility lottery also receive information encouraging subjects to purchase the insurance, such as information about the importance of regular medical exams. Then all of those in the treatment group (all the lottery winners) get this information whether or not they ultimately buy insurance. If this additional information accompanying treatment group assignment has the effect of boosting the average health care utilization by w, it will boost the estimated complier average causal effect by w/c, where c is the fraction of the treatment group that enrolls in the program. If c is small, such as one-fifth or one-tenth, then the bias will be $5w$ or $10w$, showing how even a small violation of the exclusion restriction can lead to substantial bias in the estimated treatment effect.

Finally, consider the somewhat more complicated case of two-sided non-compliance. Two-sided non-compliance occurs if some subjects assigned to the treatment group are not treated and some subjects assigned to the control group nevertheless receive the treatment. In many experimental designs, in which access to the treatment is under the control of the researcher, two-sided non-compliance is impossible. However, two-sided non-compliance arises naturally in some types of experiments. In encouragement designs, for instance, the treatment group is given an added inducement to obtain a treatment. An example of this would be a public health program that encourages subjects to get their children vaccinated. Many in the control group will vaccinate their children, and some in the treatment group will not.

Another design in which two-sided non-compliance arises is downstream experiments, which are analyses in which the outcome measure in a first experiment is recast as the treatment in a subsequent investigation. These analyses are quite common in the study of health outcomes. An example is the frequently studied natural experiment conducted during the Vietnam War–era draft lottery. To simplify, young men randomly received either a high or low draft number. For each of these randomly formed groups, a proportion, H or L, $H > L$, subsequently served in the war. The treatment effect of the lottery on whether the subject served in the military ($Y = 1$ if served in military, 0 otherwise) is estimated by the observed proportion $H - L$, and the lottery is an experiment absent of non-compliance (the treatment is the lottery number, and all subjects received the lottery number they were assigned).

Now suppose the researcher is interested in measuring the effect of military service on health outcomes. This may be thought of as a "downstream" experiment because the initial randomization has two sequential effects: an effect on military service and a subsequent effect on another outcome, health status. The setup shifts to accommodate this new use of the random assignment: Z_i is the random assignment to experimental group (the lottery group), D_i (not Y) denotes military service, and Y_i measures health outcomes. Note that we also have a situation with two-sided non-compliance: some of those assigned to the control group ($Z_i = 0$, the low lottery number group) serve in the military ($D_i = 1$), and some of those assigned to treatment (the high-number group) do not serve.

Measuring treatment effects when there is two-sided non-compliance requires modification of the formula used for the case of one-sided non-compliance. To estimate the average treatment effect among those who take the treatment if and only if they are assigned to the treatment group, we now take the average difference in Y for the treatment ($Z_i = 1$) and control group ($Z_i = 0$) and divide by the difference in the treated proportion of each group. In this example, the average difference in health outcomes among those assigned the high and low lottery numbers would be divided by $H - L$. We can now reflect on whether the downstream experiment satisfies the exclusion restriction. To interpret this ratio as an estimate of the net effect of military service on health, it must be the case that lottery group assignment does not have an effect on health outcomes through some channel other than military service. For instance, if those with a high draft number took measures to avoid induction, including leaving for Canada, changing marital or education statuses, or shooting off their toes, and these affected subsequent health outcomes, then the health effects estimates would be biased.

Non-Interference

A second key assumption is non-interference across units. This assumption requires that each subject's potential outcomes, $Y_i(1)$ and $Y_i(0)$, are not affected by which other subjects are selected at random to be in the treatment group versus the control group. Notice that this assumption is already incorporated into the notation we have used for the potential outcomes, since Y is written as a function of Z_i (or D_i) and not as a function of the treatment or control group assignments of any other subjects. A leading example of how this assumption might fail is when there are "spillover" effects from treatments. For instance, suppose the treatment is a flier informing subjects of a concert, and the outcome is attendance at the concert, or Y_i. If the flier induces conversations about the concert and some control group subjects thereby learn of the concert from their treated friends, then treating subject i (assigned to the treatment group) has affected subject j (control group) in the untreated state. If subjects in the control group show up to the concert due to the spillover treatment, then this will raise the average outcome in the control group and lower the difference between the treatment group and control group averages. Interference has caused the true effect of the treatment to be underestimated.

When non-interference is plausible, the assumption permits us to ignore any effects of the treatment given to any other subject on subject i. If this assumption does not hold, the distinction between the treated and untreated begins to break down, since a subject may be "untreated" but nevertheless have his or her outcomes be affected by the treatments being dispensed to others.

If so, the untreated subjects do not serve as a clean counter-factual for the treated in their untreated state. Back to our example, if providing more financial support for health insurance for subjects in the treatment group causes government to cut back its health expenditures on behalf of the control group, the non-interference assumption will be violated. In that case, a comparison of average outcomes in the two groups no longer gives an unbiased indication of the effect of receiving health insurance because the control group is not untreated; instead, the control group receives an adverse treatment.

The non-interference assumption is quite natural in medical interventions, since there rarely are channels for the treatment applied to one patient to have a material effect on the experience of another patient. In the context of social experiments, the plausibility of non-interference must be evaluated on a case-by-case basis. Communication, contagion, social comparisons, or displacement may cause potential outcomes for a given subject to depend on the treatments administered to other subjects.

When the non-interference assumption is false, the potential outcomes model, as written, does not accurately reflect the situation the researcher is trying to represent. There are various approaches to address interference between units. First, studies may be designed to measure the extent and pattern of interference. For example, randomly varying the density of treatment across neighborhoods and comparing those assigned to the control group across neighborhoods will measure geographic spillover within neighborhoods (Angelucci & De Giorgi, 2009; Duflo & Saez, 2003; Hirano & Hahn, 2010; Lalive & Cattaneo, 2009). Second, although the potential for contamination may prevent the measurement of individual-level treatment effects, changing the unit of observation (typically choosing a unit of observation more coarse than the individual) may reduce or eliminate the danger of spillover. If so, the non-interference assumption is satisfied for the experiment when the researcher randomizes the coarser units. To illustrate this concept, it is not difficult to imagine that the complex interactions between students, and between students and teachers, may make it impossible to measure the effect of an alternative curriculum provided to a randomly selected subset of a class. However, randomly assigning whole classes (or perhaps whole schools) to different curricula may arguably satisfy the non-interference requirement and therefore provide a credible estimate of intervention effects. Group-randomized trials are commonly used to test effects of preventive interventions, and hold great promise for advancing public health law research. This is because randomly assigning legal interventions to individual persons is typically less feasible than randomly assigning rollout of a new policy across cities, countries, districts, courts, or other organizational units. Murray (1998) provides extensive guidance on the statistical analyses of such group-randomized trials.

Interpretation and Extrapolation of Experimental Results

Finally, interpreting and extrapolating findings from a randomized trial requires care. Regarding interpretation, the measured experimental outcomes are often proxy variables for the true outcome of interest. This is very common in medical studies, in which the severity of illness and mortality is the true outcome variable of interest, but experimental treatments are evaluated on the basis of more proximal indicators such as blood test results or changes in tumor size, which are assumed to be related to more distal outcomes of interest such as reduced early mortality. The validity of any conclusions about the effect of the treatment on the true outcome of interest then rests upon the confidence with which the research can move from the proxy to the ultimate outcome of interest. In law or policy interventions, a key challenge is that subject behavior may change along many dimensions in response to an intervention. If what is measured does not provide the whole story, the results of the experiment may be misleading. For example, a recent study of the effect of advertising looked at the change in sales associated with increasing the number of clothing catalogues mailed to households by a major retailer (Simester, Hu, Brynjolfsson, & Anderson, 2009). Compared to a control group that received the normal flow of mailings, the households getting the additional catalogues ordered a substantially greater amount of clothes during the period of the experiment. Given this sales boost, additional mailings appeared to be a profitable idea. However, the researchers also measured household Internet purchases and purchasing behavior during the year after the experimental mailings had concluded. It turned out that the treatment group decreased Internet purchasing and also purchased less than the control group during the year after the experimental mailings ended. Once channel and intertemporal substitution were measured, the overall effect on sales was not large enough to cover the cost of the additional mailings.

Substitution can also occur in response to health interventions. Consider an experiment to measure the effect of posting calorie counts on lunch menus in a random selection of fast food restaurants. It is useful to know if the intervention results in more salads being ordered at treatment group restaurants during the typical lunch hour. But if the quality of the public's overall diet is the variable of interest, it would be important to know how posting calorie counts at lunch affects what people eat at dinner and whether a light lunch leads to larger afternoon snacks. Further, if overall health rather than diet is the outcome of interest, researchers should attempt to measure whether ordering in a "virtuous" way at lunch leads the subject to skip exercise in the evening. Of course, oftentimes behaviors are complements, and eating a salad at lunch might encourage the subject to build on his or her earlier good behavior and exercise. The general point is that if the experiment has only limited outcome measures, and other unmeasured behaviors of significant relevance to the outcome of interest are substitutes or complements, caution is in order when interpreting the experimental results.

A common use of experiments is to predict the effects of similar interventions applied to new subjects or in new contexts, or the effects of the same intervention scaled up from a small program to general policy. It is critical to remember that when all goes well what is obtained from an experiment is the average treatment effects for particular subjects in a specific context in response to the treatment used. Extrapolating moves us from the relatively firm ground of unbiased average treatment effect estimates secured through random assignment to theoretical conjectures about what the effects would be with modified treatments applied to a different set of subjects in other times and places. Unless the experiment includes variation in treatment or context, any extrapolation along these dimensions involves substantial guesswork, and the quality and reliability of these translations will vary from case to case. Subjects' attributes may also limit generalizability of findings when subjects are not selected randomly from some larger population. For instance, suppose the subjects in an experiment in which insurance eligibility is determined by a lottery must have very low incomes and few assets to participate in the lottery. It is possible that the results apply well to any policy aimed at the poor, but do not apply to middle-class uninsured. Because random sampling is relatively unusual in field experiments, generalizing from sample average treatment effect to population average treatment effect requires the researcher to impose additional assumptions (see Aronow & Sovey, 2011).

To shorten the distance between experimental intervention and real-world program, researchers sometimes design "place-based" experiments in which communities, school districts, or regions are assigned as units to treatment or control. Although this design sacrifices some of the statistical power that comes with the random assignment of large numbers of individuals, it has the advantage of allowing the researcher to evaluate a realistic package of treatments using natural administrative units. School districts, for example, might ordinarily administer a healthy eating initiative, and assigning entire school districts to this intervention allows researchers to study the net effect of an entire school district—students, teachers, administrators, and parents—working together in pursuit of this goal. (See Boruch, 2005, and Bloom, 2009, for reviews of place-based studies across a wide array of disciplines.)

Even when one's evidence base consists of place-based studies, there are also reasons for caution when using the results of a small-scale intervention to predict the effects of a large-scale version of the program. While third parties will ignore a small pilot study, a larger-scale intervention (or interventions that look to be long term and not just "pilot" programs) may trigger responses from individuals, groups, or organizations not directly treated by the intervention but who are affected by the program. For example, a small-scale private school voucher experiment may be ignored by the local public schools, but a large-scale voucher program might trigger a competitive response, such as an effort to improve the public schools. This potential effect of the large-scale intervention will go unmeasured by the initial randomized experiment. Similarly, if a substantial percentage of the uninsured in a neighborhood are given insurance, this may lead to crowding of local medical resources, unless additional clinics or practices open in response to the program. In addition, holding the actions of third parties fixed, the effect of the treatment may vary with the scale of the program. In a neighborhood in which everyone has health insurance, residents may discuss medical appointments and local doctors as topics of common interest, and so information might spread freely. This may not be the case when only a few insured "lottery winners" live in a neighborhood with a low rate of insurance participation. By expressing this note of caution, we do not mean to set an impossibly high standard of evidence; rather, our point is that answering big policy questions requires thoughtful designs and extensive replication across an array of settings.

Applications of Randomized Controlled Trials to Law and Health

Randomized controlled trials (RCTs) have become pervasive in program evaluation and social science investigations of policy-relevant theories. In this section, and summarized in Table 13.1, we provide readers with a sense of how RCTs have been used in five areas that are directly or indirectly related to health: institutions, disease prevention, education, migration, and health care.

Institutions

A common critique of RCTs is that they cannot be used in many issue areas due to logistical and practical difficulties. For example, in research exploring effects of institutions on health and development, it could be argued that independent variables of interest simply cannot be randomized. At first glance, an analysis of the effects of variables such as democracy, type of institution, property rights, civil liberties, and corruption on health outcomes certainly seems impervious to experimental manipulation. As a result, researchers have produced a plethora of observational research designs in this area, but these have been plagued with problems such as reverse causality, omitted variables bias, and measurement error. For example, democracy may cause development, or perhaps development causes democracy. These types of problems resulted in a failure to produce conclusive evidence (Boix & Stokes, 2003; Przeworski & Limongi, 1997).

Recently, scholars have begun to design clever RCTs in this area, which are able to overcome such problems through the use of random assignment. In a prominent study of the effect of democratic institutions on the choice of public

Table 13.1. Examples of Randomized Controlled Trials in Health Law and Policy.

Issue Area	Citation	Manipulation	Outcome Variable
Institutions	Olken (2010)	Direct democracy	Proposal type and satisfaction
Institutions	Bertrand, Djankov, Hanna, & Mullainathan (2007)	Individual versus social incentives	Bureaucratic response
Institutions	Humphreys and Weinstein (2009)	Reconstruction programs	Money raised
Disease Prevention	Kremer & Miguel (2007); Cohen & Dupas (2010); Ashraf, Berry, & Shapiro (2010); Ashraf, Aycinena, Martinez, & Yang (2011); Thornton (2005); Banerjee et al. (2010); Kremer, Miguel, Mullainathan, Null, & Zwane (2009)	Price of deworming program; water disinfectant; mosquito nets, chlorine treatment; vaccine, HIV counseling	Purchase, usage, health
Disease Prevention	Devoto, Duflo, Dupas, Parienté, & Pons (2011)	Access to tap water	Health outcomes
Disease Prevention	Jalan & Somanathan (2008)	Information about water quality	Purchase
Education	Howell & Peterson (2002); Mayer, Peterson, Myers, Tuttle, & Howell (2002); Krueger & Zhu (2004)	Voucher allocation	Test scores, satisfaction, feeling safe
Education	Schultz (2004)	Cash grants for education	Total schooling, enrollment
Education	Kremer & Vermeersch (2004); Kremer, Moulin, & Namanyu (2003); Kremer, Miguel, & Thornton (2009)	Subsidies for school meals; school uniforms; reduced school fees based on merit	Total schooling, enrollment, attendance
Migration	McKenzie, Gibson, & Stillman (2010); Stillman, McKenzie, & Stillman (2009); Clemens (2010)	Visa lotteries	Income, mental health

(continued)

Table 13.1. *(continued)*

Issue Area	Citation	Manipulation	Outcome Variable
Migration	Gibson, McKenzie, & Stillman (2010)	Migration policy rule	Income, consumption
Migration	Ashraf, Berry, & Shapiro (2010)	Control over savings accounts	Remittances, health, nutrition
Migration	Chin, Karkoviata, & Wilcox (2010)	ID card for bank use	Savings accounts, remittances
Migration	Beam, McKenzie, & Yang (2012); Bryan, Chowdhury, & Mobarak (2010)	Provision of information; cash or credit; assistance with migration process	Migration decisions
Migration	Liebman, Katz, & Kling (2004); Kling & Liebman (2005)	Housing vouchers	Mental and physical health
Health Care	Bhattacharya, Bundorf, Pace, & Sood (2011)	Health insurance coverage	Obesity
Health Care	Kim, LeBlanc, & Michalopoulos (2009)	Encouragement for mental health service	Depression severity
Health Care	King, Gakidou, Ravishankar, et al. (2007)	Health care subsidies	Health, satisfaction
Health Care	Björkman & Svensson (2009)	Monitoring of health providers	Health care provision quality
Health Care	Wansink (2006), Detweiler, Bedell, Salovey, Pronin, & Rothman (1999)	Framing of health information, eating environment	Usage of health product, food intake

health policy, Olken (2010) randomized forty-eight villages in Indonesia to use either an elite meeting or a village plebiscite to decide on two project proposals related to infrastructure and public health (roads and bridges, water and sanitation, health and education, or irrigation). One project was proposed by the village and the other was proposed by only the women in the village. Outcome measures were the closeness of proposed projects to elite preferences, proximity of proposed projects to wealthier areas of the village, and villager satisfaction with the proposals. Olken found that while the treatment had little effect on projects proposed, it had a large effect on villager satisfaction. He concludes that direct democracy can increase satisfaction and legitimacy. Olken demonstrates that variables previously thought out of reach, such as democracy, can be randomly assigned.

Other interesting examples of the randomization of institutional variables abound. Communities in post-conflict Liberia were randomly assigned to receive a community-driven reconstruction program to determine the effect of the program on money raised for a collective project (Fearon, Weinstein, & Humphreys, 2009). The researchers conclude that these types of institution-building projects can increase social cohesion. For comprehensive summaries of this literature see Humphreys and Weinstein (2009), De La O and Wantchekon (2010), and Moehler (2010).

Disease Prevention

RCTs have been used extensively in the disease prevention literature. RCTs have been important, for example, for the debate about whether policy makers should charge fees for preventive services. On the one hand, those who advocate charging fees argue that fees increase the value of the service in the minds of consumers, people may be more likely to use the product because they have already sunk a cost in it, and fees may encourage providers to provide the service. Thus many organizations, such as the nonprofit social marketing organization Population Services International, charge fees for items such as mosquito nets and water disinfectant (Population Services International, 2003). On the other hand, other organizations such as the World Bank have moral qualms about charging for health products and therefore tend to give products away (World Health Organization, 2007).

To help resolve these conflicting views, RCTs have been run in many countries to assess the effects of charging for a variety of health products. These studies conclude that usage of health products is highly responsive to price. For example, Kremer and Miguel (2007) investigated the effect of charging for a deworming program in schools. In a prior study, Kremer and Vermeersch (2004) showed that deworming programs boost school attendance and prevent worm infections. Therefore, understanding the factors that cause students to partici-pate in the program is important. They randomly assigned schools to share in the cost of the program at an average rate of thirty cents per student, and found that 75 percent of students assigned to free treatment schools participated while only 19 percent of students assigned to cost-sharing schools participated. Other RCTs showing that lower prices lead to greater usage include studies of the

effect of cost changes for mosquito nets (Cohen & Dupas, 2010), water disinfectant (Ashraf, Berry, & Shapiro, 2007), HIV results and counseling (Thornton,
2005), and vaccines (Banerjee, Duflo, Glennerster, & Kothari, 2010). (See Holla,
Kremer, & Center for Global Development, 2009, for a review)

RCTs have also been used to evaluate alternative intervention strategies.
Access to clean water is a central public health challenge in the developing
world, and policy makers must sometimes decide whether to spend limited
resources on efforts to improve the quality of water or increase the availability
of water. Observational studies have a difficult time distinguishing between the
marginal benefits of either increasing quantity or increasing quality in water
provision (Gamper-Rabindran, Khan, & Timmins, 2010; Watson, 2006). On the
basis of observational research, many researchers believed that improving
water quantity was crucial because it would encourage subjects to wash hands
and bathe more frequently (Curtis, Cairncross, & Yonli, 2000; Esrey, 1996).

Recent RCTs however, have called this finding into question. For example, Devoto and colleagues (2011) find that increasing quantity without
altering quality has no effect on health outcomes. Among villagers in Northern
Morocco without access to tap water in their homes, the authors randomly
assigned an offer to buy a household connection to tap water on credit. The
tap water was of the same quality as the water which was publicly available
to all villagers, so the intervention altered the quantity of water without
changing the water quality. Although 69 percent of treated households were
willing to purchase the household tap water access, the authors found no
change in the health of the subjects from the intervention. Even as questions
of external validity remain, further RCTs are a promising avenue for research
in this area.

Though RCTs have cast doubt on the hypothesis that water quantity is
crucial for improved health, they have confirmed that improved quality, through
filtration or chlorine treatment, can improve health quite dramatically (see Ahuja,
Kremer, & Peterson-Zwane, 2010; Harrell & Smith, 1996; and Waddington &
Snilstveit, 2009, for a review of this literature). However, RCTs have also shown
that subjects may not be willing to pay much for increased water quality.
Kremer and colleagues (2009) and Holla and colleagues (2009) randomly
assigned discounts for chlorine treatment to villagers in Kenya and showed that
purchase of the treatment is highly sensitive to price. While over half of
households use it when it is delivered to their home for free, less than 10 percent
use it when it is only thirty cents a month. Demand changes little when
households receive half-price coupons, have young children, or know a peer
who uses the treatment (although hiring local promoters of the treatment does
boost usage). In addition, Kremer and colleagues (2009) show that there is little
evidence of spillover. That is, knowing someone who uses the system does
not appear to increase usage. Other RCTs have confirmed Kremer's findings

(Ashraf, Aycinena, Martinez, & Yang, 2011), adding that information effects are small compared to price effects (Jalan & Somanathan, 2008).

The conclusion from this strand of literature seems to be that although health is most improved by increasing water quality, households are most willing to pay for increased water quantity. Taken together, this body of research shows how initial RCTs and subsequent follow-up experiments can produce a more nuanced view of the relative strengths of alternative public health policies.

Education

Recent research has strengthened the positive link between educational attainment and individual health (Cutler & Lleras-Muney, 2006). Randomized trials have been used to evaluate alternative strategies for improving schools, including requiring remote schools in Africa to provide photographic evidence of school and teacher attendance (Duflo, Hanna, & Ryan, 2008) and paying teachers and schools various bonuses if their students do well on standardized tests (Fryer, 2011). A hotly debated topic in this area is the effect of school vouchers on improving school quality. Vouchers fund students to attend schools other than those they would be assigned on the basis of geographic proximity. Voucher programs have become increasingly popular and vary in their design and administration; programs differ in the types of students they favor, the way in which they are funded, the amount of aid given, and the period during which aid is given. Examples of publicly funded programs include the EdChoice Scholarship Program in Ohio, the A+ Opportunity Scholarship Program in Florida, the Cleveland Scholarship and Tutoring Program in Ohio, and the Milwaukee Parental Choice Program in Wisconsin. Examples of privately funded programs include the Washington Scholarship Fund in Washington, D.C., and the School Choice Scholarships Foundation in New York.

While observational studies suggest that voucher programs are highly effective, confounding factors may bias the results. Although students self-select into private schools, many studies rely on comparisons between private and public school students. If students who self-select into private schools differ systematically from those who do not, the results will be biased. Other observational studies that compare voucher recipients to non-recipients can be similarly confounded because students who apply for vouchers may be more motivated than those who do not apply.

To overcome potential biases, analysts have made use of privately funded voucher programs whereby applicants are randomly selected to receive vouchers. Because vouchers are randomly assigned to applicants, the pool of applicants who apply for vouchers and receive them should not differ systematically from the pool of applicants who apply for vouchers and do not receive them. In contrast to observational studies, experimental studies typically find limited effects of vouchers on test scores, though parents of students who received vouchers reported increased satisfaction with their children's educations and felt their schools were safer (Howell & Peterson, 2002; Wolf, Silverberg, Institute of Education Sciences, & National Center for Education Evaluations and Regional Assistance, 2010).

Another closely related debate in the education literature is the effect of educational subsidies. Mexico's Programa de Educacion, Salud y Alimentacion (PROGRESA) was a pioneer in this area. The program gave poor mothers cash grants if their children attended school 85 percent of the time, and increased the amount of the grant with the child's grade level in school. Cash grants were also given for participation in a variety of health and nutrition programs. For the first two years, the program was administered in randomly selected poor areas of the country, after which it was expanded to all regions. The use of random assignment allows researchers to evaluate the program, which was found to increase enrollment by 3.4 to 3.6 percentage points in grades one through eight and increased total schooling by 0.66 years (Schultz, 2004). Given the success of the program, similar programs have been implemented in almost thirty other countries, many of which use random assignment. In addition to cash transfers, merit-based subsidies have been found to increase enrollment and attendance when given for school meals (Kremer & Vermeersch, 2004), school uniforms (Kremer, Moulin, & Namanyu, 2003), or school fees (Kremer, Miguel, & Thornton, 2009).

Migration

Researchers in the social sciences are interested in the impact of migration on a variety of outcomes, including health, nutrition, and income, and in designing migration policies that promote these outcomes. However, studying effects of migration is inherently difficult due to the fact that migrants typically choose whether to migrate. If those who choose to (or are able to) migrate are different from those who do not, estimates from observational research may be biased. RCTs remedy this problem by using random assignment. One source of randomization that has been effectively exploited is visa lotteries, which randomly select applicants for receipt of visas. Each year, the Pacific Access Category program in Tonga randomly chooses 250 applicants to relocate to New Zealand. By comparing those randomly chosen to migrate with those randomly chosen not to migrate, researchers have found that the average income of those who migrate increases by 263 percent within one year of moving (McKenzie, Gibson, & Stillman, 2010) and that mental health of migrants improves (Stillman, McKenzie, & Gibson, 2009). Interestingly, McKenzie and colleagues (2010) used a sample of the total population and compared estimates from their RCT to those they would have obtained from an observational study and found that the observational study would have exaggerated the income effect by 27 to 35 percent. Other policy experiments have exploited randomized designs in clever ways. Gibson and colleagues (2010) used the rule that a person selected to migrate often may bring only a spouse to assess the effect of migration on remaining household members. They found that remaining members had lower incomes and consumption. Clemens (2010) looked at effects of migration on a particular firm by using the lottery for an H1-B visa designed to admit high-skilled workers into the United States. However, as McKenzie and Yang (2010) point out, if wages for non-migrants within the firm increase as a result of migrants leaving, then non-interference would be violated in the Clemens study.

Rather than rely on governments to randomize policy implementation to individuals, organizations, or communities, some researchers study migration by conducting their own RCTs. For example, Ashraf and colleagues (2011) offered Salvadoran migrants who migrated to Washington, D.C., the opportunity to exercise control of their remittances by channeling them into savings accounts in El Salvador. The researchers randomly varied the amount of control over the accounts, so that migrants were offered savings accounts that were either owned by their spouses, owned jointly, or owned by the migrant. They found that the degree of control had a large effect on remittances, and are currently investigating effects on other outcomes such as health and nutrition. Researchers are pursuing other RCTs in this area, such as Chin, Karkoviata, and Wilcox (2010), who randomly offer an ID card to Mexican migrants that can be used at banks in the United States. The ID card leads migrants to open more savings accounts in the United States and to send fewer remittances home. In addition, some scholars are now running RCTs to study barriers to migration by randomizing the provision of information about jobs in the host country, cash or credit assistance, or assistance in filling out applications (Beam, McKenzie, & Yang, 2012; Bryan, Chowdhury, & Mobarak, 2010).

RCTs exploring the effects of migration have looked at both domestic and international migration. On the domestic side, a major area of research has explored effects of neighborhood income levels on physical and mental health. For example, researchers assessed the effect of the Moving to Opportunity program (MTO), which was implemented in five major cities in the United States. Families living in public housing were randomly assigned to one of three groups: the control group remained eligible to live in public housing, the first treatment group received vouchers to move to their neighborhoods of choice, and the second treatment group received vouchers to move to low-income neighborhoods. Large effects on mental and physical health are reported (Kling & Liebman, 2005; Liebman, Katz, & Kling, 2004).

Health Care

Studying the effects of health care laws and regulations can be difficult because subjects participate in the choices; those choosing the lowest amount of insurance may be the healthiest subjects. RCTs have been able to overcome this obstacle. For example, to investigate whether receiving greater health insurance coverage increases obesity, researchers analyzed data from the RAND Health Insurance Experiment, which was conducted in the early 1970s in six regions in the United States. The experiment randomized subjects to receive varying amounts of health insurance coverage and found that more insurance coverage had no effect on body weight (although moving from uninsured to insured may have increased body weight) (Bhattacharya, Bundorf, Pace, & Sood, 2011). Similarly, data from the U.S. Working Toward Wellness program revealed that randomized encouragement to seek mental health services had mixed results on depression severity (Kim, LeBlanc, & Michalopoulos, 2009). Or, as another example, low-income people who were randomly assigned opportunities to apply for Medicaid were found to have higher self-reported mental and physical health, more frequent use of health facilities, and lower health-related expenditures (Finkelstein, Taubman, Wright, et al., 2011).

Health care RCTs have not been confined to the United States. In 2003, the Mexican government passed a modification to Mexican health policy called "Seguro Popular," which provides free and subsidized health care to lower-income Mexicans. To analyze effectiveness of the program, Mexico was divided into 12,284 regions called "health clusters." Health clusters were randomly assigned to receive encouragement to participate in the program in thirteen of the thirty Mexican states where the government agreed to participate in the experiment. Outcome measures included survey responses indicating how citizens felt about the quality of their health care as well as actual measures of health such as blood pressure (King, Gakidou, Ravishankar, et al., 2007). A randomized trial in Uganda found that community-based monitoring of health care providers improves quality of health care provision (Björkman & Svensson, 2009).

Another interesting strand of research that falls into this category includes RTCs that investigate the psychology behind how people choose to care for their own health. For example, Wansink has conducted a variety of experiments whose overall implication is that the amount of food people eat is greatly influenced by factors other than hunger. His innovative experiments include random assigning the size of popcorn buckets for moviegoers, whether diners receive bottomless soup bowls, whether diners are allowed to refill their plates, and whether diners are told their wine is from North Dakota or California. If people made decisions about the amount of food to consume solely on the basis of their hunger, these seemingly unrelated factors should have had no influence on their food intake. However, those who received larger popcorn buckets, received bottomless soup, were allowed to refill their plates, and were told they received California wine all ate significantly more food (for summaries of these experiments, see Wansink, 2006).

Or consider the series of experiments that are designed to assess the effects of public service announcements on behavior (Banks, Salovey, Greener, et al., 1995). The researchers investigated a variety of message frames encouraging mammography utilization (Banks, Salovey, Greener, et al., 1995), tobacco smoking cessation (Schneider, Salovey, Pallonen, et al., 2001), sunscreen usage (Detweiler, Bedell, Salovey, Pronin, & Rothman, 1999), and improved diet (Williams-Piehota, Cox, Silvera, et al., 2004). A prominent finding to come from this line of research is that gain-framed messages were more effective in promoting healthy behaviors such as sunscreen usage, while loss-framed messages were more effective in promoting detection of problems, such as mammography utilization. The policy relevance of this broad conclusion is bolstered by the fact that this hypothesis has held up in a wide array of settings.

Conclusion

The randomized trial is widely accepted as the most reliable method for measuring causal effects. A striking development of the past decade is the rapid spread of randomized experiments from medical and pharmaceutical trials to the social sciences, public health, and beyond. It is now common to exploit naturally occurring random assignments or design experimental interventions, and this shift in research strategy has enormous implications for how we assess causal claims about the effects of law and policy. As demonstrated by the brief review of some recent literatures, an experimentally based literature on the effect of alternative institutions and policies is not just theoretically possible but experiencing active development.

Our brief review of a portion of the emerging experimental literature shows how pioneering applications of experimental methods to the study of public policy have already produced important achievements. Nevertheless, some caution is in order. Although random assignment overcomes one of the most significant barriers to evaluation of an intervention, namely that the intervention may be correlated with observable and unobservable differences related to the outcome, the results of experiments must still be interpreted with care. For the reasons outlined earlier, it is important to keep in mind how difficulties such as interference between experimental units, or violations of the exclusion restriction, may affect estimates from RCTs. To be sure, this is not an argument against random assignment or any reason to dampen enthusiasm for the method; standard observational research typically has all of the difficulties experiments face, and the selection problem as well.

The growth and development of experimental research in the social sciences may be viewed as a process by which threats to inference attract attention and inspire increasingly sophisticated and robust research designs. Concerned that experiments that administer deworming treatments individually to Kenyan schoolchildren might produce misleading results if applied to entire schools, researchers have studied the effects of village-level interventions (Miguel & Kremer, 2004). Concerned that the health effects of cash transfer programs might be underestimated if one focuses solely on the low-income beneficiaries, researchers have investigated the downstream effects on those living in proximity to low-income beneficiaries (Schultz, 2004). Much the same goes for the investigation of policy-relevant mechanisms. A policy of free distribution of disinfectants and anti-malaria products may provoke critics who argue that the psychology of "sunk cost" means that people will not value and use products that they do not pay for. In response, a series of field experiments have been launched to assess both the sunk-cost hypothesis in general and the usage and subsequent purchase of health products in particular (Ashraf, Aycinena, Martinez, & Yang, 2011; Cohen & Dupas, 2010). The broader point is that researchers are becoming increasingly adept at formulating experiments that address threats to core assumptions, replicating experiments in ways that address concerns about generalizability and crafting experiments in ways that illuminate the role of policy-relevant causal mechanisms (see Ludwig, Kling, & Mullainathan, 2011).

Summary

The randomized controlled trial (RCT) research design has transformed medical research and is now accepted as the most reliable method for measuring the effects of drugs and other specific medical interventions. In this chapter we described how randomized trials can be used to evaluate broader issues related to public health laws and policies. The distance between a medical study and evaluating a public policy appears vast. The unit of observation in medical studies is almost always the individual patient, and interventions are usually simple, clearly defined treatments, such as alternative drugs or protocols. In contrast, to evaluate laws, policies, or programs experimentally involves randomly exposing people or communities to multifaceted interventions that are often implemented on a grand scale. To study effects of a poverty relief program on health, for example, scholars randomly raise the incomes of selected households or regions. To assess effects of alternative political processes for selecting public works projects, some regions are randomly assigned one method of voting and other regions randomly assigned an alternative.

The appeal of random assignment is clear in principle. A core question is whether it is feasible for investigating the effects of laws, policies, and programs.

Although random assignment of laws to communities is understandably rare (see Forster, Murray, Wolfson, et al., 1998, for a more noteworthy exception), one can readily imagine how implementation of policies and programs might lend itself to random allocation. In this chapter we show that, in fact, the use of randomized experiments to study public policy and institutional design not only can be done, but is in fact already underway and gaining momentum. We began by introducing a basic system of notation for defining and analyzing treatment effects, known as the potential outcomes model (Rubin, 1990; Splawa-Neyman, 1923). We then reviewed basic properties of the RCT and assumptions that are required for randomized experiments to produce unbiased estimates of treatment effects. Randomization alone does not ensure that a comparison of experimental groups will yield estimates of useful quantities. Assumptions are required for group comparisons to yield estimates of the treatment effect of interest, and further assumptions are required for generalization from the particularities of a given trial, an especially important issue when experiments are used to forecast a policy's effect in a different setting. Typically, RCTs must be conducted on a much smaller scale than the law or policy they are intended to evaluate, and so a critical issue is whether an RCT can accurately foretell effects of a scaled-up version of the intervention. After discussing assumptions that are required for the use of experiments to measure effects of interest, we then described recent applications of the RCT to questions of public policy and institutional design. A brief review of the recent literature shows a range of applications of randomized experiments on issues related to health and social policies. We concluded with reflections on the direction of recent research and prospects for future work.

This chapter is restricted to a discussion of field experiments and naturally occurring real-world randomizations, that is, interventions conducted in naturalistic settings in which the treatments and outcomes are those relevant in real-world contexts. Social science laboratory experiments (Webster & Sell, 2007) also contribute in important ways to PHLR by illuminating specific micro-level mechanisms of regulatory effects on behavior. However, the question of whether results obtained in laboratory settings apply in real-world settings remains an open one, and so we focused on field experiments, in which the gap between the experimental setting and the policy setting is as small as possible.

Further Reading

Haynes, L., Service, O., Goldacre, G., & Torgerson, D. (2012). *Test, learn, adapt: Developing public policy with randomized controlled trials*. Report for the Cabinet Office of the United Kingdom. Retrieved August 30, 2012, from http://www .cabinetoffice.gov.uk/sites/default/files/resources/TLA-1906126

Murray, D. M. (1998). *Design and analysis of group-randomized trials*. New York: Oxford University Press.

Chapter 14

Natural Experiments

Research Design Elements for Optimal Causal Inference Without Randomization

Alexander C. Wagenaar   Kelli A. Komro

Learning Objectives

- Understand advantages of time-series data, with many repeated observations before and after a change in law, for evaluating the law's effects.

- Create a nested multiple comparison group study design for evaluating the health effects of a law.

- Combine several time-series design elements in a single study to strengthen causal inference.

Evaluating the health effects of a law or regulation, or any treatment or intervention, most fundamentally requires a comparison of the experience *with* the law to the experience when everything is the same but *without* the law. Imagine the pure counterfactual, which involves the same people at the same time in the same place experiencing a law, compared to the same people at the same time and same place not experiencing the law (Rubin, 1974). The counterfactual requires the same people at the same time and place in the two conditions—with and without a specific law—to ensure that everything is identical between the two conditions, except the specific law. If everything but the law is identical, the difference in health outcomes of interest then directly represents the effect of the law. But such a comparison is impossible, since the same people at the same time cannot experience both conditions. Thus the fundamental quandary of scientific research—how do we know that the difference in outcomes observed is really caused by the law, since the difference might be due to something else and not be a true effect of the specific law under study?

Random assignment was a major advance in creating the counterfactual (Fisher, 1935). Relying on the law of large numbers, randomly selecting sets of people from the whole population, randomly selecting times of intervention implementation, and randomly selecting from the set of all places or settings creates groups of people, times, and settings that *on average* are expected to be equivalent in every way but for the law or intervention we exposed one set to but not the other set. Thus any single experiment might be wrong, because the treated and untreated groups might simply, by chance, differ in some unknown way and that difference might be the true cause of an observed difference in outcome. But, on average, over many replications of the randomized experiment, the two sets of people, times, or settings compared are expected to be the same, and any difference in outcome can be confidently attributed to the effects of the one planned difference between the two conditions—one is exposed to the law under study and the other is not.

Despite its appeal, randomly exposing treatment groups and control groups is rarely possible when evaluating most new laws and regulations. Most laws are implemented at particular times and settings and, obviously, passage and implementation are not under the control of researchers. They are therefore commonly called *natural experiments*. When laws are changed, they of necessity immediately apply to everyone in the given jurisdiction. Characteristically, there are few units in the study—for example, one or a few cities or states pass an innovative law, and the entire population within the unit is exposed to the new law all at once. In short, randomization is rarely available as a strategy or *design element* to improve the likelihood of correctly assessing a law or regulation's effects.

There is an unfortunate tendency by many scientists and others to dichotomize studies into strong "experimental" studies (which use random assignment to treatment groups and control groups), which are assumed to provide clear evidence regarding the effects of an intervention, and weak "observational" studies (not using random assignment) that are assumed to provide ambiguous and often inaccurate evidence of effects (Benson & Hartz, 2000; Concato, Shah, & Horwitz, 2000; Guyatt, DiCenso, Farewell, Willan, & Griffith, 2000). This is a false dichotomy. Random assignment is only one of a dozen or more design elements that increase confidence in a causal interpretation of an observed difference (Shadish, Cook, & Campbell, 2002). When evaluating the effects of local, state, or national laws and regulations, under which random assignment is rarely feasible, careful attention to full use of many other design elements is warranted. Moreover, effectively combining many design elements into a single study can produce real-world legal evaluations with higher overall levels of validity and strength of causal inference than randomized trials, which are typically limited to special circumstances or artificial environments. The objective of this chapter is to review design elements of particular importance when evaluating laws and regulations that naturally occur in the field, and improve the quality of empirical studies of public health law by illustrating their use.

Design Elements for Strong Legal Evaluations

There are several design elements for strengthening causal inference of particular importance for PHLR when random assignment to treatment conditions is not possible.

Many Repeated Measures

A fundamental criterion for inferring whether a given law or regulation caused a change in outcomes is that the cause preceded the effect. For this reason, we measure the outcome before the law is implemented and again after. But having just one observation before and one observation after produces weak inference, because any difference observed might simply reflect the natural variation in the outcome over time. Figure 14.1 illustrates a situation in which a simple before-and-after design shows a major effect of the law, but that effect is no longer considered real when seen in the context of more observations both backward and forward over time further away from the effective date of the law.

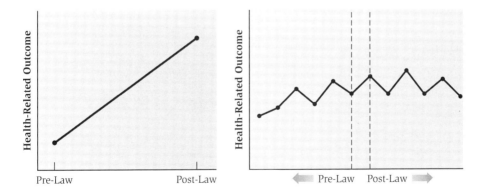

Figure 14.1. Observed Effect: Simple Pre-Post Design Versus Time-Series Design.

Collecting dozens or hundreds of observations in a *time series* before and after a new law takes effect makes it easier to see whether changes in the outcome of interest right around the time of the new law are larger than typical variation over time, and enhances confidence an observed difference occurring just at the time a new policy legally takes effect is due to that law. Any time series of observations can be viewed as a single sample (one window) from a time series that runs infinitely back in time and infinitely forward in time. The larger the time window observed around the time of a change in law, the easier it is to reliably assess that law's effects.

Beyond collecting many repeated measures, one must choose an appropriate *time resolution* for the observations. Are the observations a measure every minute, day, week, month, or year? Selecting the optimal time resolution is a complex tradeoff of multiple considerations. First is the speed by which a new law is expected to show effects. If the effects are expected to show up within weeks of the law's effective date, using weekly or monthly observations will make that effect easier to discern than using annual observations (Figure 14.2).

A second consideration when selecting the best time resolution to measure is the variation in the outcome over time at each time resolution. If there is little to no variation week by week in an outcome a new state law is meant to improve—say, math ability of teens—then monthly or even annual measures might be more appropriate. Consideration of the variation in the outcome over time interacts with a third important dimension, whether the underlying phenomenon being measured is *continuous*, or a *count*. For example, math ability, air pollution levels, water quality—like the temperature—all are continuous. The outcome is always there, we just choose intervals when we check the level. For continuous outcomes, the most important basis on which to choose the time

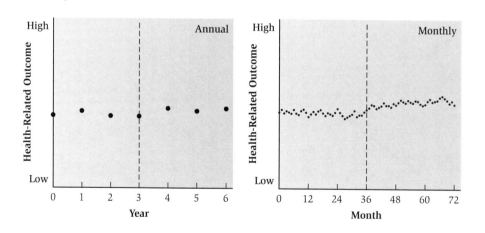

Figure 14.2. Observed Effect: Annual Versus Monthly Measures.

resolution of the measures is theory regarding the mechanism of a law's effect—when is the law first expected to show a difference in the outcome, and when (that is, at what interval) are further improvements expected?

Many public health outcomes are not continuous, but are counts or frequencies of new infections or disease cases, counts of injuries, or counts of deaths. For count outcomes, the time resolution must roughly match the frequency of the event. If there is only, on average, one or two infections, injuries, or deaths per month in the geographic unit under study, choosing a daily or weekly time resolution is not appropriate, since it will not help discern a law's effect on that outcome. Conversely, for example, if there are fifty or a hundred car crash deaths per month, lumping those data up to the yearly level for evaluating a new law's effects impairs the ability to accurately measure the law's effects. At the extreme, the problem of low counts expresses itself as numerous observations that are all zeros. Anything more than a very small fraction of zero-count observations complicates statistical analyses and makes discerning policy effects difficult or impossible. Thus, when the study design is being finalized, one must be aware of the expected outcome frequencies, and if numerous zero counts are expected at the preferred time resolution, the typical practical solution is moving to the next lowest resolution (for example, moving from monthly to quarterly counts).

Selecting the best time resolution for count data presents a tension between the desire for high-time-resolution observations and the resulting time series being "well-behaved," that is, exhibiting smooth regularities, cycles, or trends and not dominated by random unpredictability. In any study, minimizing the random, unpredictable variation from one observation to the next is important for maximizing the ability to detect the underlying "signal" of the law's effects. This is also known as maximizing statistical power (Cohen, 1988).

A fourth factor affecting the best time resolution to measure is exactly when the law took effect—a January 1 effective date works well with annual data, but typical effective dates of public health laws are distributed throughout the year. Using annual data with laws that take effect mid-year requires assumptions that the effect is going to be, say, half the size of effect in the subsequent full-year implementation (if the effective date is July 1), but those annual data will not permit the investigator to evaluate the validity of that assumption. Sometimes anticipatory effects of a new law are seen starting a couple of months before it takes effect, or there are lagged effects that do not start until a few months after it legally takes effect. Perhaps the short-term effects are much larger than long-term effects, a situation common with laws that require public attention and active enforcement. Or the longer-term effects might be larger than the short-term effects, a situation common with laws that require construction of or refinements in an implementation structure before the full effects are seen. All these situations are obscured by selecting outcome data at too coarse a time resolution (for example, annual rather than monthly).

Finally, when designing a study with lower time-resolution measures of continuous outcomes, it is critically important to take the measure at exactly the same time each year. This is because most physical, behavioral, and social phenomenon are characterized by seasonality—a nonrandom cycle within the time unit of observation. Pollution levels, dietary vegetable intake, infection rates, injuries, and most other health-relevant outcomes exhibit cyclic or other systematic differences across hours of the day, days of the week, weeks of the month, or months of the year (Figure 14.3).

So if one is surveying individuals once per year, or inspecting restaurants or schools once per year to collect an outcome for evaluating a public health law, it is important to do the data collection the exact same month of the year. This applies at all time resolutions of measurement—if one is collecting data once per month, measure the same day each month (for example, first Wednesday of the month). If one is collecting data weekly, measure on the same day and same time of day each time. The further the data collection procedures diverge from measurement at the exact same time within the time unit, the less confident one can be in interpreting observed differences from before to after a new law is implemented as representing the effect of the law—it might be just because the measures were taken at a different point in the cycle.

In summary, a strong public health law evaluation has as many observations as possible before and after the law takes effect—a lengthy time series— and uses the highest time resolution possible, constrained by the nature of the hypothesized effect, the frequency of underlying outcome counts, and feasibility limits due to resources or data available.

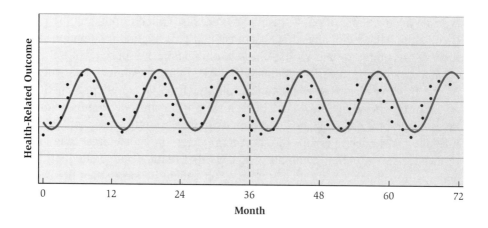

Figure 14.3.   Time Series Illustrating Seasonality.

Functional Form of Effects

High-time-resolution data have another important advantage furthering the quality of a policy evaluation. On the basis of a theory regarding mechanisms of a law's effects, one has an implicit or (even better) explicit hypothesis on the expected pattern of the effect over time (Figure 14.4).

Imagine one's theory of legal action is based on deterrence. In that case, one may expect a lag before effects are seen due to enforcement taking time to ramp up and news about enforcement actions taking time to spread in the relevant population. Alternatively, if one's theory focuses more on normative

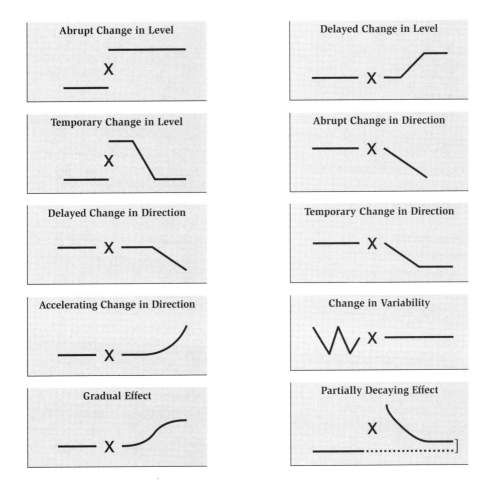

Figure 14.4. Possible Patterns of Policy Effects Over Time.

Note: **X** equals policy change.

Source: Adapted from Glass, Wilson, & Gottman, 1975.

compliance, initial timing of expected effects is based on when the relevant population first hears about the new law, suggesting that effects might be observed even before it legally takes effect, due to attention gained by hearings on the proposed law or to publicity surrounding a governor's signing the law.

Hypothesizing particular functional forms for legal effects leads to the following types of questions that shape the design of the study and the nature of the data to be collected. Is the effect expected to show up immediately when the law takes effect? Or is a delay of weeks or months expected, as enforcement or other implementation systems are developed and ramped up? Might there be an anticipatory effect before the legal effective date, due to publicity and attention to the issue surrounding debate on the new legislation, or widespread media reports at the time the law is passed? Is the effect expected to emerge gradually, as various implementation systems change or norms and behaviors gradually change? Or is the effect hypothesized to be temporary, dissipating over time as organizations and individuals adapt to the new law in ways to maintain previous conditions or behaviors?

Most public health laws are designed to affect the *level* of relevant outcomes, but there may be rare situations in which the expected effect is on another dimension, such as the *variance*. For example, laws and regulations might affect the amount of health care utilization by individual citizens, when the optimal public health objective might be to reduce both over-utilization and under-utilization—reducing the variance—while not affecting the overall level of services provided. Another example might be policies designed to reduce variance in caloric intake among children eating school lunches—some children overeating and others undereating both represent health and school performance risks. Thus the objective of regulations may be to reduce variance in calories consumed at school with no effect on overall level of calories or amount of food consumed at the school.

The bottom two panels in Figure 14.4 illustrate common patterns of effect of public health laws. The first illustrates the conventional "S-curve," when change starts slowly until reaching some "tipping point" at which change accelerates, followed by a leveling off at the (new) long-term level (Granovetter, 1978). The last panel of Figure 14.4 illustrates a sizable, fairly immediate effect that then partially dissipates over time (perhaps due to reduced attention to the issue), resulting in a much smaller, but often still important, long-term effect. One can see this in effects of strengthened driving-while-intoxicated laws, which often receive considerable media attention around the time they are passed or implemented, sometimes magnified by advocacy groups such as Mothers Against Drunk Driving, substantially raising the perceived probability of being detected and punished for driving impaired. As the short-term publicity declines, the magnitude of effect on driving behaviors also declines. But as the strengthened laws are integrated into ongoing enforcement efforts, the real and perceived probabilities of detection and punishment remain higher than base-line before the law, with a more-modest but still important long-term effect.

In short, decisions on time resolution of outcome data to collect and their analyses should be informed by expected patterns of effect over time. Important to note is that if the observed pattern of effect closely matches the hypothesized pattern that is based on a particular theory regarding the operating legal mechanism, the level of confidence in causally attributing the observed effect to the change in law or regulation is substantially strengthened.

Comparison Jurisdictions

With many repeated observations correctly measured and analyzed, it is possible to determine with a high degree of accuracy whether a change in the outcome coincides with the time of implementation of a new law or regulation—a change that is larger than expected from normal variation over time, and a change that matches the theoretically expected pattern. However, we still have the problem of the counterfactual—what if the same change in outcome would have occurred regardless of whether the new law was implemented or not? The observed change might have been caused by something else happening at the same time. A fundamental way to further improve causal inference—to assess whether the law caused the change in outcome or whether something else caused it—is to use comparison jurisdictions that did not implement the law under study. One collects the same outcome data for another city or state that did not change their law, and examines whether the observed change in the "experimental" jurisdiction is also seen in the comparison jurisdiction. If no similar change is seen in the comparison, one is more confident that the observed change at the time of the law is in fact due to the law, and not to some other factor occurring in common across jurisdictions. On the other hand, if a similar change is seen in the comparison, the observed change in outcome in the experimental site cannot be attributed to the change in law.

A key design consideration is selecting an appropriate comparison site. This is most commonly described as a site that is similar to the experimental site. Typically, evaluators select a site with broadly similar sociodemographic profiles of the population, or similar counts or rates on the key outcome variables. There are many dimensions on which one might assess degree of similarity, so it is important to consider the underlying reason why one seeks similar jurisdictions. Choosing a site with similar counts or rates on the outcome is a helpful but relatively minor consideration—it makes it easier to determine whether the comparison site experienced a change in outcome that is similar to the change observed in the experimental site. In other words, it helps ensure approximately equal statistical power to estimate change in the outcome in both the experimental and comparison sites.

The fundamental criterion for comparison site selection has much deeper significance, since it is directly connected to achieving the best possible counterfactual. The fundamental criterion for selection of a comparison site is that all the *causes* of the outcome variable are similar across the two sites. Thus the conventional approach to choose sites of similar demographics might be appropriate, *if* demographics are a key influence on the outcome under study. But in many cases, other factors are more important in any particular study. For example, if car crashes are the outcome, similar urbanization and climate are likely more important than demographics, with the exception perhaps of proportion of young drivers, since they are at such elevated risk.

Stratification before selection of comparison sites optimally is based on multiple characteristics. For example, in policy research focused on promoting healthy food environments, it may be important to find comparison sites based on urbanity, sociodemographic factors, and the overall food environment, all of which are generally associated with outcomes of interest. The goal is to achieve two groups as similar as possible in an attempt to mimic the counterfactual—what a particular outcome would look like with or without a particular policy among the same group of people at the same time in history. Selecting an optimal comparison group is an attempt to rule out competing alternative explanations for the outcomes observed post-intervention. The goal is to be able to attribute any difference between the jurisdictions to the legal intervention of interest, and rule out any other plausible explanations as best as possible. For example, if the goal was to evaluate effects of a new food policy, it would be critical to select comparison sites with similar socioeconomic and food environments prior to the new policy to help rule out alternative explanations for change in outcomes. If data for a longer baseline period with many observations are available (as is recommended), a useful tactic is to examine the correlation of the outcome variables between the experimental site and candidate comparison sites during the baseline period only; then select comparison sites with the highest correlations.

Of course, a perfect comparison jurisdiction is unachievable, because no two jurisdictions are identical in every way but for the law under study. For this reason, it helps improve inference by including multiple comparison jurisdictions. If a clear change in outcome is observed in the one with the law change, but no such change is seen in several other similar jurisdictions that did not change their law, inference that the law caused the change in the first site is enhanced.

Comparison Groups

The notion of incorporating comparisons not expected to be affected by the law under study can be fruitfully extended in other directions. If a law or regulation is targeted to particular groups of people or organizations within a jurisdiction, effects on that focal group targeted should be compared with other similar groups within the jurisdiction that are not likely to be affected. For example, consider a new state regulation intended to reduce worker injuries in auto repair shops. The injury rate can be tracked before and after the new regulation, and an observed reduction in injuries among auto-repair shop personnel is suggestive of an effect of the law. But inference of a causal effect would be strengthened by tracking similar measures of injuries among workers in the state that work in types of workplaces other than auto-repair shops. If similar declines in injuries were observed, then the observed auto-repair injury reductions are likely due to some other broader factor, and are not an effect of the new regulation specific to auto-repair shops. On the other hand, an observed reduction in injuries *only* for the specific group covered by the new law, with no reduction for workers in other settings not covered by the law, substantially strengthens the inference that the new law caused the reductions in auto-repair injuries. Most laws and regulations are inherently targeted in some way, opening important opportunities for enhancing causal inference regarding the law's effects by incorporating relevant comparison groups. For example, zoning rules that prohibit elementary schools from being sited adjacent to major highways (as a means to reduce air pollution exposure and asthma) can be evaluated by incorporating comparisons consisting of preschool, or middle- and high-school students not covered by the law.

Comparison Outcomes

Additional options for comparisons are provided by outcome variables. Appropriate comparison outcomes are related to the primary outcome, but, of importance, are not affected by the law or policy under study. For example, to evaluate the effect of New York City's regulation to post calorie information in chain restaurants, one might compare sale receipts for food purchased at chain restaurants compared to receipts from non-chain restaurants. To evaluate effects of motorcycle helmet laws, comparisons of car to motorcycle fatality and injury rates have been conducted (Sosin & Sacks, 1992). To evaluate effects of a graduated driver's license for teen drivers that forbids night-time driving, comparisons have been made between day-time and night-time teen driver fatalities (Morrisey, Grabowski, Dee, & Campbell, 2006). The difference between labeling a comparison a "group" or an "outcome" is sometimes just a matter of convention. The central importance of the notion of comparison outcomes is to expand one's thinking and highlight the many comparisons, even within the jurisdiction enacting a new law or regulation, that can be effectively used to create strong research designs for evaluating the law's effects.

Replications

A fundamental way to strengthen causal inference regarding a law's effects is to replicate the evaluation across jurisdictions. If similar effects are observed in each place a similar law is implemented, confidence in inference is clearly enhanced. If the effect is not seen in subsequent replications, suspicion increases that some other idiosyncratic or uncontrolled factor accounts for the observed effect in the first jurisdiction, and the law under study may have had no effect. It is often better to evaluate each instance of a law, rather than the all-too-common practice to lump all similar laws together into a single group and estimating the average effect across all specific instances. Consider the situation in which such a pooled analysis hints that a law might have small effects, but the effect is too small to be reliably measured (that is, is not statistically significant), leading to the conclusion that the regulatory approach is ineffective. Now imagine that in that pooled analysis lurk five states with large clear beneficial effects but ten other states with no effects. The pooled analysis might prematurely discredit the regulatory approach and miss the opportunity for more in-depth analyses of the individual states to better understand why the law works in some cases and not in others, leading to improvements in implementation and further replication of effective approaches.

Replications occur not only across sites but also over time. As jurisdictions change the law on a particular subject in different years or decades, evaluation designs incorporating those replications ensure that observed effects are not due to other factors specific to a given era, again increasing confidence the observed effects are caused by the law under study. A whole area of research design in general involves manipulating the timing of a treatment or intervention. As expected, random assignment of a treatment to a particular time of implementation is a great strategy, just like randomly assigning a treatment to groups or jurisdictions, but it is rarely feasible. However, even without random assignment, naturally occurring (that is, induced by legislatures, courts, or administrators) variation over time in law in a single jurisdiction can be used effectively to dramatically strengthen the evaluation.

Psychologists call these "ABAB" designs, in which a treatment is applied, then removed, then later reapplied, and they can support strong causal inference (Kratochwill, Hitchcock, Horner, et al., 2010). Thus we know with little doubt the causal effects of compulsory motorcycle helmet laws, since some states implemented such laws, later rescinded them, then still later reinstated them, creating an ABAB design (an "A" period without compulsory helmet law, then a "B" period with, then an "A" period without, followed by another "B" period with the law, all within one jurisdiction). The match between the legal changes and morbidity or mortality outcomes in both directions supports strong causal inference (deaths decline abruptly when helmets become compulsory and abruptly return to the higher levels again when the law is rescinded [Mertz & Weiss, 2008; Ulmer & Preusser, 2003]).

Dose Response

The notion of replications, when a similar law is implemented in multiple jurisdictions, and reversals, when a law is implemented and then removed, can be straightforwardly extended to replications in which the dose of a particular regulatory approach varies by jurisdiction or within jurisdiction over time. Dose can represent many different dimensions, tied to theory on the mechanism of the law's effects. All good legal evaluation studies should be based on a clear understanding of the underlying theory regarding legal mechanisms. This is especially true for designing a good dose-response study, because what constitutes different "doses" of the law is inherently tied to how one thinks the particular law works. It could be the size and speed of application of a penalty in a deterrence-based statute, for example, or many other dimensions of breadth, strength, or reach of a law. After effects of the law are assessed within each jurisdiction, jurisdictions are arrayed in order of low to high "dose" of the law. If the magnitude of observed effect tracks the dose—low-dose jurisdictions have small effects and high-dose jurisdictions have large effects—the causal attribution of the observed effects to the laws is substantially strengthened.

Dose-response studies substantially strengthen causal inference, but can have complications. Because the dosages are not randomly assigned to different jurisdictions and different times, it is possible the dose applied in a particular situation is correlated with some other characteristic of that situation or that time period. For example, if all high-dose locations are highly urbanized areas, and all low-dose locations are rural, perhaps dose does not truly affect the magnitude of legal effect and the observed dose-response relationship is really due to urbanism. The risk of such misattribution of effect is lowered by examining the pool of jurisdictions with differing doses for other differences that plausibly might explain the pattern of effects observed.

Multiple Design Elements

Evaluating effects of laws on public health outcomes should be guided by optimum use of multiple design elements for constructing experiments and quasi-experiments. For most cases, when randomization is not feasible, the use of matched comparisons (jurisdictions, groups, and outcomes) in combination with many repeated measures is recommended. Keep in mind that comparisons need not be matched one for one. One jurisdiction implementing a new law is typically compared with a similar jurisdiction that has not. Causal inference is often enhanced by using several jurisdictions in comparison with the one implementing a new law rather than just one. And comparisons of different kinds nested in a hierarchical fashion substantially strengthen the design. Finally, when multiple sites pass new laws, replications can be built directly into the design.

An illustration of such a combination of design elements that produced strong causal inferences about a law's effects can be seen in studies of the legal drinking age (Figure 14.5).

Two states that changed the legal age for possession and consumption of alcoholic beverages (Maine and Michigan) were compared to two states with, at that time, unchanged drinking age (New York, with a consistent legal age of

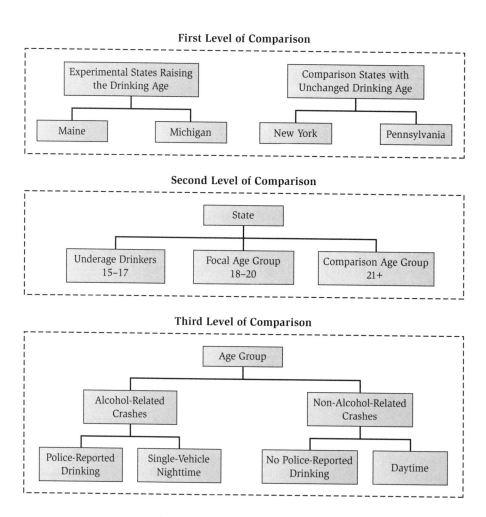

Figure 14.5. Hierarchical Multilevel Time-Series Design: Legal Drinking Age Example.
Source: Wagenaar, 1983a.

eighteen since Prohibition ended, and Pennsylvania, with a consistent legal age of twenty-one). Experimental states versus comparison states constituted the first level of comparison. Second, nested within each state, the focal age group affected by the change in law (eighteen- to twenty-year-olds) was compared to younger and older age groups. Third, nested within each age group, frequencies and rates of alcohol-related car crashes were compared to frequencies and rates of non-alcohol-related crashes. Fourth, to avoid the possibility that the law changed reporting of alcohol involvement perhaps more than the actual incidence of such crashes, two measures of alcohol-related crashes were observed—one based on normal crash reports by police officers regarding drivers' drinking, and an alternative that did not rely on officer reports of drinking (single-vehicle nighttime crashes, which are well-known from other research to have a high probability of involving a drinking driver). These two measures were compared with crashes with no police report of drinking and crashes occurring during the day—providing two measures of non-alcohol-related crashes.

For each cell in this hierarchical design, outcomes were measured monthly for many years before and after the legal changes. The pattern of observed effects—reductions in crashes beginning the first month after the new law, only in the "experimental" states that raised their legal drinking age (and not in the comparison states), only among teenagers (not among drivers twenty-one and over who were not affected by the change in legal age from eighteen to twenty-one), only among alcohol-related crashes (and not among non-alcohol-related crashes, and confirmed with two alternative measures of alcohol-related crashes)—together produced an inference with high levels of confidence that this particular law caused a change in car crashes. Replications in other states that raised the legal age confirmed this pattern of effects. Moreover, a look back to reports and studies from a decade earlier in the 1970s, when twenty-nine states lowered their legal age for drinking, produced an implicit ABAB or intervention reversal design. After many states lowered the legal age for drinking in the early 1970s, teen car crashes increased; when a decade later the legal age was returned to twenty-one, crashes decreased, reversing the earlier increase.

Despite periodic renewed attention to the legal age issue, with various individuals and organizations occasionally arguing in favor of returning again to a lower legal drinking age, the fundamental findings from the decades-earlier research has not been seriously challenged by scientists or most evidence-based review panels. In fact, the U.S. National Highway Traffic Safety Administration (2010) estimates the age-twenty-one law continues to prevent about nine hundred teen crash fatalities per year, saving more than twenty-five thousand lives since the 1970s (Fell, Fisher, Voas, Blackman, & Tippetts, 2009; Voas, Tippetts, & Fell, 2003). Empirical legal evaluations that creatively took advantage of numerous design elements for strong causal inference produced important empirical results that have continuing policy relevance decades later.

Conclusion

Given the number of design elements available to strengthen empirical evaluations of public health laws and regulations, opportunities for continued improvement in the science on public health laws is clear. Awareness and understanding of available research designs for use in the real world outside the laboratory, where random assignment to both treatment and control conditions is often difficult, is important not only for scientists and legal scholars but also for policy makers, public health professionals, and advocates as well. Advancing the effectiveness of heath policy requires differential weighting of the evidence coming from various studies based on the quality of the research design—how well a given study incorporates multiple design elements and thus produces high-confidence causal conclusions. A simple before-and-after design should get little weight in policy deliberations compared to a high-time-resolution, time-series study that includes a hundred or more repeated observations. A single-state study with no comparisons should get less weight than one that incorporates multiple comparison states and multiple comparison outcomes within each state.

High-quality and consistently implemented monitoring systems of relevant population-level health outcomes is critical for increasing the number of well-designed time-series evaluations. These ongoing data-collection efforts are the "management information systems" for population health, facilitating the monitoring of health status, evaluation of changes in laws, regulations and implementation procedures, and achievement of expected standards of health and safety for the population as a whole. Continuing outcome-monitoring systems are necessary for "continuous quality improvement" in the health and well-being of the population. A great example of the role of such information systems is the Fatality Analysis Reporting System, which collects hundreds of detailed data elements on every fatal car crash in the entire United States. The system was carefully designed and tested by a large community of scientists and engineers inside and outside the federal government in the 1960s and early 1970s. Then, full implementation began in 1975, and has continued ever since. The complete data in analysis-ready formats are publicly and easily available. This data system resulted in an explosion of research on the causes and prevention of car crash deaths, and each year as additional longitudinal data are added, more high-quality time-series evaluations are possible. Because of the knowledge gained from thousands of studies using these data over the past few decades, we have saved hundreds of thousands of lives and millions of injuries. This is a truly phenomenal public health achievement (Hemenway, 2009). For decades, each time a state innovates with laws and regulations designed to further reduce crash injuries, investigators can simply access the data system and build well-designed multistate time-series studies evaluating the effect of the change.

There are many other examples of emerging data systems that will facilitate the use of strong time-series research designs to evaluate the effects of laws and regulations. The dissemination of electronic medical records (Hillestad, Bigelow, Bower, et al., 2005), including records on health risk behaviors recorded routinely in primary care practices (Hung, Rundall, Tallia, et al., 2007), will provide population-level daily, weekly, or monthly indicators of health-relevant behaviors and outcomes. Continuing improvements in the breadth, quality, consistency, and availability of continuous monitoring data systems will facilitate further well-designed evaluations of the effects of laws and regulations.

Combining many design elements in a hierarchical multiple time-series research design represents the best approach for evaluating the effects of public health laws and regulations, in many ways providing better knowledge of effect than that gained from randomized controlled trials (RCTs). Randomization to treatment condition is a useful design strategy in many fields (for example, testing specific treatments such as new pharmaceuticals), but has more limited utility in the field of public health law research. RCTs can be used productively to study the effects of specific "micro" mechanisms found in many theories of legal effect, and those results help design better laws and regulations. But RCTs, of necessity, are almost always conducted in small, localized, and unnatural laboratory-type settings, with small samples of people. Natural experiments with public health relevant laws, in contrast, are implemented in real-world settings, use the actual legal tools and implementation processes widely available in society, and apply to very broad or universal populations. And results from actual field implementations of laws and regulations are more persuasive to policy makers, public health practitioners, and citizens, facilitating diffusion of successful approaches to other jurisdictions, resulting in major improvements in population health.

Summary

Most changes in laws and regulations affecting population health represent natural experiments, in which scientists do not control when and where these changes are implemented and thus cannot randomly assign the legal "treatments" to some and not to others. Many research design elements can be incorporated in evaluations of public health laws to produce accurate estimates of the size of a law's effect with high levels of confidence that an observed effect is caused by the law:

- Incorporate dozens or hundreds of repeated observations before and after a law takes effect, creating a time series.

- Measure outcomes at an appropriate time resolution to enable examination of the expected pattern of effects over time that is based on a theory of the mechanisms of legal effect.

- Include comparisons in the design, such as multiple jurisdictions with and without the law under study, comparison groups within a jurisdiction of those exposed and not exposed to the law, and comparison outcomes expected to be affected by the law and similar outcomes not expected to be affected by the law.

- Replicate the study in additional jurisdictions implementing similar laws.

- Examine whether the "dose" of the law across jurisdictions or across time is systematically related to the size of the effect.

Combining design elements produces the strongest possible evidence on whether a law caused the hypothesized effect and magnitude of that effect. Well-designed studies of public health laws in natural real-world settings facilitate diffusion of effective regulatory strategies, producing significant reductions in population burdens of disease, injury, and death.

Further Reading

McCleary, R., & Hay, R. A. (1980). *Applied time series analysis for the social sciences.* Beverly Hills, CA: Sage.

Shadish, W. R. (2010). Campbell and Rubin: A primer and comparison of their approaches to causal inference in field settings. *Psychological Methods, 15*, 3–17.

Shadish, W. R., Cook, T. D., & Campbell, D. T. (2002). *Experimental and quasi-experimental designs for generalized causal inference.* Boston: Houghton-Mifflin.

Shadish, W. R., & Sullivan K. (2012). Theories of causation in psychological science. In H. Cooper (Ed.), *APA handbook of research methods in psychology* (Vol. 1, pp. 23–52). Washington, DC: American Psychological Association.

Chapter 15

Qualitative Research Strategies for Public Health Law Evaluation

Jennifer Wood

Learning Objectives

- Identify and distinguish the key qualitative methods of public health law research.
- Compare and contrast standards of research quality for quantitative and qualitative research.
- Describe the role of qualitative research in a causal pathway from lawmaking to population health.

The field of PHLR occupies a rich space where interdisciplinary theoretical perspectives meet rigorous empirical methods to examine law as an independent variable and population health as the ultimate outcome of concern (Burris, Wagenaar, Swanson, et al., 2010). Systematic qualitative research strategies can help form our understanding of relationships between and mechanisms influencing law, legal practices, and public health. Qualitative research can shed light on the nuanced ways in which law works; how human decision makers, organizations, and whole environments may act or behave differently as a direct or indirect response to legal constraints; and how these changes, in turn, can reshape the physical and social landscape of health risk and well-being for populations.

Because of its inductive nature, qualitative research can generate insight into previously unstudied (or understudied) mechanisms of legal effect (see Chapter 9). It can explore new theoretical ideas, identifying previously uncharted terrain that may not be found through deductive hypothesis testing. Qualitative research often dominates the initial phase of research on a new PHLR topic, building a foundation of understanding for later quantitative studies. Qualitative methods help uncover ways in which laws have effects that lie outside existing theories and models, and for which standardized quantitative measures do not exist. It can also inform the study of law's implementation, peering into the gap between "law on the books" and law in action. Those charged with the administration or enforcement of law can be vital sources of empirical data, as can populations and subgroups that are targeted by law. Understanding how law is applied and in some cases contested in various real-life situations is an integral piece of the puzzle that seeks to explore law's effects on public health, including unintended consequences. Understanding the factors that drive and shape lawmaking is also an important aspect of PHLR, and the texts capturing legislative debates, including testimonies and committee reports, provide the empirical material for qualitative analysis.

The purpose of this chapter is to situate qualitative research on the wider stage of PHLR and describe ways in which it can be rigorously and effectively used in PHLR. It outlines examples of broad research strategies and data-collection methods they employ, both alone and in combination. The utility and appropriateness of each method will be discussed in relation to examples of PHLR questions or studies. The chapter closes with a discussion of core criteria for guiding high-quality empirical research.

Qualitative Research in Context

Qualitative research is centrally concerned with the study of *meaning*, including people's understandings of and beliefs about aspects of their experiences. The focus of qualitative studies can range from a few people to small social networks to large groups that are defined by a shared characteristic, experience, or institutional membership. Based on the definition of *empirical* as "relying on direct experience and observation" (Janesick, 2004, p. 18), the task of qualitative research is to provide an authentic account of how people think about the world and act within it. Human thought and action are shaped by social, cultural, organizational, political, and geographic conditions or contexts. Such contexts can be seen, or rendered visible, through various representations including written text (such as laws, policies, or procedures), oral texts (including personal narratives or stories), researcher field notes, and video or audio recordings (Denzin & Lincoln, 2005, p. 3).

Qualitative research is vital to empirical legal studies of "law in the real world" (Genn, Partington, Wheeler, & Nuffield Foundation, 2006, p. iii), including the realities of enforcement and compliance behaviors (McBarnet,

Voiculescu, & Campbell, 2007). Sociolegal or "law and society" scholars care about the effects or consequences that law in action may have on populations and social institutions (McBarnet, Voiculescu, & Campbell, 2007; see Unger, 1983; Fitzpatrick & Hunt, 1987, on the field of "critical legal studies"). In bridging law and social science, law and society scholarship treats law not as neutral or purely technical, but rather as "meaning-making" in the way that Stryker describes (see Chapter 4). As such, qualitative inquiry has long been integral to the study of law (Jabbari, 1998).

Many theoretical frameworks and methodological approaches are being advanced and refined as the field of PHLR advances. Taken together, these frameworks and approaches provide a comprehensive toolkit for answering questions of *whether* and *how* law influences population health. Beyond revealing the patterns, nature, and distribution of laws, qualitative tools can produce evidence to support causal inference, enhancing what we know about the theoretical mechanisms of law. Robust causal inference obviously is vital to evaluations of law's effectiveness, and qualitative tools can help assess both the intended *and* unintended effects of a law, including such effects on particular groups, by exploring the causal mechanisms and identifying potentially important but previously undetected effects.

Data-Collection Methods and Sources

Qualitative research typically involves analyses of written texts and the collection of data from, and in conjunction with, human subjects. At the outset, one must determine the nature of one's data sources and their accessibility. Documents capturing processes of lawmaking or law's implementation may be searchable on the Internet or made available by public agencies. Access to human subjects can in some cases be challenging, particularly in studies of a law's effects on vulnerable or protected groups, such as people affected by mental illnesses, or prisoners. Of course, access is only the first consideration. Depending on the characteristics of interview respondents (are they members of an elite professional group, or do they have language or literacy challenges?), the content of interviews and the manner in which interviews are performed affect the ethics and difficulty of the research.

Interviews

The purpose of an interview is to elicit peoples' knowledge and perspectives that might otherwise remain unknown, simply because they weren't asked before. Such individuals might include those involved in lawmaking or in the implementation of the law, or those who experience law's enforcement. Interviews are a useful vehicle for tapping into people's experiences, assuming such individuals are comfortable sharing information with researchers and through two-way verbal communication.

Researchers must decide how much structure to impose on interviews, and whether interviews should be with one individual at a time (one on one) or with groups. Semistructured interviewing is most useful to PHLR because it is both systematic and flexible, allowing for the generation of rich qualitative data. A researcher directs an interview by following an interview guide containing general questions to which interviewees can respond with as much detail as is relevant. The researcher strives for depth in responses, using general, open-ended questions that make sure to avoid "yes" or "no" answers. As the interviewee replies, the researcher actively listens for insights. This may prompt the interviewer to ask new questions in order to gain a deeper understanding of the initial response (see Miller & Crabtree, 2004).

The semistructured approach therefore aims to strike a balance between guiding the interview to cover preplanned topics while asking unplanned questions that cover new, previously unexplored ground. Therefore, it is an approach that is appropriate when a topic is partially understood and some key research questions are known in advance. Yet "the best probing is that which is responsive, in the moment, to what the interviewee is saying" and having an interview guide allows for comparison of answers to key questions across interviews, therefore ensuring that data gathering is systematic (Cohen & Crabtree, 2006). This semistructured approach stands in contrast to highly structured interviewing, or survey research, in which respondents must choose from a list of answer options provided in a set of preordered questions (Willis, 2007), and the data generated are numerical and subject to quantitative analyses.

When law is a topic of exploration, care must always be taken not to bias responses through questions that assume law is important. Sociolegal research has shown that law often influences behavior and attitudes at a deep or unconscious level, defining options and setting bounds of possibility. It may be at work defining norms that are not recognized as coming from law, or people may have folk beliefs about what the law is that are not factual. So when an interview is designed to explore how the law influences behavior, it may be useful to allow law to emerge in a semistructured interview rather than prompting people to define their legal knowledge or explain how law influences them. An example of this more patient but revealing process is Engel and Munger's work on how disability rights law has changed the lives of people with disabilities. In their "autobiographical" approach, they asked interviewees to tell their life stories, waiting for the law to emerge, or not, in the narratives of their subjects (Engel & Munger, 1996).

A semistructured approach was used by Dodson and colleagues (2009) to better understand the various conditions influencing the development and passage of childhood obesity laws and regulations. The researchers argued that knowledge was lacking on the complex dynamics of the policy-making process, and that those involved directly in this process would be best placed to help deepen and extend existing knowledge. To this end, the team conducted semistructured interviews with legislators and staffers from various states with different political climates. The researchers used interview guides that contained questions on basic demographic information (for example, respondents' educational backgrounds) as well as open-ended questions designed to probe respondents on their perceptions and experiences of the legislative process. The interviews elicited information that served to validate existing knowledge about lawmaking dynamics in general, while illuminating factors specific to the area of childhood obesity prevention. For example, the research affirmed that concerns with the costs of legislation can serve as a barrier to enacting law, while having wide stakeholder support is an enabling condition. At the same time, interviewees illuminated factors specific to the childhood obesity debate, namely the influence of lobbyists representing companies in the production of obesogenic foods, as well as the problem of misinformation among constituents, such as the assumption that school districts would lose money with the passage of legislation.

The Dodson study used one-on-one interviews with people involved in lawmaking. Interviews are also useful for tapping into the knowledge and experiences of people targeted by law. For instance, a study carried out by Cooper and colleagues (2005) set out to examine whether and how a police drug crackdown shaped the health-risk behaviors of injection drug users in New York City. Drug users themselves are obviously the most direct source of information on this topic because they can express how policing tactics influence their thought and actions, and, in particular, whether such tactics serve to alter their daily health risk habits and routines. Although previous research revealed that police crackdowns can undermine healthy behaviors (by, for example, discouraging users from obtaining or using sterile syringes), Cooper and colleagues wanted to generate an in-depth understanding of users' thoughts and habits in relation to crackdowns. As part of this, they wanted to see whether specific police tactics had differential impacts on the health risk behaviors of individuals with different demographic and social characteristics (race or ethnicity, gender, age, socioeconomic status, enrollment in a syringe exchange program). To this end, the lead researcher recruited a diverse sample of individuals who lived in and around a police precinct that was the site of a police crackdown.

In addition to a brief survey (highly structured interview), the researcher undertook an open-ended, semistructured interview that addressed core issues such as community-police relations, contributions of police to public safety, the ways in which the sociodemographic characteristics of users influenced police interactions, and drug use behaviors. These individual interviews provided an opportunity for respondents to describe their thoughts and actions—as they were shaped by police crackdown tactics—through stories of daily struggles and rituals. The research revealed both commonalities and differences in experiences and practices of drug users across different subgroups of the sample. For instance, poorer users—particularly those without homes or access to private spaces—were more likely than users with more resources to resort to high-risk drug use practices, such as injecting hastily (to avoid being caught) without proper regard for safe injecting practices (for example, failing to clean their injection site, not heating up the drug adequately). In this research, semistructured interviews were essential to drawing out details and nuances of these struggles and rituals as shaped by users' individual life circumstances. Interviews were carried out on an individual or one-on-one basis, but in some cases a semistructured approach with groups—commonly referred to as focus groups—can be used as well.

Focus Groups

A focus group is a type of group interview designed to facilitate a social process in which interaction and sharing of views among people produce valuable information. Sometimes this information emerges through a new awareness of shared understandings that no single individual group member could provide alone if interviewed separately. In simple terms, "participants relate their experiences and reactions among presumed peers with whom they likely share some common frame of reference" (Kidd & Parshall, 2000, p. 294). One common frame of reference could be an occupational position. For example, Eman and colleagues (2011) conducted focus groups with family doctors in Canada—as well as administering a short questionnaire—in order to better understand the nature of doctors' concerns about disclosing patient health information in the interests of public health. Previous research had identified privacy issues as a critical barrier, but the researchers wanted to learn more about the legal and extra-legal factors shaping doctors' perception and application of privacy principles, in specific relation to the 2009 pandemic H1N1 influenza outbreak.

With groups of people sharing the same occupation position, the focus group method was able to draw from a common pool of knowledge, eliciting the experiences of people facing similar challenges as medical practitioners, such as protecting patient-physician relationships and maintaining confidentiality, while dealing with larger public health obligations. Focus groups can also serve as an efficient means of gathering information from people who might otherwise be difficult to access on a one-on-one basis. In the case of this study, research participants were recruited from a sample of doctors who were going to attend a family medicine conference, and thus the focus groups were held in private meeting rooms at the conference venue.

Focus groups have other advantages by virtue of bringing together people who have circumstances, characteristics, or experiences in common. Focus groups create opportunities for participants to build on others' insights, contradict them, or refine them (Kitzinger, 1994). Participants may have to explain or justify what they mean by a given statement when prompted by their peers. This may then cause them to explicate or refine their statements; doing so may cause others to do the same. This iterative engagement does not serve to falsify previous statements, but rather helps add nuance and precision to the researcher's understandings of a group's norms or shared experiences, especially in cases when the researcher is working with a group for the first time (Kitzinger, 1994; Morgan, 2004).

Focus groups also help give a voice to participants who otherwise may have little opportunity to offer their knowledge, helping them to have greater control over the research conversation than they would otherwise have in an interview situation (Morgan, 2004). That being said, it is important for researchers, as focus group facilitators, to steer the focus group and ensure that it addresses the key issues of the study. Otherwise, the objectives of the study might get lost. Similar to those conducting individual semistructured interviews, focus group facilitators follow a general question guide while giving participants the opportunity to provide detailed answers and to draw from relevant personal stories. In a group dynamic though, different strands or insights may emerge in quick order, and it is up to the researcher to keep track of these insights and to follow up with them as is relevant to the study's questions of interest. As in the case of individual stories in interviews, law in focus group discussions may hide in the background, shaping how members understand a notion such as privacy without becoming explicit in the discussion.

Some suggest that focus groups could potentially inhibit participants from speaking fully about their experience, because doing so can involve acts of highly personal self-disclosure in front of others. However, a group setting can create a safe environment for people who share a common life experience or set of risk factors and who might otherwise be less likely to discuss "taboo" subjects in a one-on-one interview (Kitzinger, 1994; Morgan, 2004). Focus groups, for example, have long been an important tool in HIV research (Joseph, Emmons, Kessler, et al., 1984). As part of a larger study on the effects of using criminal law as a tool to reduce HIV transmission, a recent Canadian study used focus groups with people with HIV to elicit information on how they perceived and responded to the legal obligation to disclose their HIV status prior to engaging in sexual activity that posed "significant risk" (Mykhalovskiy, 2011, p. 669). The researcher wanted to better understand how people with HIV interpreted and applied the specific provisions of the law, and in particular the law's rather ambiguous legal conception of "significant risk" (which didn't necessarily align with public health-based understandings of risk). Focus groups in this case brought together people with a common characteristic (HIV-positive status) who—through active participation, listening to others, refining and explicating views—generated a multifaceted understanding of a shared phenomenon.

While focus groups are useful for discussing sensitive topics, it is nonetheless important to consider factors that might serve to silence certain participants in a group setting. In studies of occupational groups, such as law enforcement personnel, for example, it is important to ensure there are no power dynamics that allow certain participants to dominate. Holding focus groups with officers that share the same rank (or gender or both) can avoid this, especially if the topic centers on the informal decision-making norms that guide officers' arrest decisions in sensitive areas of concern to PHLR (for example, management of people with mental illness, or arrests of drug users).

Researchers may choose to use focus groups in conjunction with interviews. Doing so can combine the depth achieved in interviews with the breadth achieved in focus groups. Focus groups can be used to validate previous findings from interviews while expanding the sample of people involved in a study. Alternatively, focus groups can generate ideas that can be explored in more depth through one-on-one follow-up interviews.

Field Observations

Sometimes direct observations of people's behavior and informal conversations *in situ* are the most appropriate method to address a special topic in PHLR. When people are asked—in the case of interviews and focus groups—to "talk" about what they do, there's a good chance that their narratives mask aspects of what they actually do. It is human nature to want to be perceived as a good person making sensible choices. People may not always be consciously aware of what they do; they may not reveal some of the minutia of their daily lives that for them is not worth mentioning, but for a researcher may be profoundly insightful. Direct observations provide the opportunity for researchers to judge for themselves what is significant.

Levels of participation in an observation setting can vary, and may change over time (Bailey, 2007). Unobtrusive observations may be most appropriate, in a relatively public setting, such as fast food restaurants or a school cafeteria, if one is interested in observing how healthy foods are explained on menus or displayed on buffet tables, or whether people ask questions about calories or nutritional content. It may, though, be preferable to join a group, or to become an honorary member of it. Doing so helps build trust between the researcher and the group, which is important when the behavior of interest is largely hidden from public view, and one needs to be physically close to the actors under study to observe what they are doing. Becoming a semi-participant, or even a full participant, has been used in research on the police, where the focus is on the "practical reasoning" of front-line workers in bureaucratic organizations (Brewer, 2004).

Without placing oneself in the group, and building rapport, the researcher may have the figurative door closed to them by organizational gatekeepers, or have the observed behaviors "stage managed" when the outsider is present.

Observations can be used for different purposes. Researchers may be interested, for example, in understanding how something is done, such as the implementation of an intervention. Observations were used by Frattaroli and Teret (2006) as part of a case study on the implementation of the Maryland Gun Violence Act of 1996, which authorizes judges to issue protective orders requiring batterers to surrender their firearms. To see whether and if judges were making use of this authority the researchers observed protective order hearings in a court that specialized in domestic violence cases. The researchers took detailed notes of these hearings and subsequently categorized the judicial activity they observed. These observations revealed that some judges were stricter than others in making sure that that the surrender of firearms—as one "relief" option for protective orders—was reviewed with the petitioner. These direct observations of judicial behavior therefore helped the researchers to gauge the degree to which the law was being implemented in practice.

Observations can be used as a tool for understanding the meanings, rules, and norms that guide the behaviors and everyday routines of groups. Such observations can be useful to PHLR when one is concerned with understanding the norms guiding health risk behaviors, or the norms guiding the practices of those implementing or enforcing the law. This use of observations is central to ethnographic research, which seeks to gather data on culture and cultural practices. What people say or how they talk while they are being observed is just as important as what they do, because their everyday talk can reveal a deeper logic or sensibility that explains actions being observed. Depending on the study, what people wear, how they talk, and their body language could all reveal power relationships, or interpersonal dynamics, that illuminate how a culture operates. The ethnographer documents this social world in as much rich detail as possible. All of these observations then form the data for the analysis of the meaning-making practices of a group.

Written Textual Analysis

In addition to peoples' words and actions, written texts are another valuable source of qualitative data. For instance, a researcher may be interested in gathering and analyzing texts that help us understand how and why a particular lawmaking effort was successful or how it was implemented. As part of understanding lawmaking, it may be important to examine the nature and extent of arguments used either in support of, or against the passage of a particular piece of legislation. Written texts produced as part of legislative debates can provide detailed information on this argumentation, and because they were produced at the time of the legislative process, can be considered accurate and not subject to the failures of human memory. Written texts, such as standard operating procedures or guidance documents, can also help us understand implementation practices.

As an example of textual analysis, Apollonio and Bero (2009) set out to examine which arguments were used in the passage of workplace smoking legislation. They also wanted to weigh this evidence, seeing how much certain arguments were used more than others. The researchers were particularly interested in discovering whether arguments that deployed research evidence, or scientific discourse, ultimately were associated with the passage of workplace smoking legislation that had strong protections for public health. To this end they performed a content analysis of materials including written and oral testimony, the text of proposed and passed bills and amendments, audiotapes of committee hearings, meeting minutes, and public commentary. Content analysis is a common form of textual analysis that involved, in this case, coding text segments according to argument types and counting the number of times certain arguments were used. Content analysis therefore produced both qualitative data (descriptions of different argument types, categorized by reading and analyzing the narratives) and quantitative data (the number of times different arguments were used). The researchers discovered varying types of argument in the texts, such as those centered on science and health effects and those stressing ideological positions. After analyzing and weighing different forms of argumentation, the authors concluded that "an emphasis on scientific discourse, relative to other arguments made in legislative testimony, might help produce political outcomes that favor public health" (Apollonio & Bero, 2009, p. 1).

Texts can serve as an important data source for PHLR because they capture arguments and discourse that are so much a part of legislative and adjudicative processes. They help us understand thoughts and actions of people, both historically and in present times. Written texts provide good clues into how issues are framed and articulated. They can capture forms of reasoning that help in understanding human practices.

Research Strategies

The data-collection methods I have described can be deployed, singularly or in combination, for different purposes depending on one's legal or health topic, research question, and broader research strategy. This section briefly describes some common qualitative research strategies of use for PHLR.

Ethnography

Ethnographic studies are ideal for understanding the behavioral or cultural norms or rules (both formal and informal) that guide practices of groups or organizations. They help describe and explain everyday activities and logics of groups, about which little may be known. Direct observation of behaviors and practices is the tool of choice in ethnographic studies, but it is common to deploy interviews or focus groups as well. Regardless of how one mixes data-collection tools, an ethnographic study focuses on a group or a collective—its norms, traditions, everyday behaviors, and forms of "practical reasoning" (Brewer, 2004)—as its primary unit of analysis. "Ethnographers," writes Herbert, "unearth what the group takes for granted, and thereby reveal the knowledge and meaning structures that provide the blueprint for social action" (2000, p. 551).

One example of ethnographic research comes from India, where researchers set out to uncover the ways in which an HIV prevention nongovernmental organization (NGO) and female sex worker community-based organizations (CBOs) worked to transform the legal and normative environment in which sex workers were being policed. In a context in which law enforcement practices were arbitrary, corrupt, and a significant threat to the physical and mental health of sex workers, an NGO (with funding from an international donor) worked with CBOs to alter power dynamics. Through extensive community mobilization efforts, sex workers were given tools to identify police abuse and to set new standards of police behavior, thus transforming the "regulatory space" of police work (Biradavolu, Burris, George, Jena, & Blankenship, 2009). An ethnographic approach, involving prolonged engagement in the field, made it possible for researchers to understand this community transformation process, and in particular the sophisticated legal, political, and normative strategies deployed by the various actors to make this transformation happen. The researchers collected data through detailed observations of NGO and other activities, as well as through interviews with sex workers, intimate partners, police, and others. These data were gathered over a two-year period, by four trained observers. The researchers used this extensive time in the field to understand not just what was being done but how all of the activities observed were understood by participants.

Case Study Research

Case studies help illustrate a process, an action, or an event (Creswell, 2007). In PHLR, a case study approach might be best suited for answering questions related to how a law was crafted and passed, or how it was implemented at the administrative level. Methods of data collection include observations; interviews; and analyses of laws, policies, or other guidelines for action. A strong case study uses as many data sources as possible, including individuals involved in the process or event under study and documents that help elucidate what unfolded (for example, media articles, meeting minutes, court decisions).

All of these sources shed light on "how things get done" (Cohen, Manion, & Morrison, 2000; Stake, 2005, p. 444).

The case study researcher has to make a choice about parameters of the empirical "case," including a beginning and end time period for an observed process, and size of the subject population or institution involved in the phenomenon (an occupational subgroup, a whole organization, a community). Both of these "time and size" choices determine the scope of the study. Given the need for multiple data sources in a case study, researchers must determine whether they have sufficient time and resources to study multiple sites or whether it is more feasible to focus on a single case. Frattaroli and Teret (2006) focused their research on the single case of Maryland's Gun Violence Act, a law that authorized judges to order batterers to surrender their firearms and police to remove firearms from the scene of an alleged act of domestic violence. Within this case, they studied implementation of these provisions by both judges and police, drawing on three key sources of data: observations of protective order hearings, semistructured interviews with key informants including judges and law enforcement officers, and documents related to the implementation process, such as training materials. Given the finite resources of the project, the researchers selected four study sites covering urban, suburban, and rural areas within the state, and defined an observation period of one year.

Grounded Theory

The purpose of a grounded theory approach is to inductively produce a theory of a process, behavior, or interaction through the research, rather than to apply an existing theory at the outset (Glaser & Strauss, 1967). Proponents of grounded theory have provided clear guidelines for using the approach. A central text is *Basics of Qualitative Research*, written by Corbin and Strauss (2008). A grounded theory project starts with a general research question, which guides the start of the data collection. The researcher then moves back and forth between data collection and analysis. Analysis is aided by coding, in which emerging concepts or ideas are linked to segments of the data. Through the coding process, the researcher works to establish tentative relationships between concepts. The researcher then engages in more focused data collection and analysis in a process of "constant comparison," which involves comparing new data with previously collected data in order to discover similarities or differences in their conceptual properties or relationships. The process of constant comparison allows the researcher to refine concepts and identify higher-level concepts (often referred to as categories or themes). Theory emerges through this refinement of concepts and conceptual relationships. The researcher continues this cyclical process of data collection and analysis until no new concepts or conceptual relationships emerge. At this point, described as the stage of "theoretical saturation," the theory developed is determined to be robust enough to explain all of the data gathered, and there are no negative cases (that is, actions or behaviors that cannot be explained by the theory). In other words, the theory is considered to be "grounded" in the data (Corbin & Strauss, 2008; Eriksson & Kovalainen, 2008; Lacey & Luff, 2001).

A grounded theory approach can be used with one or more sources of data, such as narratives from interviews, observations from field notes, written texts such as media clippings or correspondence, or all of the above. Cooper and colleagues (2005) used the grounded theory approach in analyzing interview data on drug injectors' health risk behaviors in the wake of a New York Police drug crackdown. "Throughout the analysis," they write, "the authors discussed emerging concepts, categories, and their inter-relationships; negative cases were sought to extend and enrich our findings" (p. 677). Using the grounded theory approach, they developed a theory of the relationships between specific policing tactics and drug users' sense of sovereignty over their bodies and the spaces in which they lived, and users' abilities to practice harm reduction. Their theoretical model was general enough to explain experiences of all of the users they interviewed, while providing enough specificity to distinguish between experiences and practices of users with different sociodemographic characteristics or circumstances.

Action Research

In an action research approach, researchers and practitioners (or members of a community of interest) work hand-in-hand in all stages of a research project, from conceptualizing the problem to identifying a needed change to developing ways to improve practice (and ultimately human well-being) (Brydon-Miller, Greenwood, & Maguire, 2003; Stringer, 2007). Action research involves collapsing traditional boundaries between researchers and subjects. Research teams include members of a targeted group, such as a mental health consumer working with research investigators who are studying a legal intervention to improve community mental health, or HIV-positive individuals providing ideas for a more promising legal intervention that assists in prevention. The assumption is that such participants possess unique insights into the relevant risk behaviors and environments, and how best to study them (Schensul, 1999). Action research therefore centers on "change *with* others," serving as a strong critique of, and alternative to, "ivory tower" research (Reason & Bradbury, 2008, p. 1).

Within PHLR, an action research method called rapid policy assessment and response (RPAR) has been developed recently to bring together researchers and community stakeholders to improve the working of law on the ground. Community-based researchers, together with a Community Action

Board, gather and interpret data about the implementation of law in the community and its effect on local health. Researchers and the action board use facilitation techniques such as "power maps" and a "root causes" exercise to analyze who is wielding power in the community, how law relates to practice, and where there might be "pressure points" for healthy change (Temple University, Beasley School of Law, 2004). This approach has been deployed especially in relation to drug and sex-related behaviors, but the method applies to any regulatory problem (Sobeyko, Leszczyszyn-Pynka, Duklas, et al., 2006; Vyshemirskaya, Osipenko, Koss, et al., 2008).

Models such as RPAR can benefit marginalized populations whose experiences with laws have been unfavorable or whose ability to influence lawmaking has been limited or even nonexistent. While incorporating the knowledge and experience of such groups is key to the research process, participants also benefit by acquiring skills in data collection and analysis. The purpose of action research is precisely to link researchers and the research process to stakeholders in the locale who are in a position to translate knowledge into action.

Mixed Methods

Qualitative research may also form part of a mixed-methods study that integrates numeric and text-based data to offer complementary or a richer set of answers than provided by either quantitative or qualitative research on its own. Mixed-methods researchers adopt the pragmatic view that quantitative and qualitative approaches to research are compatible, with each compensating for limitations of the other (Johnson & Onwuegbuzie, 2004). At the design phase, getting the right mix involves determining the ordering of different research strategies (whether one component should precede the other, or whether data collection should occur simultaneously) (Creswell & Plano Clark, 2007). For example, a focus group study exploring health risk behaviors could assist in refining hypotheses to be tested by a survey of a representative sample of the population. Alternatively, an experimental or quasi-experimental evaluation might produce evidence that a law is connected to a specified public health outcome. Direct observations combined with key informant interviews might then shed light on the mechanisms that "tell us why interconnections . . . occur" (Pawson, 2006, p. 23), as could ethnographies that are nested in randomized controlled trials (Sherman & Strang, 2004).

The term *mixed methods* therefore applies to studies that use both quantitative and qualitative tools and sources, and respective quantitative and qualitative analyses. Various combinations of data sources, tools, and analyses can be used depending on the research questions (see recent guidance on this by Creswell, Klassen, Plano Clark, Smith, & The Office of Behavioral and Social

Sciences Research, 2011). One might choose to conduct two parallel studies of the same thing, such as a random sample survey combined with key informant interviews, comparing or integrating the results. In such a case, qualitative data are interspersed with results from the quantitative analysis as a way to unpack, interpret, or confirm what the numbers are indicating.

Standards of Research Quality

Scholars vary in their views as to whether qualitative research is more of an art (demanding the skills of improvisation) or a science (demanding structure and rigid adherence to procedures).

The former view suggests that researchers need to be flexible, ready to change aspects of their designs as they go along (for example, sampling). Researchers may experience such profound "ah ha" moments that the course of the research must change in order to pursue a potentially groundbreaking finding. Howard Becker, a seminal American sociologist and ethnographer, is a particularly vocal advocate of this improvisational orientation, arguing that "researchers can't know ahead of time all the questions they will want to investigate, what theories they will ultimately find relevant to discoveries made during the research, or what methods will produce the information needed to solve the newly discovered problems" (2009, p. 548). The research process is not linear, nor is the process of designing it. But this does not mean, Becker points out, that it isn't "systematic, rigorous, [and] theoretically informed" (2009, p. 548).

Notwithstanding Becker's view, researchers require guidance as they embark on the most systematic and rigorous study that they can achieve within the scope and resources of their project. From the perspective of funders who support research (quantitative or qualitative), it is important for researchers to justify their financial support by giving careful consideration to every aspect of their research, factoring in the chance that certain design elements may change or expand, and ensuring that such changes along the way can strengthen the research and advance its goals. Institutional review boards may also insist on a well-defined research plan and set of objectives.

Undoubtedly, qualitative researchers can't or shouldn't "imitate" guidelines designed for deductive, hypothesis-testing research, but the paradigms of quantitative and qualitative research do share core concerns about quality of data, appropriateness of data-collection tools, validity and generalizability of findings, and robustness of the analytical process. Although some prominent qualitative researchers choose not to use such terms (because they align too closely with positivist research) and use others (for example, *confirmability, authenticity*), we use the more traditional language here, in a qualified manner, to provide consistency, as well as a source of comparison, with the other chapters in the book. The considerations that follow are particularly complex in the design of mixed-methods research. Fortunately, this complexity is recognized by the National Institutes of Health, which recently commissioned a guidance document from prominent authorities on mixed methods (Creswell, Klassen, Plano Clark, Smith, & The Office of Behavioral and Social Sciences Research, 2011).

Sampling

Researchers must decide on the particular characteristics of people or texts that make up their sample as well as how large the sample should be. For example, if someone wants to interview injection drug users about their health behaviors, it's important to determine which set of drug-user characteristics should be captured in the sample (for example, people living in certain areas, people of a certain age, males, females, people who are wealthy, or people with few resources). The research question will determine whether a diverse or homogeneous sample is required. Determining how many people to recruit for interviews is equally important, and it is possible that this number can increase or decrease over the course of the research, depending on emergence of new insights or questions. Qualitative researchers aim to reach a point at which additional data collection (increasing the sample) would not generate new insights. The point at which this occurs depends on the research question. There could be little variation in views among a sample of family physicians in terms of their concerns with health information privacy, but there may be huge variation among injection drug users in their experiences of targeted policing, depending on whether users are living in certain parts of a city, or are wealthy or poor, or have access to support networks and social services. Researchers must think carefully about their level of access to the people or to the texts that will allow them to answer their question comprehensively, with depth, and with confidence that there are not parts of the question that have remained unanswered.

Different approaches to sampling in qualitative research can be used alone or in combination. Probability sampling, most commonly found in quantitative research, seeks to make sure that the sample represents the broader target population. This approach can be suitable for large-scale qualitative studies, although higher levels of generalizability can compromise depth, especially in projects with limited resources to collect detailed data (Lamont & White, 2005).

There is a variety of purposeful sampling strategies, and some common ones are highlighted here. Criterion sampling involves selecting participants who meet one criterion or more of interest, such as a legislator working in the area of childhood obesity prevention. Maximum variation sampling consists of choosing sites or participants that differ along various dimensions or criteria, such as injection drug users that differ in terms of levels of wealth, gender, ethnic background, or some combination. Homogenous sampling refers to selecting participants or cases that are similar in some ways, such as judges who work in specialized domestic violence courts in the State of Maryland. Snowball or chain sampling refers to the process of expanding one's sample by asking previous participants to nominate other potential participants (Bailey, 2007). For instance, a police officer involved in a targeted foot patrol intervention in a violent area of a city might refer a researcher to another police officer from a gang unit who has extensive knowledge about drug market dynamics associated with the violent behaviors.

Respondent-driven sampling (RDS) is a relatively new approach used in the study of hidden or "hard to reach" populations, such as drug users, sex workers, gay men, or people experiencing homelessness. RDS was developed to help overcome the challenges of achieving probability samples with such groups. Depending on the research question, having a probability sample or random sample is important when the goal is to measure the effect of a law or its enforcement on *all* members of a wider population of interest, not simply those who are most visible or accessible. With hidden populations, however, the sampling frame can be unknown; there is no clear under-standing of the extent of such populations or the varying characteristics of their members (Heckathorn, 1997). The RDS approach uses respondents to recruit their peers (as in snowball sampling), while researchers keep track of peer-to-peer referrals. This snowballing occurs through "waves" (with one wave having been recruited through the previous wave). RDS deploys a mathemat-ical model that helps calculate the non-randomness of the sample, while implementing techniques for reducing bias, including lengthening referral chains and rewarding recruiters (Heckathorn, 2008; see Salganik & Heckathorn, 2004, and Heckathorn, 2007, for further information on the RDS process).

Validity

In qualitative research, the representation of data is very much a product of a researcher's own interpretation of meaning (Creswell, 2007, pp. 206–207). "Qualitative data," write Corbin and Strauss, "are inherently rich in substance and full of possibilities. It is impossible to say that there is only one story that can be constructed from the data" (2008, p. 50). There are, however, several strategies that researchers can employ to make sure that findings are valid, which in the context of qualitative research refers to findings that are credible (capturing the truth of peoples' experiences and perceptions), transferable (applicable to other contexts), and neutral (not distorted by researcher bias) (Cohen & Crabtree, 2006; Lincoln & Guba, 1985).

"Negative case analysis" (Creswell, 2007, p. 208) involves identifying or collecting data that might not be explained by one's existing analysis, and may even contradict it (Cohen, Manion, & Morrison, 2000). A related form of analytical scrutiny is "communicative validity," a process in which researchers subject their claims to other researchers with relevant content and theoretical expertise. Entering into such a dialogue with one's intellectual community can create an opportunity for one's interpretation to be refuted or refined (Hesse-Biber & Leavy, 2006).

In ethnographic research, the validity of one's findings is strengthened when one commits a sustained period of time in the field, and offers a reflective account of the ways in which one gained access to a setting, developed trust with participants, and made sure that one's own cultural predispositions did not distort or skew one's interpretations (Creswell, 2007, pp. 207–208). "Pragmatic validity" is particularly important in action research, and is important to PHLR more generally. Pragmatic validity is the ability of a research study to enable participants to better understand and navigate their environment, thus enhancing their ability to effect change, either to the lives of participants or to the contexts in which people live and work (Hesse-Biber & Leavy, 2006; Marks, Wood, Ali, Walsh, & Witbooi, 2010).

Regardless of sampling strategy or size, it is important to be very clear about the ways in which one's findings may have relevance beyond the individuals, cases, or sites studied. Although generalizability to the whole population, in the sense claimed by quantitative researchers, is usually not the goal of qualitative research, it is nonetheless important to discuss whether and why one's findings could be more widely applied to other groups, institutions, or processes (Lamont & White, 2005). Researchers can help readers judge this transferability by providing as much detail as possible on the research setting and characteristics of one's data and sample. With this information, others can compare with the characteristics of other potential research sites or settings.

Reliability

A reliable study is one in which findings would be consistent if the data were to be collected for a second time or if the study were to be repeated. In qualitative research involving observations and interviews, it's not really possible to collect the same data twice (Trochim, 2005). For instance, if a researcher is observing people's behavior, there is no single instance when a behavior will be exactly the same as it was in a previous moment (although there are presumably common and repeated patterns in the behavior). An interview respondent could answer the same questions differently from one day to the next. Nonetheless, it is important to guarantee the reliability of the procedures for data gathering and analysis. This involves providing transparency into how the data were collected and analyzed. This transparency is important not only to the outside world but to members of teams that have different people collecting and analyzing data.

In large projects, it is critical to ensure that data are collected in the same way by different team members, and that the processes of data organization and coding are the same. In ethnographic or other observational studies, for example, observers should be similarly trained and should be producing the same quality of field notes. Being a good note taker is not a trivial skill, and it is a true craft (Emerson, Fretz, & Shaw, 1995). If interviews are being carried out by multiple researchers, it is important for each person to follow the same general guide. Assuming there are open-ended components in such interviews, all researchers should be trained on interviewing techniques that elicit as much relevant information as possible from respondents.

Finally, if there are multiple people coding data, it is important that there be constant dialogue in the development and definitions of codes and emerging themes so that there is a shared overall interpretive framework and process. Doing so promotes inter-rater reliability. Team members must discuss their analysis regularly, particularly as new codes and themes emerge. It is also useful in the beginning of an analysis phase for two people to code the same piece of data to ensure that they do not differ fundamentally in technique or in the interpretation of codes. For very large, multisite projects involving teams of qualitative researchers, it is useful to seek guidance on specific techniques for achieving high inter-rater reliability.

Analysis: Inductive-Deductive Engagement

Qualitative research requires the researcher to cyclically engage particular descriptive data and higher levels of abstract understanding (Janesick, 2004). In conducting one's analysis, researchers must engage in a meaningful and iterative dialogue between theory and data. This analysis begins while the researcher is collecting data. Analytical insights gleaned from initial data can drive researchers to collect more or different data as the study progresses, meaning that the qualitative research processes we have described tend to be more fluid than quantitative research. Research findings along the way can inform further sampling procedures, or choices about which elements or phenomenon in the data will become center stage as one works to form a story from the empirical material.

It is common for researchers to take advantage of qualitative analysis software that can assist with the organization and coding of data. Software such as *Atlas.ti* or *NVivo* (see Creswell, 2007) does not, however, serve to replace the analytic work of the researcher. The software helps enhance efficiency of the analysis process and provides useful tools for presenting data, such as charts and visual diagrams, including network views of relationships between concepts. The software also makes it easy for researchers to code text segments as well as to write and organize memos or reflections on those segments. Technology helps analysts become more efficient in an otherwise labor-intensive task.

Conclusion

When evaluating the effectiveness of law it is critical for researchers to design studies that can help support causal inferences (see Chapters 13 and 14). Thinking in causal terms both depends on and contributes to a fundamental understanding of mechanisms, or the ways in which law has effects. In tracing causal pathways beginning with lawmaking and ending with health, qualitative research helps answer questions along the way that are important to practice and essential to theory. Moreover, it can help identify law's unintended consequences on health behaviors and risk environments.

As a complement to quantitative research, qualitative research strategies and methods help answer important questions about what law means to people, how it is experienced, and how law's agents might do a better job in furtherance of public health. Advancing the field of PHLR therefore depends in part on advancing qualitative research that is empirically rich, theoretically innovative, and pragmatically useful. Exactly how this is done in practice requires careful consideration by academics in partnership with agencies and communities intended to benefit from, and ideally contribute to, the design and conduct of research that matters.

Summary

Qualitative research helps form our understanding of relationships between law, legal practices, and public health. Because of its inductive nature, qualitative research generates insight into previously unstudied (or understudied) mechanisms of legal effect. Its various methods and strategies help uncover ways in which laws have effects that lie outside existing theories and models, and for which standardized quantitative measures do not exist.

Different data-collection tools can be used alone or in combination. Semi-structured one-on-one interviews involve open-ended questions that generate detailed narrative data on an individual's unique knowledge and experience. Focus groups create opportunities for participants to build on others' insights, contradict them, or refine them, generating insight that would not emerge through individual interviews. Direct observations help in understanding how an action is carried out, and can reveal cultural norms that guide behaviors. Collection and analysis of written texts help us understand how issues are framed and articulated, and capture forms of reasoning that help us understand human practices.

Qualitative tools can be deployed within broader research approaches or strategies. Ethnographic studies are ideal for understanding the behavioral or cultural norms that guide the practices of groups or organizations. Case studies illustrate a process, and are suited to answering questions of how a law was crafted, passed, or implemented. A "grounded theory approach" produces a theory of a process, behavior, or interaction—generating theory inductively from the data. Action research involves researchers and practitioners (or members of a community of interest) working hand-in-hand in all stages of a research project, from conceptualizing the problem to identifying a needed change to developing ways forward to improve practice. Qualitative research is often part of mixed-methods research that integrates quantitative and qualitative data to offer a richer set of answers than either could provide alone.

Regardless of research strategy, studies must be designed with appropriate sampling strategies, and researchers must ensure validity and reliability. Purposeful sampling strategies are common in qualitative research, and their choice depends on the research question, types of data-collection methods deployed, availability of participants, and resources of the researcher. There are several strategies that researchers employ to ensure that findings are valid, including use of "negative case analysis" or "communicative validity" processes in which researchers subject their claims to other researchers with relevant content and theoretical expertise. It is important to guarantee the reliability of qualitative research by using consistent and systematic procedures for gathering and analyzing data. Finally, good qualitative research involves a robust cyclical engagement between descriptive data and higher levels of abstract understanding, which is facilitated by a process of coding (assigning concepts to segments of data).

Further Reading

Apollonio, D. E., & Bero, L. A. (2009). Evidence and argument in policymaking: Development of workplace smoking legislation. *BMC Public Health, 9,* 189.

Corbin, J. M., & Strauss, A. L. (2008). *Basics of qualitative research: Techniques and procedures for developing grounded theory* (3rd ed.). Los Angeles: Sage.

Creswell, J. W., & Plano Clark, V. L. (2007). *Designing and conducting mixed methods research.* Thousand Oaks, CA: Sage.

Chapter 16

Cost-Effectiveness and Cost-Benefit Analysis of Public Health Laws

Ted R. Miller   Delia Hendrie

Learning Objectives

- Plan and construct an analysis that compares costs and benefits of a public health law.
- Identify special issues in applying economic analysis to public health laws.
- Appraise relative cost-effectiveness of competing public health laws, enforcement, and sanctioning.

Understanding costs and benefits of public health laws helps decision makers and the general public understand likely effects on different sectors of the community. Inherent tensions exist when laws or regulations restrict activities that are harmful to health, with tradeoffs required between the good of the whole community and the good of a single individual. For example, wearing a helmet is well known to substantially decrease a motorcyclist's risk of death or severe injury in a crash and decrease the associated costs, most of which are not borne by the motorcyclist. Legislation mandating helmet wearing while motorcycling, however, restricts freedom of choice and deprives motorcyclists of the perceived pleasure of riding without a helmet.

All decisions involve some degree of weighing anticipated costs and expected future benefits of courses of action. While in everyday decision making costs and benefits may not all be explicitly considered, or mental shortcuts may be used to speed decision making, what differentiates economic evaluation is its systematic investigation of costs and benefits of alternative options for meeting an objective such as safeguarding the public's health. Although uncertainty may exist in quantifying costs and benefits, the key questions addressed in economic evaluation of a public health law are whether its benefits, as measured by health outcomes or cost savings, exceed its costs; secondarily, there is the question of the distribution of those costs and benefits across stakeholders. Data on cost-saving benefits that arise from changing a public health law can be a rallying point in the battle to pass or preserve a public health law. The press, legislators, and the public all care about costs a law can reduce. Cost savings are concrete and understandable benefits, and they provide a single compact measure that captures wrecked cars, stolen statues, fractured arms, even deaths.

This chapter provides an introduction to the economic evaluation of public health law. It begins by briefly reviewing ten key steps in a typical economic evaluation (Miller & Levy, 1997). It illustrates these steps with an analysis of costs and benefits of *voluntary* use of a motorcycle helmet. The second section then elaborates on issues that arise in applying economic evaluation to public health laws, including an explanation of the complex steps required to modify the motorcycle helmet estimate to evaluate passing or enforcing a *law* that mandates motorcycle helmet use. The third section discusses the issue of how to compare cost-outcome estimates and provides a table of benefit-cost and cost-effectiveness estimates for a variety of public health laws. The fourth section addresses the complexity of communicating economic evaluation results to policy makers.

Steps in Conducting an Economic Evaluation

There are ten main steps to conducting an economic evaluation.

Step 1: Define the Intervention

The first step in conducting an economic evaluation is to carefully define the intervention to be evaluated. This includes deciding on objectives of the evaluation, alternatives to be compared, target population, the setting of the intervention, and the time horizon over which costs and outcomes will be calculated. As our example, we take the objective of computing the return on voluntary investment in a motorcycle helmet by a motorcycle operator. The two alternatives evaluated are to ride one's motorcycle in the United States helmeted and to do the same unhelmeted. We estimate that a helmet has a five-year useful life. This initial analysis assumes a helmet use law is not in force.

Step 2: Choose a Type of Economic Evaluation

The type of economic evaluation is determined by how health outcomes are measured. If naturally occurring outcome measures are selected, then the type of economic evaluation is a cost-effectiveness analysis. Naturally occurring outcomes include generic outcomes that can be compared across all interventions (for example, fatalities prevented, life years gained) or more specific outcomes that can only be used to compare interventions with the same objective (for example, the number of assaults prevented). The economic evaluation results are reported as the cost per life year saved or the cost per assault prevented. Cost-utility analysis is a special form of cost-effectiveness analysis in which the outcomes are measured using multidimensional measures of health outcomes such as quality adjusted life years (QALYs) that incorporate both quality and survival information. A QALY is a health outcome measure valued at 1 for a year in perfect health and at 0 if someone is dead, with values less than 0 (fates worse than death) allowed. In cost-utility analysis, the evaluative measure is the cost per QALY gained or saved. Benefit-cost analysis is a different type of economic evaluation in which all of the health outcomes are measured in monetary terms, with the results reported either as a benefit-cost ratio or as net benefits (that is, benefits minus costs). In our motorcycle helmet example, we will illustrate both a benefit-cost analysis and a cost-utility analysis.

Step 3: Determine the Perspective

The next analytic decision is to choose a *perspective*. The perspective determines whose costs and whose benefits count. For example, discomfort associated with wearing motorcycle helmets is a cost to wearers but a benefit to health insurers as fewer injuries to helmeted motorcyclists will reduce the costs paid out for medical and related treatment. Any cost savings attributable to a public health law represent a benefit to the agency or individual who would otherwise pay these costs. The broadest perspective for an economic evaluation is the societal perspective, which incorporates all costs and benefits regardless of who incurs the costs and who obtains the benefits. This is the perspective recommended by the U.S. Panel on Cost-Effectiveness in Health and Medicine (Gold, Siegel, Russell, & Weinstein, 1996). Other perspectives include those of the government, the health care sector, health insurers, health care institutions, employers, and individuals. Choice of perspective depends on the objective of the study, and more than one perspective can be adopted if appropriate. Whatever perspective is adopted, it is important that it is clearly stated and justified.

Public health laws often reflect tension between what maximizes utility of individual participants in an activity versus the utility of non-participants who are affected by that activity. Legislatures may attempt to protect both interests.

For example, Texas requires motorcyclists who choose not to wear a helmet to show proof of health insurance that would partially cover the medical care cost of any traumatic brain injury that could result from a motorcycle crash. Examining costs and benefits to those who are regulated by public health laws versus those affected by problem behaviors corresponds to the distinction between adopting an internal or an external perspective. The individual or internal perspective—costs and benefits to those who are regulated—provide insight into the likely intensity of opposition to a law. Risk misperception often causes people to underestimate costs of their behavior. An analysis showing that people choose a behavior because they under-perceive their risks—for example, because they think the risk of being in a motor vehicle crash is half of the actual risk—strengthens the case for regulatory action. An analysis of individual costs requires estimating discomfort, inconvenience, and psychic losses associated with behavioral controls. When evaluating minimum drinking age laws, helmet use laws, gun control, and other laws that interfere with personal freedom, economists often focus on the *external perspective*—costs and benefits of problem behavior accruing to people other than the person whose behavior is constrained. High external costs justify public intervention. To justify public health laws that interfere with personal freedom of adults, the record needs to show that the behavior being regulated unduly burdens members of the public who do not engage in that behavior.

The definition of external costs presented here is not universal (Miller, 2001). Consistent with our definition, the highway safety literature defines external crash costs as costs that one group of road users involved in crashes impose on another group of crash-involved road users or on people who were not crash-involved (Elvik, 1994; Lave, 1987). Elvik (1994) clarifies this definition, arguing that all costs borne by the drinker's own family due to injuries to a drinking driver or pedestrian should be treated as internal and all other costs including costs of injuries to other members of the drinker's family and to unrelated individuals who might have been injured in the crash as external. This external cost definition is the relevant one for most public policy decisions.

Another perspective issue, and a second definition of external costs, arises when costing illegal acts. From a societal perspective, many economists believe stolen money is an involuntary transfer payment, not a cost. The total money in circulation remains constant, so society does not experience a loss. Taking this reasoning to its extreme, some economists might argue that the sadist gained pleasure from an assault, a gain that offset some of the suffering costs to the victim. Trumbull (1990) suggests a better alternative, stating that lawbreakers lack standing in societal costing. He and Zerbe (1991) both recommend not counting gains criminals get illegally as societal benefits, and not viewing the prevention of criminals from reaping those gains as a loss. In proscribing these actions, legislatures implicitly state that the gains are ill-gotten and ipso facto do not benefit society. Trumbull's rule underpins a definition of external costs used by both Cohen (1998, 2000) and Rajkumar and French (1997) in analyzing substance abuse and related crime costs:

> An external cost is a cost imposed by one person onto another, where the latter person does not voluntarily accept the negative consequence (through monetary payments or otherwise). For example, the external costs associated with a mugging include stolen property, medical costs, lost wages, and pain and suffering endured by the victim. The victim neither asked for, nor voluntarily accepted, compensation for enduring these losses. Moreover, society has deemed that imposing these external costs is morally wrong and against the law [Cohen, 2000, p. 272].

In Cohen's work, the definitional line blurs, with the money stolen by the criminal not counted as a cost but the wages that the criminal lost while in jail counted. Again on the cusp, Cohen (1998) counts the money spent on illicit drugs as a cost of substance abuse.

Often one displays costs and benefits (that is, cost savings) from multiple perspectives, as in Figure 16.1, which shows costs and benefits from a sustained compulsory breath-testing program in New Zealand. Showing costs and benefits from multiple perspectives provides a more complete representation of the costs and benefits of a law or program.

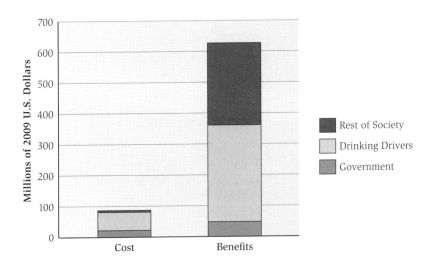

Figure 16.1. Costs and Benefits from a Sustained Compulsory Breath-Testing Program in New Zealand by Perspective.

Source: Miller & Blewden, 2001.

In our motorcycle helmet example, we analyze the investment from two perspectives: a societal perspective, which means that everyone's costs and benefits count, including the motorcyclist, his family, his employer, his insurers, and the government and its taxpayers, and the individual perspective, examining the decision to voluntarily wear a helmet from the motorcyclist's viewpoint.

Step 4: Decide How to Adjust for Differential Timing

Costs and benefits of many interventions extend over years. Inflation results in price changing over time even though the amount of resources used (or saved) and their opportunity cost remains the same. An economic evaluation measures all costs and benefits in inflation-free dollars stated in a base year. Costs of an intervention incurred in the future and benefits received in the future, however, are of lesser value than immediate ones, because money can earn interest when invested and the future is uncertain. For example, a motorcyclist could be killed by a drunk driver while strolling about on the day after his helmet allowed him to emerge from a motorcycle crash unscathed. Conversely, a scientific breakthrough three years after he buys his helmet could reduce the consequences and costs of a brain injury. Therefore cost-outcome analyses reduce or *discount* future cost and benefit streams to reflect their present value. The further in the future a cost or benefit will be, the less weight discounting gives it in the present.

In our motorcycle helmet example we state all costs and benefits in 2010 dollars. We use the 3 percent discount rate that the Panel on Cost-Effectiveness in Health and Medicine (Gold, Siegel, Russell, & Weinstein, 1996) recommends using in analyses of health policy. In a full study, we also would compute estimates at other discount rates to see how sensitive the findings are to the choice of discount rate.

Step 5: Estimate Costs of Alternative Options

Intervention costs should be comprehensive. They include costs of program startup and operation. If staff will be involved, one includes their wages, fringe benefits, and overhead expenses. Volunteer time is priced at the amount it would cost to hire someone to do the volunteer's work.

In our helmet example, an Internet search in August 2011 located U.S. Department of Transportation–approved and Snell-certified helmets for $50 including shipping, a good selection below $100, and some priced as high as $750. We analyze a $100 helmet, with sensitivity analysis estimating the savings for a $50 and a $200 helmet. We add an hour's wage of $19 to shop for the helmet (the national average wage according to the 2010 U.S. Current Employment Survey).

Step 6: Select Relevant Effectiveness Measures

Ideally, effectiveness measures should be final outcomes such as impaired driving crashes averted, not measures such as reductions in alcohol outlets that sell to minors, or worse, changes in vendor attitudes about the harm caused by selling alcohol to minors. The choice of effectiveness measures often will be driven by available data and the underlying purpose of conducting the economic evaluation. In our example, we estimate how much motorcycle helmets reduce deaths and non-fatal brain injuries.

Step 7: Estimate Effectiveness

In prospective analyses of regulatory strategies previously evaluated through small-scale experiments or demonstration programs in selected locations, it is wise to assume effectiveness in jurisdiction-wide replication will be 25 percent lower than the efficacy achieved by a program developer in a focused research trial (see Aos, Lieb, Mayfield, Miller, & Pennucci, 2004; Caulkins, Pacula, Paddock, & Chiesa, 2002; Miller & Hendrie, 2009). Developers are highly motivated. Early experiments often operate under ideal conditions in terms of fidelity and resources (see Chapter 13). Replications almost never reach the same level of effectiveness as they move to a broad society-wide scale. On the other hand, if effectiveness was previously estimated in jurisdictions where whole populations in natural settings were exposed to the regulatory strategy (see Chapter 14), there is no need to reduce the expected magnitude of effect.

Let's go back to our helmet example. Deutermann (2004) uses 1993–2002 data and a very robust evaluation design to estimate that a motorcycle helmet reduces fatality risk by 37 percent for motorcycle operators and 41 percent for passengers. For simplicity, we assume operators never ride as passengers. A meta-analysis (Liu, Ivers, Norton et al., 2008) estimates from six higher-quality studies that a helmet reduces non-fatal brain injury risk by 69 percent.

Table 16.1 uses those effectiveness figures to estimate lives saved by helmets. The first row of data in Table 16.1 shows a complete count of all motorcycle operator deaths in crashes in 2008 (National Highway Traffic Safety Administration, 2011). The second row shows the estimated number of deaths if helmets were not worn. The third row shows the formulas used to compute the numbers of deaths that would occur if nobody wore a helmet. For those not wearing a helmet, that simply is the current number of deaths. For those wearing a helmet, we compute the number of deaths without helmets by dividing the number of deaths while helmeted by the percentage of deaths that helmets do not prevent, in this case by 63 percent (100 percent – 37 percent helmet effectiveness). The fourth column in Table 16.1 estimates deaths avoided among riders with

Table 16.1. 2008 Motorcycle Fatalities in the United States and Predicted Fatalities Without Helmet Use.

Actual and Predicted Scenarios	Helmet Used?			
	Yes	No	Unknown	Total
Actual Operator Deaths	2,855	1,990	130	4,975
Deaths If Nobody Wore a Helmet	4,532	1,990	175	6,697
Calculation of Number of Deaths If Nobody Wore a Helmet	2,855/ (1−.37)		130* (1,990 + 4,532)/ (1,990 + 2,855)	

unknown helmet use. This estimate assumes that helmet use was comparable among cyclist fatalities with unknown and known helmet use. In that case, the number of deaths that would have occurred if no one in this group wore a helmet equals the number of deaths with unknown use times the deaths if none of the riders with known helmet use had worn a helmet divided by the actual number of deaths of riders with known helmet use.

Risk is computed as the number of deaths or injuries divided by exposure. To translate the gains from helmet wearing displayed in Table 16.1 into estimates of risk reduction per helmet, we divide by the number of helmets. To do that, we need to estimate the number of helmets in use. A 2008 survey estimated that 10.4 million motorcycles were in use in the United States with 25 million regular or occasional riders (Motorcycle Industry Council, 2009). If we assume one regular operator per motorcycle, with a helmet shared if a cycle has multiple operators, then 10.4 million helmets were in use. In that case, the annual fatality risk of unhelmeted operation is 6,697 deaths if nobody wore a helmet divided by 10,400,000 helmets. If everyone wore a helmet, helmets would prevent 37 percent of the deaths, so the risk reduction from helmet use is 37% * 6,697/0,400,000 = .000238.

We can make similar estimates for non-fatal brain injuries. Johnson and Walker (1996) reported the ratio of hospitalized non-fatal brain injuries to fatalities as 135/132 among unhelmeted motorcyclists in six states during the 1990–1992 time period. Multiplying the fatality count times this ratio suggests 6,849 brain injuries would have occurred if no one used a helmet in 2008 (6,697 * 135/132). Recall that helmets prevent an estimated 69 percent of non-fatal brain injuries. Thus the annual brain injury risk reduction from wearing a helmet would be 0.000454 (6,849 * 69%/10,400,000). Keep in mind these risk levels are averages and vary with miles ridden, both because exposure increases and because more experienced or regular riders may have lower risks. And a rider who avoids death may be non-fatally injured instead.

Step 8: Calculate and Value Benefits

The type of economic evaluation selected for a given study determines how benefits are calculated and valued. In cost-effectiveness analysis, the benefit measure (for example, the gain in health-related outcomes) can be the increase in a final outcome measure (that is, the benefits may be the number of lives, life years, or QALYs saved) or in an intermediate measure (that is, the percentage of cigarette vendors who refuse to sell to minors or the number of motorcycle riders who begin wearing helmets). The cost-effectiveness measure is computed by dividing the cost of the intervention by this non-monetary benefit measure. When evaluating public health programs, typically some portion of the benefits are reductions in resource costs such as medical costs, property damage, police response, or attorney fees in liability lawsuits. For prevention of illegal acts such as violence, impaired driving, and serving alcohol to underage patrons, reduced adjudication and sanctioning costs add to the resource-cost-saving benefits. Decision makers are interested in how much of the cost of the intervention is offset by resource cost reductions, which represent tangible financial benefits. For example, when the Consumer Product Safety Commission estimated baby walkers that had been redesigned to prevent stairway falls cost $4 more than traditional baby walkers and resulted in benefits that included medical cost savings averaging $17 per walker (Rodgers & Leland, 2008), it was easy to understand why the Commission required the redesign. For this reason, it is preferable for a cost-effectiveness analysis to subtract benefits that can be expressed as resource cost savings from the intervention costs before dividing by the non-monetary outcome measure. When conducting a cost-effectiveness analysis, it thus is desirable to separately estimate financial benefits that can be expressed as resource cost reductions as well as measure non-monetary benefits.

In cost-utility analysis, the most commonly used benefit measure is a final outcome, the number of QALYs gained or saved. QALYs are routinely used as benefit measures by many regulatory agencies that incorporate economic evaluation into their decision-making processes, and in clinical trials of pharmaceuticals and medical treatment protocols. QALYs are calculated on the basis of two factors: the gain in quality of life and the number of life years over which the gain is sustained (Miller & Hendrie, 2012). Several generic quality-of-life instruments have been developed to use in measuring quality of life (McDowell, 2006) or alternatively, techniques are available to measure quality of life directly. An alternative comprehensive measure of health outcomes is disability adjusted life years (DALYs), which are primarily a measure of disease burden but are also commonly used in economic evaluation studies. A DALY typically equals one minus a QALY.

Benefit-cost analysis expresses health outcomes in monetary values, so the overall analysis of the costs and benefits of an intervention can be conducted in dollars or other currency values. The generally preferred method to place monetary values on health gains in benefit-cost analysis is called *willingness to pay*. The willingness-to-pay approach involves assessing what people actually pay or say they would pay for changes in their health status or for small changes in the risk of injury or death. Thus it values the fatality risk reduction resulting from passage or enforcement of a public health law, not the preservation of a known life. If one makes an unrealistic assumption that the value of a QALY is independent of a person's age (that is, that the loss of six months of quality of life is valued the same at age eighteen and at age eighty-eight) and independent of the type of risk involved (for example, cancer versus heart attack), one can monetize the QALY gains so that they can be treated as benefits in a benefit-cost analysis. The QALY includes health-related work loss, but it may be preferable to value that wage-related loss separately and explicitly in a benefit-cost analysis—the approach we take in our examples in this chapter. Doing so reduces the impact of the age-independence assumption because the wage loss can be tailored by age. This chapter presents both monetized QALY gains for use in the benefit-cost analysis and non-monetized gains for use in the cost-effectiveness analysis. (For details on QALY measurement and valuation methods, see Drummond, Sculpher, Torrance, O'Brien, & Stoddart, 2005; Miller & Hendrie, 2012).

Four ethical issues arise in valuing fatality risk, work losses, and QALY losses averted by public health laws. All are fraught with significant political hazard. They require delicate handling in economic analyses of public health laws and regulations. First, although wages, household work, and lifespan vary by age, sex, and race, these are differences resulting, in part, from discrimination. White males earn more than women or minority males, but that does not mean government should place a higher value on the life of a white male than on another citizen. The U.S. Department of Transportation, for example, decided against placing a higher value on the lives of air travelers than automobile drivers, because the value difference results from an income difference. Government, they reasoned, should not place a higher value on a wealthy citizen than on a pauper (Ackerman & Heinzerling, 2004; McCormick Jr. & Shane, 1993; Sunstein, 2004; Viscusi, 1994). Remaining lifespan varies with age simply as a result of basic biology, not discrimination. Analysts, therefore, often use a constant value per life-year, which implicitly places lower values on elderly than young lives (Johansson-Stenman & Martinsson, 2008). Nevertheless, a firestorm erupted when the U.S. Environmental Protection Agency (EPA), at the U.S. Office of Management and Budget's (OMB) urging, made that relationship explicit in analyzing a regulation that would avoid respiratory deaths of elderly people (Seelye, 2003; Viscusi, 2009). The public reaction forced EPA to return to using the same value for the life of any adult citizen, regardless of age.

The second ethical issue arises from the discounting of future costs and benefits. Because death and permanent disability create a lifetime's worth of work and QALY losses, these losses are reported as present values. Discounting reduces the value of future losses below the value of current losses. An environmental regulation that addresses global climate change is concerned with outcomes over the centuries. At a 3 percent discount rate, the present value of losses a century from now is 5.35 percent of the actual loss. The ethical question is whether we have the right to significantly harm future generations in order to avoid making small sacrifices now. In analyzing public health laws and actions with lasting consequences, a number of authors suggest that the discounting clock start as those affected are born (Cowen, 1992; Cowen & Parfit, 1992; Schelling, 1995). Cowen (2001) argues convincingly that intragenerational and intergenerational discount rates should be the same. In other words, just because they are further out into the future, the health and well-being of future generations should not be discounted more than future benefits that accrue to those currently alive.

The third ethical issue is related to the role of national borders. People disagree on responsibility to illegal immigrants and people living in countries other than their own. They debate whether illegal immigrants who pay taxes should be entitled to government services including medical care and education. Environmental regulatory analyses often include separate estimates of the domestic and world impacts (U.S. Interagency Working Group on Social Cost of Carbon & Government, 2010). When the United States tightens a workplace toluene exposure law, for example, it may merely shift the exposure to an Asian or Mexican worker rather than achieving a net worker health gain. Regulatory analyses in the United States typically ignore this risk migration.

Finally, valuation inherently involves a mix of science and ethical judgment. No clear line divides better regulatory analysis values from advocacy-driven values. The EPA, for example, always has chosen a higher willingness-to-pay value than other agencies for fatal risk reduction. It is unclear to what extent this reflects better science versus enthusiasm for justifying environmental regulation. Or, people may object more to risk of disability from ambient air pollution they feel they cannot control, compared to risk of disability from a car crash they feel they can control. Some analysts suggest valuing the risk reduction of death from dreaded causes more than other causes, with nuclear accidents and terrorism leading candidates. In this vein, the EPA suggested doubling the value of fatal risk reduction for cancer (Interagency Working Group on Social Cost of Carbon & Government, 2010). This decision would greatly reduce allowable levels of toxic pollutants. John Graham, who headed OMB's regulatory oversight during the Bush administration, questioned the wisdom of the "cancer premium . . . in light of the reluctance of citizens to monitor for radon in their homes, enroll in cancer screening programs, and eat their fruits and vegetables on a daily basis" (Borenstein, 2011).

Table 16.2. Estimated Costs and Benefits per Year by Riding Helmeted.

	Medical	Other Resource	Work	Quality of Life	Total Dollars	Quality Adjusted Life Years	Annual Risk Reduction if Helmeted
Costs							
Fatality	$36,786	$208,119	$1,202,809	$2,685,269	$4,132,983	20.98	.000238259
Hospitalized Brain Injury	$135,087	$71,985	$111,595	$409,102	$727,769	3.20	.000454423
Annual Benefits							
Societal Perspective	$70	$82	$337	$826	$1,315	0.0065	
Internal Perspective	$10	$0	$160	$826	$996	0.0065	
External Perspective	$60	$82	$177	$0	$319	0	
Government Perspective	$17	$1	$33	$0	$51	0	

Note: All costs and benefits are in 2010 dollars. Benefits are costs avoided by helmet use from each perspective.

Now we'll return to our helmet example. We tabulated costs and QALY losses per motorcycle death from the database underlying the work of Miller and colleagues (2011). Similar estimates for a hospitalized brain injury came from Miller and colleagues (2009). We adjusted the costs to 2010 dollars using three indices: two Consumer Price Indexes (CPIs), one for all items and the other specific to medical care, and the Employment Cost Index for total compensation for all private workers. These price indexes are published monthly by the U.S. Bureau of Labor Statistics. For example, the medical cost per critical brain injury = $249,356 * CPImedical2010/CPImedical2002 = 249,356 * 388.25/260.8 = $371,213. Table 16.2 shows the estimated costs by cost category.

Given these costs of death and brain injury and the annual risk reduction estimates, the average motorcycle operator's helmet was estimated to avert $1,315 in injury costs annually. We computed the benefits from internal, external, and government perspectives using payer matrices (Blincoe, Seay, Zaloshnja, et al., 2002; Miller & Hendrie, 2012). A rationale for a public health law mandating helmet use is that citizens other than the rider pay a total of $319 per year (from "external perspective" row in Table 16.2) in medical, other resource, and wage replacement costs for the average rider who does not wear a helmet (Miller, 1994).

Earlier we assumed a helmet has a five-year life. Statistical tables are available that provide the present value factors of a given monetary amount received each year. A present value factor is the "multiplier" that when multiplied by the amount received each year gives the present value of the cash flows. The present value factor for five years at a discount rate of 3 percent is $1 + 1/1.03 + 1/1.03^2 + 1/1.03^3 + 1/1.03^4 = 4.717$. The average present value of the benefits stream from using a motorcycle helmet thus is $6,205.

Step 9: Compute the Cost-Outcome Measure

Cost-outcome measures are the metric used in economic evaluation to compare benefits of an intervention such as a public health law with its costs. In calculating cost-outcome measures, an incremental approach is typical, with the additional net costs that one alternative imposes over another compared with the additional benefits provided. The ratio of the additional costs over the additional benefits is termed the incremental cost-effectiveness ratio (ICER). For example, results of a cost-effectiveness analysis evaluating the introduction of a law reducing the times of sale of alcohol could be reported as the additional net cost (that is, the intervention costs minus the financial benefits resulting from resource cost reductions) per additional injury averted. If QALYs were being used as the health outcome measure, then the ICER would be reported as the additional net cost per additional QALY gained. If the financial benefits from resource cost reductions following the introduction of the law exceed the costs involved in implementing and enforcing the law, no ICER needs to be calculated and the *net cost savings* (that is, the costs minus the financial benefits) and injuries averted or QALYs gained can be reported separately.

In the case of benefit-cost analysis, a choice of measures can be used to determine which option provides the best value for money. The first measure, the benefit-cost ratio, equals the benefits divided by the costs. It shows the return per dollar invested. For example, the All Stars substance abuse education program for middle schools has a benefit-cost ratio of 34, while its competitor Project Northland has a benefit-cost ratio of 17 (Miller & Hendrie, 2009). Thus All Stars returns twice as many benefits per dollar spent. The second measure, net benefits, equals the benefits minus the costs. This measure is important to consider in conjunction with the benefit-cost ratio when using an economic analysis to guide a choice among alternatives. In our example, All Stars costs $140 per pupil and returns $4,760 in benefits for a net benefit of $4,620 per pupil. Project Northland costs $400 per pupil and yields $6,800 in benefits for a net benefit of $6,400. All Stars offers the largest return per dollar invested, but Project Northland produces a larger reduction in youth substance abuse and yields a larger net benefit per person. If a school system can afford Project Northland, it will yield a larger reduction in the underlying problem and greater net benefits.

A benefit-cost ratio or net benefit calculation needs to value quality-of-life gains in dollar terms (Gold, Siegel, Russell, & Weinstein, 1996). These gains measure the good health preserved. Ignoring them provides a distorted underestimate of the return on investment that should never be used in allocating resources between competing interventions. For example, suppose the government is deciding whether to mandate bumpers that will withstand higher-speed impacts without damage. Those bumpers will reduce vehicle repair costs but will increase injury severity when cars hit pedestrians. To justify the mandate, the analysis must show the repair cost reduction is larger than the quality-of-life losses as well as the more tangible injury costs.

In our helmet example, we compute the discounted cost-outcome measures from the helmet cost of $25.33 per year for five years ($119/4.717) and the benefits per helmet per year from Table 16.2. Table 16.3 shows formulas used to compute the cost-outcome measures and the associated estimates. From a societal perspective, the net cost of a helmet is less than zero. The financial benefits from reduced medical and other resource costs save society more than the helmet costs; the helmet offers a net cost savings. Moreover, from the internal perspective of the helmet user, the cost per QALY gained is only $2,286, and thus only a small fraction of the estimated $127,989 monetary value of a QALY. This figure is inflated to 2010 dollars, and used when valuing quality of life in the crash costs in Table 16.2.

Society saved money when a motorcyclist rode helmeted. The rider also realized an excellent return on investment in the helmet. Note that on average,

Table 16.3. Cost-Outcome Estimates for Voluntary Motorcycle Helmet Use from Various Perspectives.

Measure	Benefit-Cost Ratio (Benefits/ Costs)	Net Benefit (Benefits − Costs)	Cost per QALY Saved (Costs − Medical Savings − Other Resource Savings)/QALYs Gained
Societal Perspective	$1,315/ $25.33 = 51.9	$1,315 − $25.33 = $1,290	$25.33 − $70 − $82 is less than $0; net cost savings
Internal Perspective	$996/ $25.33 = 39.3	$996 − $25.33 = $971	($25.33 − $10)/0.0065 = $2,286
Adjusted for Perceived Risk	$319/ $25.33 = 24.1	$319 − $25.33 = $584	($25.33 − .612 * $10)/ (0.0065 * .612) = $4,827

people underestimate their risks of crash injuries. Blomquist (1982) estimates that perceived risk is only 61.2 percent of the actual risk, so motorcyclists will perceive a smaller benefit from wearing a helmet than they actually get. From the last row of Table 16.3, a benefit-cost ratio of 24 based on perceived risk means that the average rider will perceive that voluntarily wearing a helmet will return more than $24 per dollar invested, while the actual benefit ratio (from the second row of Table 16.3) is 39.

Step 10: Conduct a Sensitivity Analysis

Every economic evaluation suffers from uncertainty. Cost estimates, effectiveness estimates, and benefit values are imprecise. More important, cost-outcome analyses involve assumptions (for example, we chose to use a 3 percent discount rate) and controversial methods with alternative approaches (for example, the way to value QALYs). Sensitivity analysis deals with uncertainty; it tests whether plausible changes in selected estimates or assumptions affect results of the analysis. Sometimes cost-effectiveness analysts also use statistical bootstrapping methods to estimate a confidence interval around cost-effectiveness measures (Drummond, Sculpher, Torrance, O'Brien, & Stoddart, 2005).

Sensitivity analysis is especially important in analyses assessing proposed public health laws. Effectiveness of legislated interventions varies with enforcement and media coverage. As Figure 14.4 illustrates, effects can decay over time or slowly ramp up. A U.S. law requiring that cars sense when tire inflation is low, for example, yielded no benefits until the Federal government developed implementing regulations, allowed public comment on them, issued them, and allowed auto manufacturers more than a year to implement them. Even when implemented, the auto fleet's safety only improved as people replaced old cars with new ones. The replacement rate was affected by the economy, as was the number of miles driven per vehicle-year. When driving intensity changed, the rate of benefit accrual changed too. Finally, changes in medical care and in other safety features (for example, addition of side airbags) reduced the frequency and consequences of the crashes that the sensors were projected to prevent.

In our helmet example, we tested sensitivity of the results to helmet costs. Excluding time spent buying a helmet from the costs raised the benefit-cost ratio from 51.6 to 61.6. Assuming a four-year helmet life lowered the ratio to 41.8.

Special Issues in Economic Evaluation of Public Health Laws

Economic evaluations of public health laws involve decisions and challenges that rarely arise in economic analyses of health care programs and practices. They include methods to value a variety of subtle intangible costs that a law imposes on people by shaping their behavior directly; costs of passing and implementing a law; costs of enforcement and sanctioning; unanticipated costs and benefits; and non-health benefits such as employment or educational benefits.

Intangible Costs

Laws shape or restrict personal choices. They put the common good above individual desires. Public health laws sometimes impose discomfort and inconvenience. They can reduce mobility, increase travel time, impinge on freedom of choice, or deny access to accustomed pleasures. These largely intangible effects count as societal costs. Some are easier to value than others.

INCONVENIENCE AND DISCOMFORT

Inconvenience tends to be either extra expense or extra time spent in completing a task. For example, it can be the four seconds spent putting on a safety belt, or the time and money spent on a way to securely store a motorcycle helmet when parking a cycle away from home. The value of time has been widely studied, so these savings can be valued. In particular, around the world, the value of travel time is deemed to be 50 to 60 percent of the wage rate and of unplanned delay time to be 60 to 90 percent of the wage rate (Kruesi, 1997; Waters & William 1996). Thus one can value most inconveniences in dollar terms. Seemingly irrational choices to not use safety devices with benefits that exceed the purchase price result from the failure to value discomfort and inconvenience, meaning these intangibles can be valued by analyzing usage decisions.

In terms of our helmet example, many motorcyclists do not wear helmets even though the individual benefits they think they will get from a helmet (based on their perceived risk levels) show a helmet would clearly save them money or quality of life. This seemingly irrational behavior results because the analysis has not priced the intangibles, the costs of discomfort, inconvenience, and loss of freedom associated with helmet use. We estimated values for the intangibles from Blomquist and colleagues' (1996) analysis of usage decisions. They estimate that the inconvenience costs of putting on and taking off a helmet each trip equal $48/year (1.3481 hours/year * $22.23/hour in 1991 dollars * 1.601 inflator to 2010 dollars). Blomquist and colleagues developed a formula to combine with survey interview data to support an estimate of the combined value of discomfort and inconvenience costs. With the current 48 percent probability that a rider wears a helmet in states without helmet laws (National Highway Traffic Safety Administration, 2010), the combined value is $540.

The calculations involved are quite complex. Blomquist's estimate is (willingness to pay of $1,333,000 per death averted * .0002264 lives saved/helmet/year − .05 * $355.18 net benefit from helmet use) * 1.601 inflator to 2010 dollars, where the coefficient − .05 is the probit score that corresponds to a 48 percent probability. As a check on these costs, our estimates in Table 16.3 ignored the costs of discomfort and inconvenience associated with a helmet that someone wore voluntarily. A rational rider would not wear a helmet if those costs exceeded the benefits. Since 52 percent of riders travel unhelmeted in states without helmet laws, the $584 in perceived net benefits of helmet use should closely approximate the median discomfort and inconvenience costs. And indeed, they are reasonably close to our $540 estimate of these costs. Blomquist and colleagues (1996) also provide a way to value the freedom lost when helmet use is mandated. From the helmet use choices of motorcyclists, it estimates they value fatality risk at $1,333,000 per death (in 1991 dollars). It estimates that motorists' choices about safety belt use suggest a higher value of $2,213,000 per death. If we assume motorcyclists value their lives as highly as anyone else, the difference between these values results from the value motorcyclists place on the discomfort, inconvenience, and loss of freedom when a law mandates helmet use. The annual loss is valued at $915 per person whom a law forces to wear a helmet (estimated with the formula above and the higher value of life). Thus the inconvenience is an estimated $48, the discomfort cost $492 ($540 − $48), and the value of lost freedom $375 ($915 − $540).

An unresolved issue about these estimates is their duration, in that inconvenience costs will persist. Conversely, the discomfort costs are likely to decline over time. Most drivers become so accustomed to a safety belt that they eventually feel uncomfortable driving without its light pressure. Similarly, the discomfort of a motorcycle helmet on a hot day may be offset by the warmth and protection it provides on a cold or breezy day. In the analyses that follow, we assume that a new user's helmet discomfort costs fall by 25 percentage points per year to a stable level equal to 25 percent of the initial loss. We treat loss of freedom resulting from a law as a one-time loss due to a legislated change in standing.

MOBILITY

Mobility is much easier to value than inconvenience or discomfort. We could value the miles foregone at the federal reimbursement rate per mile driven in a personal vehicle inclusive of vehicle maintenance and amortization. In valuing the cost of raising the age for a driver's license, for example, we first could estimate what portion of travel would be foregone and what portion would be provided by older family and friends. We could value transportation by others by assuming average suburban travel speeds and pricing driver time at the average value for household work (Grosse, Krueger, & Mvundura, 2009). That approach represents a lower bound. If failing an eye exam at license renewal forces an elderly person to stop driving, the person loses not only mobility but independence. As another example, single-trip mobility losses for when an intoxicated person does not drive home are generally priced at the cost of alternative transportation, including the trip to retrieve the car.

JOY OF INTOXICATION

A particularly difficult, yet important intangible loss is the loss of the joy of intoxication. Alcohol is the only legal intoxicant. Because no similar legal goods exist, forced reductions in alcohol consumption can cause far larger consumer losses than restricting consumer access to goods for which close substitutes exist (Jonathan Caulkins, personal communication with Ted Miller, January 2011). Raising alcohol taxes or limiting promotion pricing or volume pricing such as happy hours shifts the price of alcohol. As Chapter 7 explains, it shifts the supply curve. Consumers incur virtually the same expense as before but get to consume less alcohol. Economics has relatively straightforward ways to estimate the resulting loss in consumer surplus if one can estimate the shape of the supply and demand curves.

The situation is different if one artificially restricts supply by limiting sales hours, outlet density, or alcohol advertising. In that case, consumers buy less alcohol than they want to at the offered price. Unlike interventions that raise prices, these restrictions leave money in consumers' pockets. They spend that money on second-best substitute goods or buy their alcohol at less convenient times and places. To the extent that they buy less alcohol, the loss is the difference in utility of alcohol versus the substitute good. The question then becomes how much of the enjoyment from drinking alcohol cannot be replaced by instead eating an ice cream cone or watching a movie or playing with a puppy. Because alcohol is the only readily available legal intoxicant, we conservatively suggest assuming that the loss is quite high, 50 percent of the retail price of the alcohol they did not buy (in the United States, a loss of $0.60 per drink foregone in 2010 dollars). The choice of 50 percent has political appeal. Half of the retail sales price of a drink equals the profits realized above production costs by producers, wholesalers, and retailers (Miller Brewing Company, 2000). Using this value ensures that the cost estimate used for the law accounts for all profits foregone by the alcohol industry. This value is an overestimate of producer and seller losses because it ignores the increased profits of the industries that sell the substitute goods. The 50 percent estimate probably is high, and thus conservative, from the consumer's perspective as well. If the reduction results from constraints on alcohol outlet density, for example, then the consumer chose to forego the alcohol purchase rather than travel to a less convenient outlet. The value of the alcohol foregone was less than the added travel cost.

CHILD DISCOMFORT AND INCONVENIENCE

As parents, we are quite comfortable ignoring child comfort and convenience when regulating child welfare. Unlike restrictions on adult choices, therefore, laws that regulate child behavior tend to be viewed as cost-free protection of those not mature enough to make wise choices. We put health and safety first. For example, almost all bicycle helmet laws and many motorcycle helmet laws apply only to children and youths. In costing a child car safety seat, one would consider shopping time, purchase price, the time spent putting the child into and out of the seat, the safety gained, and possibly the greater ease of driving without a child crawling around the car. One would not consider whether the child would be happier if unrestrained and count that loss in happiness as a cost of the law requiring child restraints.

Costs of Passage and Implementation

Analysis of the passage of a law requires choosing a *counterfactual*. The counterfactual is the scenario that is compared with the scenario if the law passes. It may simply be the status quo, but it could be a non-legislative approach to problem reduction. In the latter case, the analysis needs to consider the probability that the law will pass and how long it will take before it becomes effective. Regardless of the counterfactual, the analysis should include passage and implementation costs.

Downing (1981) estimates the costs of passing a law and issuing any required implementing regulations. The estimated costs of approving mandates are 2.9 to 7.1 percent of the first-year direct costs imposed on the public. Variation within this range depends on how many vertical legislative and administrative levels must act on the program, how controversial the program is, and how many groups it will adversely affect. These same factors affect probability of passage and delay before the law is enacted and implemented. If one takes a national perspective, the cumulative adoption rate of a model law is likely to resemble an S-shaped or cumulative normal curve (Gray, 1973; Rogers, 1962). Initially a few states will pass the law; then passage will gather speed; finally it will taper off, with some states possibly never passing the law. Discussions with legislators, government legislative liaisons, and lobbyists can yield reasonable estimates of adoption likelihood and timing. Their judgment can be supplemented with data on the delay involved in passing or rejecting other legislation. The best comparison would be a legislative proposal on related subject matter, or roughly equal in scale and controversy, and likely to bring forth the same pro and con coalitions.

Downing (1981) estimates public implementation and administration will cost another 4.2 to 4.6 percent. Miller and colleagues (1985) assessed the actual public implementation and administrative costs to mandate high-mounted center rear brake lights on cars to reduce rear-end crashes. They enumerated fifteen work tasks and seventy-two comments to the regulatory docket involved in implementing this $90 million regulation and estimated the cost was $3.7 to $4.0 million, or 4.1 to 4.4 percent. Expected costs could be substantially higher if the law or regulation were challenged in court (for example, mandatory health insurance). Implementation costs for laws often are available in budget estimates provided to the legislature. When an estimate is not readily available, Downing's percentages offer a convenient and efficient way to estimate passage and implementation costs.

And now, we revisit our helmet example. Recall we estimated the first-year costs of buying and riding with a motorcycle helmet at $940, including $25 in out-of-pocket costs and $915 in intangible costs. The large intangible costs suggest the costs of passing a helmet law will be at the high end of Downing's range; conversely, implementation should be relatively easy and inexpensive. This suggests costs of passage and implementation might be 11 percent of first-year usage costs, or $101. Table 16.4 shows the total costs of a helmet law from several perspectives, including the intangible and public costs and the associated savings.

Table 16.4 shows that the motorcycle law is quite appealing from the perspective of government and of those who do not ride motorcycles. It costs them relatively little (just $101 per new helmet user) and allows them to escape paying large bills associated with motorcyclist brain injuries (benefit-cost ratios of 2.4 and 14.9). From the viewpoint of the motorcyclists whom the law forces to wear helmets, the law is at best marginally beneficial with a benefit-cost ratio of 1.4 based on the injury risk levels that motorcyclists perceive and a cost per QALY gained of more than $100,000. Given these figures, it is not surprising that

Table 16.4. Costs and Cost-Outcome Estimates per Newly Helmeted Rider for a Motorcycle Helmet Law (in 2010 dollars).

Measure	Cost per New User (Over five years)	Benefit-Cost Estimate	Net Benefit	Cost/QALY Saved
Societal Perspective	$2,125	2.9	$4,080	$46,203
Ignoring Loss of Freedom	$1,750	3.5	$4,455	$33,879
Internal Perspective	$2,024	2.3	$2,676	$64,946
Based on Perceived Risk	$2,024	1.4	$853	$107,075
External Perspective	$101	14.9	$1,404	Net saving
Government Perspective	$101	2.4	$140	$2,480

many states have repealed their helmet laws despite the life-saving benefits and taxpayer savings that these laws offer.

Enforcement and Sanctioning Costs

A public health law's cost and effectiveness also are functions of enforcement and publicity. Those efforts tend to be fairly level across laws, except possibly for laws passed in response to federal incentives. Perhaps as a result, laws requiring use of safety devices—child seats, safety belts, helmets—fairly predictably increase use by 30 to 40 percentage points (Blomquist, Miller, & Levy, 1996; National Highway Traffic Safety Administration, 2010).

A further issue in analyses of safety device mandates is the possibility of misuse. Civil disobedience and legal loopholes, for example, led to motorcycle helmets worn on knees. Discomfort leads some people to put the shoulder harness of a safety belt behind them or hold it away from their body. Misuse also can be unintentional. For example, child safety seats often are installed incorrectly; a decade of misuse campaigns and misuse-oriented seat design improvements resulted in a rise from 52 percent to 82 percent effectiveness in rear seating positions (Zaloshnja & Miller, 2007). The effectiveness estimates underlying the analysis may need to be reduced to account for misuse.

With Trumbull's rules on standing, gains from the illegal acts foregone because of enforcement unequivocally are not costs to wrongdoers. Many criminologists view the purpose of incarceration and probation as prevention, not punishment. Both fear of sanctioning and supervision of past offenders deter crime. Even if sanctioning costs borne by the government are costs of prevention rather than costs of a specific criminal incident, they count in the cost-outcome analysis. But what about sanctioning costs borne by criminals? Does the criminal's lack of standing mean that if a fine covers court costs or the drunk driver pays for the ignition interlock on his car, these payments are not costs to society? If so, they should be omitted from the cost-outcome analysis. We agree with Cohen (1998, 2000) that these costs are societal costs. Productivity would increase if government did not have to process citations and levy fines.

Whether to count the wage losses that a criminal experiences while incarcerated is less clear. Cohen counts them as costs of crime, but we suspect he errs. Because the economy rarely is at full employment, the criminal will be replaced by another worker. While the criminal's family has less income, the family of the replacement has more. The criminal's employer will experience some costs in the process, primarily costs related to hiring and training a replacement worker. Gramlich's (1981) classic work on the return on investment in government programs suggests employer costs will ripple, with a series of people getting better jobs and a low-skilled person ultimately escaping unemployment. Friction costs value the employer costs and typically are around 30 percent of the associated wage loss (Berger, Murray, Xu, & Pauly, 2001; Koopmanschapp, Rutten, van Ineveld, & van Roijen, 1995; Lofland, Pizzi, & Frick, 2004). Because friction costs are difficult to estimate, a simpler second-best approach is to estimate the costs of hiring someone to replace the criminal.

Unexpected Costs and Benefits

Laws can have unforeseen or unevaluated consequences. Economists call these *spillover costs and benefits*. For example, bicycling dropped in Australia following implementation of a helmet law (Robinson, 2006). In several places, mandatory motorcycle helmet laws reduced motorcycle theft; thieves who wanted to joyride rarely had a helmet handy and were likely to be apprehended if they rode without one (Insurance Institute for Highway Safety, 2011). At a minimum, limitations sections of economic analyses need to consider these spillover costs and benefits. Highway safety laws are especially prone to have unevaluated spillover effects. Does reducing the maximum legal driver blood alcohol content to 0.08 or 0.05, for example, shift drinking locations, in the process reducing barroom brawls but increasing domestic violence? Voas and Kelley-Baker (2008) describe a broad range of unevaluated benefits that might result from the youth driving curfews in graduated licensing laws, such as reduced drinking, drug use, risky sex, and violence.

Non-Health Benefits of Public Health Laws

Recall that the denominator used in computing net cost per QALY gained subtracts those financial benefits that can be valued in dollars from the intervention costs. The literature makes one important exception (Gold, Siegel, Russell, & Weinstein, 1996). Medical treatment and preventive health services result in improved physical and mental health that allows people to work more and earn more. The QALY gain values their improvements not only in physical and mental functioning but in role functioning and ability to work, play, and socialize. That means the health-related wage gains resulting from a public health law are included in the QALY gain; they are not separate benefits. They should not be subtracted from the intervention costs when computing cost per QALY gained. Subtracting them would double count the QALY gain (Gold, Siegel, Russell, & Weinstein, 1996).

Not all wage gains resulting from public health programs, however, are health related. Unlike medical treatment, "social policies often have effects that spill over from one domain to another, such as education and health investments that affect human capital and work effort" (Vining & Weimer, 2010, p. 4). For example, school financial assistance to orphans in Zimbabwe is designed to reduce early marriage and associated HIV transmission, but it also increases schooling and raises lifetime incomes (Hallfors, Cho, Rusakaniko, et al., 2011). Similarly, the Nurse Family Partnership intensive home visitation program to low-income mothers bearing their first child is designed primarily to improve child health outcomes (Olds, 2006). The program also provides job counseling that may increase maternal employment and earnings levels. Basing cost-effectiveness on QALYs includes the health-related earnings gains but does not include the wage gains from improved education or employment coaching. The handful of cost-effectiveness articles that have dealt with wage gains like this appropriately treat these benefits as gains over and above the QALY gains (Cheng, Rubin, Powe, et al., 2000; Frick, Carlson, Glass, et al., 2004; Miller & Hendrie, 2012). In computing cost per QALY saved, these wage gains should be treated as benefits that are subtracted from the intervention costs.

Comparing Cost-Outcome Estimates

In evaluating public health laws from an economic perspective, a comparison of benefit-cost ratios or incremental cost-effectiveness per QALY gained is a valuable aid in deciding which options represent optimum value for money invested (Miller & Hendrie, 2012). A table of comparable cost-outcome estimates is called a *league table*. Its side-by-side comparisons of economic evaluation results are most useful if the cost-effectiveness analyses have been undertaken specifically to facilitate between-treatment comparisons using standardized methods or if

(*Text continues on page 375*)

Table 16.5. League Table of Costs, Savings, Benefit-Cost Ratio, and Cost per QALY Gained for Public Health Laws, Enforcement, and Sanctioning (in 2010 dollars).

	Cost	Unit Studied	Medical	Other Resource	Work	Quality of Life	Total	Benefit-Cost Ratio	Cost Per QALY
Substance Use/Abuse Interventions									
20% Alcohol Tax	$11	Drinker per year	$5	$8	$28	$63	$104	9.5	< $0
30% Alcohol Tax	$22	Drinker per year	$6	$11	$36	$83	$136	6.2	$8,213
21 Minimum Legal Drinking Age	$207	Youths 18 to 20	$45	$83	$150	$457	$734	3.5	$22,256
Mandatory Server Training	$59	Driver	$12	$22	$46	$119	$199	3.4	$27,540
Enforce Serving Intoxicated Patron Law	$0	Driver	$3	$4	$8	$17	$31	68.8	< $0
TV Alcohol Advertising Ban	$6,253	Million population	$5,316	$3,196	$13,975	$34,719	$57,205	9.1	< $0
10% Outlet Density Reduction	$1,607	Million population	$1,329	$799	$3,494	$8,680	$14,301	8.9	< $0
Ten Fewer Sales Hours per Week	$3,933	Million population	$3,322	$1,997	$8,734	$21,699	$35,753	9.1	< $0
Retain State Stores as Sole Sellers of Beer and Wine in Pennsylvania	$0.46	Drink not consumed	$0.52	$0.31	$1.37	$3.39	$5.59	12.1	< $0

Program									
Workplace Peer Support and Drug Testing[1]	$77	Employee					$1,824	23.7	< $0
Add Alcohol Testing to Peer Support[1]	$13	Employee					$786	60.5	< $0

Crime Adjudication and Sanctioning

Youth Offender Programs

Program									
Sentence Youth to Multisystemic Therapy	$6,684	Client	$6,809	$0	$136,065	$115,938	$258,812	38.7	< $0
Sentence Youth to Functional Family Therapy	$3,045	Client	$2,535	$0	$50,663	$43,169	$96,367	31.6	< $0
Lansing Adolescent Diversion	$2,223	Client	$2,011	$0	$47,041	$37,923	$86,975	39.1	< $0
Intensive Probation Supervision, Youth	$2,211	Client	$263	$0	$5,066	$4,473	$9,802	4.4	< $0
Young Offender Boot Camp	$2,891	Client	−$837	$0	−$16,735	−$14,260	−$31,833	−11.0	Infinite

Adult Offender Programs

Program									
Drug Courts	$2,947	Client	$271	$0	$7,041	$4,716	$12,029	4.1	< $0
Optimized Sentencing of Drug Dealers	$16,920	Client	$1,412	$0	$5,751	$29,699	$36,863	2.2	$63,498
Three Strikes and You're Out Sentencing	$22,806	Client	$1,412	$0	$5,751	$29,699	$36,863	1.6	$88,376
Sentence Adults to Moral Reconation Therapy	$421	Client	$374	$0	$6,187	$6,322	$12,882	30.6	< $0
Sentence Adults to Reasoning and Rehabilitation	$436	Client	$106	$0	$2,200	$1,783	$4,089	9.4	< $0
Intensive Probation Supervision, Adult	$4,925	Client	$166	$0	$3,791	$2,714	$6,671	1.4	$47,904

(continued)

Table 16.5 (continued)

	Cost	Unit Studied	Medical	Other Resource	Work	Quality of Life	Total	Benefit-Cost Ratio	Cost Per QALY
Driving Laws, Enforcement, and Sanctions									
.08% Driver Blood Alcohol Limit	$4	Driver	$3	$6	$13	$33	$55	13.8	< $0
Zero Alcohol Tolerance, Drivers Under 21	$39	Driver	$63	$98	$207	$601	$969	24.8	< $0
Sobriety Checkpoints	$12,309	Checkpoint	$5,555	$7,033	$14,899	$55,700	$83,187	6.8	< $0
Administrative License Revocation (ALR)	$3,604	ALR	$3,861	$5,173	$10,958	$40,748	$60,740	16.9	< $0
ALR with Per Se Law	$3,384	ALR	$4,615	$6,141	$13,010	$48,471	$72,237	21.3	< $0
Alcohol-Testing Ignition Interlock	$1,200	Interlock	$309	$596	$1,213	$4,879	$6,997	5.8	$7,753
DWI Offender Auto Impoundment	$1,027	Impoundment	$423	$613	$1,248	$3,296	$5,579	5.4	< $0
DWI Offender Electronic House Arrest	$1,797	House arrest	$251	$3,026	$763	$2,017	$6,058	3.4	< $0
DWI Intensive Probation and Treatment	$1,612	Probation	$496	$1,322	$1,181	$3,122	$6,121	3.8	< $0
Provisional Licensing and Midnight Driving Curfew	$86	Driver	$45	$112	$129	$398	$683	7.9	< $0
Change Driving Curfew to 10 P.M.	$164	Driver	$26	$67	$78	$239	$410	2.5	$37,765

Occupant Protection Laws

Pass Child Safety Seat Law, Ages 0 Through 4	$59	New user	$161	$152	$390	$1,547	$2,250	38.1	< $0
Pass Booster Seat Law, Ages 4 Through 7	$40	New user	$368	$225	$579	$1,375	$2,548	63.7	< $0
Pass Safety Belt Law	$351	New user	$296	$530	$1,363	$4,010	$6,199	17.7	< $0
Upgrade Secondary Belt Law to Primary	$351	New user	$296	$530	$1,363	$4,010	$6,199	17.7	< $0
Enhanced Belt Law Enforcement	$363	New user	$296	$530	$1,363	$4,010	$6,199	17.1	< $0
Require Driver Airbag	$437	Vehicle	$142	$162	$416	$1,220	$1,940	4.4	$13,925
Require Passenger Airbag	$226	Vehicle	$38	$38	$97	$285	$459	2.0	$67,307
Pass Motorcycle Helmet Law	$2,125	New user	$331	$388	$1,591	$3,895	$6,205	2.9	$46,203
Pass Bicycle Helmet Law, Ages 3 Through 14	$14	New user	$61	$59	$152	$318	$591	42.2	< $0
Pass Bicycle Helmet Law, Ages 15 and Over	$112	New user	$37	$24	$62	$164	$287	2.6	$39,854
Fire Prevention and Harm Reduction									
Childproof Cigarette Lighter Mandate	$0.05	Lighter	$0.41	$0.54	$0.81	$1.84	$3.61	78.1	< $0
Less Porous Cigarette Paper Mandate	$0.00014	Pack	$0.006	$0.003	$0.005	$0.062	$0.076	559.2	< $0
Pass Smoke Alarm Law	$49	New user	$10	$40	$111	$670	$827	17.0	< $0
Require Sprinkler System, New Colonial House	$2,502	New home	$80	$373	$755	$4,539	$5,747	2.3	$57,770

(continued)

Table 16.5 (*continued*)

	Cost	Unit Studied	Medical	Other Resource	Work	Quality of Life	Total	Benefit-Cost Ratio	Cost Per QALY
Require Sprinkler System, New Townhouse	$2,285	New home	$80	$373	$755	$4,539	$5,747	2.5	$51,650
Require Sprinkler System, New Ranch House	$999	New home	$80	$373	$755	$4,539	$5,747	5.8	$15,385
Mattress Flammability Standard	$27	Mattress	$0.67	$2.82	$10	$61	$75	2.8	$49,146
Other									
Tetanus-Diphtheria-Pertussis Vaccination, Ages 0 Through 6	$93	Child	$498	$0	$1,817	$0	$2,315	24.9	< $0
Baby Walker Redesign Mandate to Prevent Stairway Falls	$4	Walker	$17	$1	$17	$154	$190	47.5	< $0
Impact-Absorbing Playground Surfacing	$14,588	Playground	$3,442	$5,603	$100	$19,847	$28,992	2.0	$35,750

Note: < $0 means that the financial benefits from reduced medical and other resource costs exceed the costs of the intervention. The intervention yields a net cost saving.
[1]Benefits and costs to the employer rather than to society.
Source: Miller & Hendrie, 2009; Miller & Hendrie, 2012. All estimates were computed at the same discount rate and with comparably estimated benefit values.

results of economic evaluations of treatments have been adjusted and standardized to make comparisons meaningful. This is not always done in preparing cost-effectiveness league tables, with the result that studies in the same table may take different perspectives, use different discount rates, and so on. This often makes cost-effectiveness ratios in a league table non-comparable. A notable exception is a league table maintained for injury and substance abuse (Miller & Hendrie, 2009). Miller and Hendrie's tables currently include more than 160 interventions with estimates of cost per QALY saved and benefit-cost ratios computed at a 3 percent discount rate with consistently computed costs for injury, illness, and other societal ills. A notable feature of these tables is the assumption that replications of demonstration programs and randomized trials will achieve 25 percent less effectiveness than the original programs.

Table 16.5 is a league table of estimates for public health legislation and enforcement. All the values in this table were drawn from Miller and Hendrie (2009; Miller & Hendrie, 2012) or were computed for this chapter using their benefit estimates. Many of the estimates were developed using Downing's (1981) factors to cost law passage and implementation. Because intangible costs figure prominently in the estimates for laws governing adult behavior, we show them explicitly. In the table, < $0 means that the financial benefits from reduced medical and other resource costs exceed the costs of the intervention; the intervention yields a net cost savings.

Complexity in Communicating Economic Evaluation Results

It is essential to make sure champions of a proposed law understand which savings they can spend and which costs they must fund. Intangible costs tend to dominate the costs of many laws. While information about those costs provides insight into political acceptability, they are not out-of-pocket costs. It seems important to explicitly differentiate them from the tangible costs of the law. That avoids misleading the policy debate. Similarly, only financial benefits represent immediate out-of-pocket savings in resource costs. The rhetoric of the debate needs to avoid the impression that reduced work and quality-of-life losses will result in immediate economic gains.

Although economic analysis can help guide decisions about public health laws, these laws rarely are economic panaceas. Other than sin taxes that generate revenue, public health laws are unlikely to ease a budget crisis in the short run. Government, especially state government, pays only a small fraction of the health and safety bill.

Table 16.6 shows our estimates of the societal benefit-cost ratio (with costs restricted to government investments) required for the U.S. federal government and state governments to recover their costs. Governments rarely will save much money by passing road safety laws (Miller, Bhattacharya, Zaloshnja,

Table 16.6. Minimum Societal Ratios of Benefits to Government Costs Required for Government to Break Even on a Public Health Law or Program, by Public Health Problem Addressed and Level of Government.

Problem Addressed	Government	Federal	State or Local	Source
Violent Crime	5.9	39	6.9	Miller, Cohen, & Wiersema, 1996
Property Crime	1.4	14	1.5	Miller, Cohen, & Wiersema, 1996
Road Crash	15.1	26.7	34.5	Miller, Bhattacharya, Zaloshnja, et al., 2011
Alcohol Abuse	12.7	34.9	20.0	Miller & Hendrie, 2009
Underage Drinking	12.7	36.9	21.0	Miller & Hendrie, 2009
Drug Abuse	5.8	31.5	7.0	Miller & Hendrie, 2009
Smoking	5.6	7.2	25.9	Guilfoyle, 2011

Note: Computed from societal cost estimates or payer matrices in the sources shown. The cited estimates of costs of smoking to government excluded foregone taxes, which we computed from the societal wage loss and Census Bureau data on the percentage of earnings paid as taxes.

et al., 2011) or laws that reduce tobacco use. They will save more on interventions that prevent crime, reducing adjudication and sanctioning costs (which all directly accrue to the government). The return also will be greater for programs targeted to specific populations such as Medicaid recipients, because government garners virtually all of the medical care savings and may save on other related safety net payments.

The job of the state is to protect and enhance the welfare of its citizens. Government invests in medical treatment of illness to save lives and improve quality of life. Like medical care, preventive health and safety efforts are designed to save lives and increase quality of life. Public health laws and prevention programs save life years and improve quality of life at a small cost to government compared to most medical treatments. They should not be held to a higher standard of cost-effectiveness.

Conclusion

The role of economic evaluation is to assess costs and benefits of alternative options for meeting an objective. In many fields, this involves a relatively straightforward exercise of comparing the costs of alternative options and their benefits measured using an appropriate outcome measure. Steps involved in a typical economic evaluation were outlined in the first section of this chapter, which presented an example of an economic evaluation of voluntary use of a motorcycle helmet. As the subsequent sections illustrated, evaluating costs and benefits of public health laws is more complex than evaluation of personal or infrastructure decisions, with additional issues to be considered. Several factors contribute to the added complications of conducting economic evaluation of public health laws. These include the tradeoffs involved between protecting individual freedom and serving the common good, uncertainty in the magnitude of several of the parameters included in analyses, and spillover costs and benefits of public health regulation.

Despite complexities, careful economic evaluation of public health laws has an important role to play in informing policy decisions, by providing more accurate, explicit, and transparent estimates of costs and benefits of regulatory alternatives. While decisions regarding legal measures to safeguard the health of populations are inherently political—not just technical questions weighing up costs and benefits—economic evaluation of public health laws quantifies many of the tradeoffs involved in safeguarding the health of the public. Economic evaluations also guide closely related decisions regarding implementing regulations, enforcement strategies, and appropriate sanctions.

Summary

Policy decisions can be informed by information on anticipated costs and expected future benefits of courses of action. The key questions in economic evaluation of a public health law are whether its benefits, as measured by health outcomes or cost savings, exceed its costs; secondarily, there is the question of the distribution of those costs and benefits across stakeholders. Cost savings are concrete and understandable benefits, and they provide a single compact measure that captures wrecked cars, stolen statues, fractured arms, even deaths.

Economic evaluation begins with the selection of an intervention to be studied and a type of economic evaluation to use. Cost-effectiveness analysis uses naturally occurring outcomes to compare interventions with the same objective. The results are reported as the cost per life year saved or the cost per assault prevented. Cost-utility analysis is a special form of cost-effectiveness analysis in which the outcomes are measured using multidimensional measures of health outcomes such as quality adjusted life years (QALYs) that incorporate both quality and survival information. In cost-utility analysis, the evaluative measure is the cost per QALY gained or saved. Benefit-cost analysis is a third type of economic evaluation, in which all of the health outcomes are measured in monetary terms, with the results reported either as a benefit-cost ratio or as net benefits (that is, benefits minus costs).

An economic evaluation measures all costs and benefits in inflation-free dollars stated in a base year (for example, in 2010 dollars). An estimate of the costs of the various alternative options is computed. Relevant effectiveness measures are selected, ideally final outcomes such as impaired driving crashes averted, and effectiveness estimated. The benefits of the various options are calculated and valued, and then a cost-outcome measure is computed. Cost-outcome measures are the metric used in economic evaluation to compare benefits of an intervention such as a public health law with its costs. In calculating cost-outcome measures, an incremental approach is typical; with the additional net costs that one alternative imposes over another compared with the additional benefits provided. The ratio of the additional costs over the additional benefits is termed the incremental cost-effectiveness ratio (ICER). Sensitivity analysis is then deployed to deal with uncertainty; it tests whether plausible changes in selected estimates or assumptions affect results of the analysis.

Economic evaluations of public health laws involve decisions and challenges that rarely arise in economic analyses of health care programs and practices. They include methods to value a variety of subtle intangible costs that a law imposes on people by shaping their behavior directly, costs of passing and implementing a law, costs of enforcement and sanctioning, unmeasured anticipated costs and benefits (for example, if a driving curfew reduces crime), and non-health benefits such as employment or educational benefits. In evaluating public health laws from an economic perspective, a comparison of benefit-cost ratios or incremental cost-effectiveness per QALY gained is a valuable aid in deciding which options represent optimum value for money invested. Researchers also face the challenge of explaining the limits of cost analysis to policy champions.

Further Reading

Aos, S., Lieb, R., Mayfield, J., Miller, M., & Pennucci, A. (2004). *Benefits and costs of prevention and early intervention programs for youth.* Olympia, WA: Washington State Institute for Public Policy.

Gold, M. R., Siegel, J. E., Russell, L. B., & Weinstein, M. C. (Eds.). (1996). *Cost-effectiveness in health and medicine: Report of the panel on cost-effectiveness in health and medicine.* New York: Oxford University Press.

Miller, T. R., & Hendrie, D. (2012). Economic evaluation of interventions. In G. Li & S. Baker (Eds.), *Injury research: Theories, methods and approaches.* New York: Springer.

Trumbull, W. N. (1990). Who has standing in cost-benefit analysis? *Journal of Policy Analysis and Management, 9*(2), 201–218.

Vining, A., & Weimer, D. L. (2010). An assessment of important issues concerning the application of benefit-cost analysis to social policy. *Journal of Benefit-Cost Analysis,1*(1), Article 6.

Chapter 17

The Future of Public Health Law Research

Scott Burris   Alexander C. Wagenaar

Learning Objectives

- Formulate a rationale for the future development of public health law research as a field.

- Recognize potential future contributions of public health law research in improving population health.

Public health law research (PHLR) empirically studies the complicated ways that laws and legal practices influence health. Because both *law* and *public health* encompass a vast range of heterogeneous human activities, institutions, and environments, research methods serve as an important mechanism for building unity and coherence in the field. We may study very different laws, environments, and behaviors, but all of us in PHLR build on established theory to hypothesize and measure how legal inputs contribute to levels and distributions of health in the population. We help each other, and strengthen the field, by our efforts to explicitly and transparently define the concepts of interest; reliably and validly measure the processes under study; incorporate the strongest possible research design features to maximize plausibility of causal interpretations of observed relationships; and analyze the resulting data with the most advanced qualitative and statistical methods available. Better PHLR makes the field more attractive to new entrants, facilitates interdisciplinary collaboration, increases the chances the major health research funders will support research on law, and enhances the credibility of research results in scientific and policy-making communities. The chapters in this book suggest how far the field has come, and, as we discuss in this closing chapter, how much further we have to go.

Continuing Quality Improvement

A volume devoted to methods for PHLR is an unmistakable milestone in the development of the field—and, we are confident, one that will spur debate, criticism, new ideas, and continued improvement. Our work on this volume has pointed us to three particular needs as the field moves forward: further disciplinary integration on several axes; methods improvement in terms of further development of field-specific tools and approaches; and a broad effort to make progress in PHLR within a social determinants framework.

Disciplinary Integration

We hope and expect to see more researchers who will identify themselves as primarily focused on PHLR. A core group of dedicated specialists can give the field a clear identity, serving as the stewards of its history and standards. Given the interdisciplinary nature of the field, and the breadth of both law and health, however, the field's boundaries of necessity will continue to be fuzzy. We expect that many or even most of the researchers who identify themselves with the field will not be specialists in PHLR. Moreover, we see it as essential to the development of the field that *all* researchers who work in social and behavioral health be able and willing to integrate legal questions and legal variables into their research, even if the study is not primarily focused on law. For example, while a primary PHLR researcher might investigate whether laws that require the reporting of HIV test results deter people from being tested (Hecht, Chesney, Lehman, et al., 2000), it is equally (or possibly more) valuable for studies examining the behavior of people with HIV to consider including law as one possible influence among many (Myers, Orr, Locker, & Jackson, 1993). Law is rarely the main driver of behavior, but it is very rarely absent from an individual's environment.

The need for fuzzy integration extends as well toward non-health-related empirical legal research (Mello & Zeiler, 2008). The PHLR category of incidental public health law encompasses laws passed, or legal activities conducted, with little or no consideration of possible health consequences. It follows that research on the operation and outputs of such laws can contribute to the PHLR evidence base if data on health outcomes are included in the research scope. For example, many empirical legal scholars have investigated the implementation and effects of the Americans with Disabilities Act. Studies have documented the importance of the ADA and its enforcement processes to people with disabilities, including its effect on their sense of social position and the fairness of the system (Engel & Munger, 2003; Swanson, Burris, Moss, Ullman, & Ranney, 2006). From a PHLR perspective, we would expect that a law protecting basic social and employment rights of a people with a wide range of health conditions would have affective effects on people with disabilities, and would regard health outcomes of one kind or another to be important components of its overall impact. Criminology offers another example. The study of violence and its control by the police is a matter with obvious health implications (Ratcliffe, Taniguchi, Groff, & Wood, 2011). Criminologists themselves have addressed the overlap in proposing a discipline of epidemiological criminology (Akers & Lanier, 2009). Including actual or self-reported health outcomes associated with crime within the scope of empirical legal studies would enrich both legal and public health research.

Economists, criminologists, epidemiologists and other empirical scientists evaluating legal and policy effects would be well served by incorporating improved understanding of the sociology of law from sociolegal traditions. Law is much more than a specific statute or regulation, and a more nuanced conceptualization and understanding by health and social scientists of the nature of law and its meanings and diffused operation throughout all of society's major institutions would clearly advance the field of PHLR.

Another form of integration that is important to the future robustness and impact of the field encompasses empirical researchers and lawyers, including legal scholars who do not do empirical research. Lawyers are, we believe, crucial constituents of a multidisciplinary team for a number of reasons. As we discuss in Chapters 11 and 12, lawyers are usually indispensable to the accurate conceptualization and execution of processes to collect, code, and measure legal variables that meet scientific standards of reliability and validity. Lawyers bring to bear experience and knowledge about how legal systems work, and through training and socialization are professionally suited to identifying issues—including research questions—that other lawyers and legal decision makers are likely to deem important. The combination of legal mapping skills, a good eye for policy importance, and empirical analysis can produce hybrid legal research and empirical analysis that are both conceptually elegant and policy-relevant. Consider, for example, a classic study from the early days of PHLR. Teret and colleagues (1986) analyzed and categorized state law on child car restraints to determine the population covered. These legal data were then merged with Fatality Analysis Reporting System (FARS) data, which allowed the researchers to estimate the number of child fatalities among children who would have been protected by laws with fewer exemptions or a wider range of covered ages (Teret, Wells, Williams, & Jones, 1986). Integrated cross-disciplinary teams that combine lawyers with empirical social and health scientists are essential for continued advances in the theoretical sophistication and methodological quality of PHLR studies.

Methods Improvement

The section of this volume devoted to elucidating the "mechanisms of law" reflects our belief in the importance of opening the black box that too often fills the causal diagram between law and health effects in PHLR. Theories of how law works to change environments and behaviors can support more robust hypotheses and more confident causal inferences. We hope that the contributions of our authors will support that sort of improvement. As we worked on this volume, however, we identified several topics we expect will require more coverage in a future edition: the need to develop widely accepted standards and protocols for measuring law, and norms of archiving and sharing legal datasets; the need for further conceptual and operational clarity regarding indices and scales for measuring attributes of laws such as stringency; and diffusion of optimal research designs and methods across all topics in PHLR.

The two chapters focused on coding legal variables propose a variety of good practices in conducting, memorializing, and sharing the results of legal research. Anderson and coauthors in Chapter 11 suggest that creators of legal datasets routinely include certain basic attributes (such as exact dates a law takes effect or ceases to be in effect) and use widely accepted geographic tags (such as FIPS codes). Further conventions for consistent citation of statutes and regulations could also be useful. Anderson and colleagues also propose a norm of open-source legal data, in which datasets are posted with codebooks and detailed research protocols for replication by other researchers, who in turn post updated and expanded datasets including their own contributions. The idea is conceptually attractive, but even leaving aside issues of intellectual property and authorial incentives, the mechanics of such wiki datasets—and of a related idea of collecting local law through some sort of crowd-sourcing—will require an infrastructure of conventions and technical specifications that the field will have to develop and disseminate.

As this volume illustrates, theory and methods are inextricably intertwined. Reliable and valid measurement of legal concepts is central for the advancement of scientific evaluation of the many public health effects of law. Designing a quality measurement protocol requires conceptual clarity about what dimensions of law one wishes to measure. The design of quality measures is inherently related to the specific research questions at issue in a given study. As studies accumulate, an improved understanding of the effects of law leads to further specificity about the possible components or dimensions of law needing more refined measures for the next study. Not only does theory shape measures, measurement processes also improve theory. Many PHLR studies are taking on the challenge of creating an ordered scale of strength or quality of laws in a given area, to permit improved dose-response studies of legal effects

(Woodruff, Pichon, Hoerster, et al., 2007). And working through the operational problems and complexity in reliably coding "strength" enhances conceptual clarity about the many meanings of "strength" and which of those meanings are most relevant for the current study. Increased use of scientific standards and protocols for the measurement of law will provide the opportunity then to create accessible archives of legal datasets across an increasing number of domains relevant to PHLR. Given the costs and complexity of constructing quality legal datasets, the availability of such public-use datasets will increase the number of PHLR researchers, and increase the number of PHLR studies.

The importance of high-quality public-use datasets also extends to the dependent variables in PHLR studies—measures of health-relevant exposures, behaviors, and outcomes. These include regularly repeated consistently conducted sample surveys across all states (for example, BRFSS), as well as census records on all adverse events (for example, FARS). Continuing technology and management information system improvements will result in an increasing number of very large longitudinal continuous measures (for example, uniform statewide or national electronic medical records). Such databases will create many opportunities for statistically powerful and precise evaluations of public health law effects.

Finally, increased creative use of randomized experiments and the many available design elements strengthening the validity of studies of natural experiments will further establish PHLR as a respected field of scientific and scholarly inquiry. As a recent collaborative paper between a lawyer and a statistician reminds us (Ho & Rubin, 2011), research *design* trumps statistical methods. Complex statistical methods imperfectly attempt to make up for poor design. Strong research designs (for example, long time series, multiple comparison groups, and multiple measures) have been used for many years on some topics in PHLR, such as road safety. Such strong designs, which are the studies that produce credible causal inferences, must now be disseminated across all topics in PHLR. Studies testing the links between law and health outcomes must be expanded to include a greater emphasis on proximal effects of law, including implementation processes and their fidelity across jurisdictions and across time.

Social Determinants

Research to date has made a clear case that social position, particularly income and education, matter for almost all dimensions of mental and physical health. Responding to this evidence is arguably the most important challenge we face in public health, and it is one of particular importance to law. Law clearly acts as a major force structuring our societies, defining our social positions, maintaining or altering existing distributions of resources. It follows that law has the potential to be a major domain of action to address social determinants of health. So far, however, efforts to pursue PHLR aimed at the social determinants of health have been limited.

In a 2002 paper, an interdisciplinary team of authors from PHLR, social epidemiology, and sociolegal research set out a conceptual framework for research in this area (Burris, Kawachi, & Sarat, 2002); more recent papers have elaborated on the original model (Burris, 2011a; Burris, 2011b). The basic idea advanced is that we can study law as a system that sorts people, a powerful mechanism through which social position becomes health outcome. Neither the approach in these papers, nor any alternatives, has to date led to a burst of empirical research advancing our understanding of the patterns of law's effects on the social determinants of health, nor advancing effective legal or other interventions addressing social determinants in a way that significantly improves population health. There are many opportunities for PHLR, from macro-level multinational studies of dozens of countries across dozens of years to micro-level studies of biomarkers (for example, allosatic load) as measures of legal effects.

Conclusion

Research over time approaches the truth, and gains credibility and authority, by accretion. A series of more or less coordinated studies explores a particular phenomenon, producing a body of evidence that in time can be systematically weighed and even reanalyzed to produce a confident statement of the facts. So, with law, the efficacy of interventions ranging from fluoride to safety belts to tobacco and alcohol taxes was established by years of assiduous study. In a field as new and diverse as PHLR, however, this level of sustained attention may be difficult to reach. As individual researchers, we need to keep in mind our place within a larger effort not only to assess the effects of particular laws but to determine the particular mechanisms and mediators of legal effect that are broadly generalizable across public health problems, and to illuminate the utility of law generally as a force for better public health. In turn, PHLR will have more visibility, more resources allocated to it from NIH and other health research funders, and a larger impact on population health if we have a measure of coherence and identity as a field, and some degree of consensus on major critical opportunities for research advancing the public's health. The field of PHLR asserts and demonstrates the importance of objective inquiry and rational analysis to a policy process that too often seems to undervalue both. PHLR stands for the propositions that even complicated health problems can be grasped through research and that, sometimes, collective action through social intervention can make us all better off.

Summary

The chapters in this book are points on a long arc of improvement in public health law research methods. Scientific strength is crucial to the field of PHLR in several ways. Better research makes the field more attractive to new entrants, facilitates interdisciplinary collaboration, increases the chances the major health research funders will support investigation of law, and enhances the credibility of research results among policy stakeholders. As the field moves forward, key areas for methodological improvement include disciplinary integration and interdisciplinary collaboration, development of research standards and tools, and better approaches to studying law in a social determinants framework.

As an applied research field, PHLR ultimately will be justified by the extent to which it proves useful to health policy decision makers. To this end, building the field as measured by the quality and quantity of individual studies is only part of the story. We do well, as a field, to think also in terms of our "collective impact." Individual studies can illuminate particular policy choices; a few studies will be game changers. Collectively, though, the impact of PHLR as a field must exceed the sum of the effects of particular studies. The field asserts and demonstrates the importance of objective inquiry and rational analysis to a policy process that too often seems to undervalue both. PHLR stands for the propositions that even complicated health problems can be grasped through research and that, sometimes, collective action through social intervention can make us all better off.

Further Reading

Burris, S., Kawachi, I., & Sarat, A. (2002). Integrating law and social epidemiology. *Journal of Law, Medicine & Ethics, 30*, 510–521.

Epstein, L., & King, G. (2002). The rules of inference. *University of Chicago Law Review, 69*(1), 1.

Mello, M. M., & Zeiler, K. (2008). Empirical health law scholarship: The state of the field. *Georgetown Law Journal, 96*(2), 649–702.

References

AcademyHealth. (2009). *Advancing research, policy and practice.* Retrieved October 16, 2009, from www.academyhealth.org/About/content.cfm?ItemNumber=831&navItem Number=514

Acevedo-Garcia, D., Osypuk, T. L., McArdle, N., & Williams, D. R. (2008). Toward a policy-relevant analysis of geographic and racial/ethnic disparities in child health. *Health Affairs, 27*(2), 321–333.

Ackerman, F., & Heinzerling, L. (2004). *Priceless: On knowing the price of everything and the value of nothing.* New York: New Press.

Adler, N. E., & Newman, K. (2002). Socioeconomic disparities in health: Pathways and policies. *Health Affairs, 21*(2), 60–76.

Adler, N. E., & Rehkopf, D. H. (2008). U.S. disparities in health: Descriptions, causes, and mechanisms. *Annual Review of Public Health, 29,* 235–252.

Ahuja, A., Kremer, M., & Peterson-Zwane, A. (2010). Providing safe water: Evidence from randomized evaluations. *Annual Review of Resource Economics, 2*(1), 237–256.

Ainsworth, M.D.S., & Bowlby, J. (1991). An ethological approach to personality development. *American Psychologist, 46*(4), 333–341.

Ajzen, I. (1985). From intentions to actions: A theory of planned behavior. In J. Kuhl & J. Beckman (Eds.), *Action-control: From cognition to behavior* (pp. 11–39). Heidelberg, Germany: Springer.

Ajzen, I. (2003). *Constructing a TpB questionnaire: Conceptual and methodological considerations.* Retrieved April 15, 2011, from people.umass.edu/aizen/pdf/tpb .measurement.pdf

Akers, R. L. (1977). *Deviant behavior: A social learning approach* (2nd ed.). Belmont, CA: Wadsworth.

Akers, R. L. (1991). Self-control as a general theory of crime. *Journal of Quantitative Criminology, 7*(2), 201–211.

Akers, R. L. (1998). *Social learning and social structure: A general theory of crime and deviance.* Boston: Northeastern University Press.

Akers, R. L., & Jensen, G. F. (Eds.). (2007). *Social learning theory and the explanation of crime* (Vol. 11). New Brunswick, NJ: Transaction.

Akers, T. A., & Lanier, M. M. (2009). "Epidemiological criminology": Coming full circle. *American Journal of Public Health, 99*(3), 397–402.

Albers, A. B., Siegel, M., Cheng, D. M., Biener, L., & Rigotti, N. A. (2004). Relation between local restaurant smoking regulations and attitudes towards the prevalence and social acceptability of smoking: A study of youths and adults who eat out predominantly at restaurants in their town. *Tobacco Control, 13*(4), 347–355.

Alstott, A. L. (2010). Why the EITC doesn't make work pay. *Law and Contemporary Problems, 73*, 285–314.

Altman, D. (1986). *AIDS in the mind of America* (1st ed.). Garden City, NY: Anchor Press/Doubleday.

Anderson, G., & Horvath, J. (2004). The growing burden of chronic disease in America. *Public Health Reports, 119*(3), 263–270.

Andrews, D. A., Zinger, I., Hoge, R. D., et al. (1990). Does correctional treatment work? A clinically relevant and psychologically informed meta-analysis. *Criminology, 28*(3), 369–404.

Angelucci, M., & De Giorgi, G. (2009). Indirect effects of an aid program: How do cash transfers affect ineligibles' consumption? *American Economic Review, 99*(1), 486–508.

Aos, S., Lieb, R., Mayfield, J., Miller, M., & Pennucci, A. (2004). *Benefits and costs of prevention and early intervention programs for youth.* Olympia, WA: Washington State Institute for Public Policy.

Apollonio, D. E., & Bero, L. A. (2009). Evidence and argument in policymaking: Development of workplace smoking legislation. *BMC Public Health, 9*, 189.

Ariza, E., & Leatherman, S. P. (2012). No-smoking policies and their outcomes on U.S. beaches. *Journal of Coastal Research, 28*(1A), 143–147.

Arnett, P. K. (2011). Unpublished dissertation. University of Kentucky.

Arno, P. S., Sohler, N., Viola, D., & Schecter, C., (2009). Bringing health and social policy together: The case of the earned income tax credit. *Journal of Public Health Policy, 30* (2), 198–207.

Aronow, P., & Sovey, A. (2011). From LATE to ATE: Dealing with treatment effect heterogeneity in instrumental variables estimation. Unpublished working paper. Yale University.

Ashe, M., Jernigan, D., Kline, R., & Galaz, R. (2003). Land use planning and the control of alcohol, tobacco, firearms, and fast food restaurants. *American Journal of Public Health, 93*(9), 1404–1408.

Ashley, M., Northrup, D., & Ferrence, R. (1998). The Ontario ban on smoking on school property: Issues and challenges in enforcement. *Canadian Journal of Public Health, 89*(4), 229–232.

Ashraf, N., Aycinena, D., Martinez, C. A., & Yang, D. (2011). Remittances and the problem of control: A field experiment among migrants from El Salvador. Unpublished working paper. University of Chile.

Ashraf, N., Berry, J., & Shapiro, J. (2007). Can higher prices stimulate product use? Evidence from a field experiment in Zambia. *American Economic Review, 100*(5), 2383–2413.

Ashraf, N., Berry, J., & Shapiro, J. N. (2010). Can higher prices stimulate product use? Evidence from a field experiment in Zambia. *American Economic Review, 100*(5), 2383–2413.

Autor, D. H., Manning, A., & Smith, C. L. (2010). *The contribution of the minimum wage to U.S. wage inequality over three decades: A reassessment.* London: Centre for Economic Performance.

Ayres, I., & Baker, K. (2004). *A separate crime of reckless sex.* Unpublished manuscript. Yale Law School Public Law & Legal Theory Research Paper Series.

Ayres, I., & Braithwaite, J. (1995). *Responsive regulation: Transcending the deregulation debate.* New York; Oxford: Oxford University Press.

Ayres, I., Listokin, Y., & Abramowicz, M. (2010). *Randomizing law.* New Haven: Yale Law School.

Backstrom, C., & Robins, L. (1995). State AIDS policy making: Perspectives of legislative health committee chairs. *AIDS & Public Policy Journal, 10*(4), 238–248.

Bailey, C. A. (2007). *A guide to qualitative field research* (2nd ed.). Thousand Oaks, CA: Pine Forge Press.

Baker, E. L. Jr., & Koplan, J. P. (2002). Strengthening the nation's public health infrastructure: Historic challenge, unprecedented opportunity. *Health Affairs, 21*(6), 15–27.

Baker, E. L., Potter, M. A., Jones, D. L., et al. (2005). The public health infrastructure and our nation's health. *Annual Review of Public Health, 26*, 303–318.

Bandura, A. (1977a). Self-efficacy: Toward a unified theory of behavioral change. *Psychological Review, 84*(2), 191–215.

Bandura, A. (1977b). *Social learning theory.* Englewood Cliffs, NJ: Prentice-Hall.

Bandura, A. (1986a). The explanatory and predictive scope of self-efficacy theory. *Journal of Social and Clinical Psychology, 4*(3), 359–373.

Bandura, A. (1986b). *Social foundations of thought and action: A cognitive theory.* Englewood Cliffs, NJ: Prentice-Hall.

Bandura, A. (2006). Guide for constructing self-efficacy scales. In F. Pajares & T. Urdan (Eds.), *Self-efficacy beliefs of adolescents* (Vol. 5, pp. 307–337). n.c.: Information Age Publishing.

Banerjee, A. V., Duflo, E., Glennerster, R., & Kothari, D. (2010). Improving immunisation coverage in rural India: Clustered randomised controlled evaluation of immunisation campaigns with and without incentives. *British Medical Journal, 340* (c2220).

Banks, S. M., Salovey, P., Greener, S., et al. (1995). The effects of message framing on mammography utilization. *Health Psychology, 14*(2), 178–184.

Bardach, E. (1977). *The implementation game: What happens after a bill becomes law.* Cambridge, MA: MIT Press.

Bassett, M. T., Dumanovsky, T., Huang, C., et al. (2008). Purchasing behavior and calorie information at fast-food chains in New York City, 2007. *American Journal of Public Health, 98*(8), 1457–1459.

Bauman, K. E., & Fisher, L. A. (1985). Subjective expected utility, locus of control, and behavior. *Journal of Applied Social Psychology, 15*(7), 606–621.

Bayer, R. (1989). *Private acts, social consequences: AIDS and the politics of public health.* New York: Free Press.

Beam, E., McKenzie, D., & Yang, D. (2012). *Financial and informational barriers to migration: A field experiment in the Philippines.* Working paper. Ann Arbor: University of Michigan.

Beccaria, C. (1764). On crimes and punishments. In J. E. Jacoby (Ed.), *Classics of criminology* (2nd ed.). Prospect Heights, IL: Waveland Press.

Beck, A. T., Kovacs, M., & Weissman, A. (1979). Assessment of suicidal intention: The Scale for Suicide Ideation. *Journal of Consulting and Clinical Psychology, 47*(2), 343–352.

Beck, L. F., Shults, R. A., Mack, K. A., & Ryan, G. W. (2007). Associations between sociodemographics and safety belt use in states with and without primary enforcement laws. *American Journal of Public Health, 97*(9), 1619–1624.

Becker, H. S. (2009). How to find out how to do qualitative research. *International Journal of Communication, 3*, 545–553.

Beitsch, L. M., Brooks, R. G., Grigg, M., & Menachemi, N. (2006). Structure and functions of state public health agencies. *American Journal of Public Health, 96*(1), 167–172.

Beitsch, L. M., Grigg, M., Menachemi, N., & Brooks, R. G. (2006). Roles of local public health agencies within the state public health system. *Journal of Public Health Management and Practice, 12*(3), 232–241.

Bender, K., & Halverson, P. K. (2010). Quality improvement and accreditation: What might it look like? *Journal of Public Health Management and Practice, 16*(1), 79–82.

Bennett-Carlson, R., Faria, D., & Hanssens, C. (2010). *Ending and defending against HIV criminalization.* New York: The Center for HIV Law and Policy.

Benson, K., & Hartz, A. J. (2000). A comparison of observational studies and randomized, controlled trials. *New England Journal of Medicine, 342*(25), 1878–1886.

Bentham, J. (1789). *Theory of legislation.* London: Paul, Trench, Trubner.

Berger, M. L., Murray, J. F., Xu, J., & Pauly, M. (2001). Alternative valuations of work loss and productivity. *Journal of Occupational and Environmental Medicine, 43*(1), 18–24.

Berkman, L. F., & Kawachi, I. (2000). *Social epidemiology.* New York: Oxford University Press.

Bero, L. A., Montini, T., Bryan-Jones, K., & Mangurian, C. (2001). Science in regulatory policy making: Case studies in the development of workplace smoking restrictions. *Tobacco Control, 10*(4), 329–336.

Bertrand, M., Djankov, S., Hanna, R., & Mullainathan, S. (2007). Obtaining a driving licence in India: An experimental approach to studying corruption. *Quarterly Journal of Economics, 122*, 1639–1676.

Berwick, D. M., & Brennan, T. A. (1995). *New rules: Regulation, markets, and the quality of American health care.* San Francisco: Jossey–Bass.

Bhandari, M. W., Scutchfield, F. D., Charnigo, R., Riddell, M. C., & Mays, G. P. (2010). New data, same story? Revisiting studies on the relationship of local public health systems characteristics to public health performance. *Journal of Public Health Management and Practice, 16*(2), 110–117.

Bhattacharya, J., Bundorf, K., Pace, N., & Sood, N. (2011). Does health insurance make you fat? In M. Grossman and N. H. Mocan (Eds.), *Economic aspects of obesity* (pp. 35–64). Cambridge, MA: National Bureau of Economic Research.

Biradavolu, M. R., Burris, S., George, A., Jena, A., & Blankenship, K. M. (2009). Can sex workers regulate police? Learning from an HIV prevention project for sex workers in southern India. *Social Science & Medicine, 68*(8), 1541–1547.

Björkman, M., & Svensson, J. (2009). Power to the people: Evidence from a randomized field experiment on community-based monitoring in Uganda. *The Quarterly Journal of Economics, 124*(2), 735–769.

Black, J. (2008). Constructing and contesting legitimacy and accountability in polycentric regulatory regimes. *Regulation & Governance, 2,* 137–164.

Blackenship, K. M., Friedman, S. R., Dworkin, S., & Mantell, J. E. (2006). Structural interventions: Concepts, challenges and opportunities for research. *Journal of Urban Health, 83*(1), 59–72.

Blader, S. L., & Tyler, T. R. (2003a). What constitutes fairness in work settings? A four-component model of procedural justice. *Human Resource Management Review, 13*(1), 107–126.

Blader, S. L., & Tyler, T. R. (2003b). A four-component model of procedural justice: Defining the meaning of a "fair" process. *Personality and Social Psychology Bulletin, 29*(6), 747–758.

Blankenship, K. M., & Koester, S. (2002). Criminal law, policing policy, and HIV risk in female street sex workers and injection drug users. *The Journal of Law, Medicine & Ethics, 30*(4), 548–559.

Blau, P. (1964). *Exchange and power in social life.* New York: John Wiley & Sons.

Blincoe, L. J., Seay, A., Zaloshnja, E., et al. (2002). *The economic impact of motor vehicle crashes, 2000* (DOT HS 809 446). Washington, DC: U.S. Department of Transportation, National Highway Traffic Safety Administration.

Blomquist, G. (1982). Estimating the value of life and safety: Recent developments. In M. W. Jones-Lee (Ed.), *The value of life and safety* (pp. 27–40). New York: North-Holland.

Blomquist, G., Miller, T. R., & Levy, D. T. (1996). Values of risk reduction implied by motorist use of protection equipment: New evidence from different populations. *Journal of Transport Economics and Policy, 30*(1), 55–66.

Bloom, H. S. (2009). The core analytics of randomized experiments for social research. In P. Alasuutari, L. Bickman, & J. Brannen (Eds.), *The Sage handbook of social research methods* (pp. 115–133). Thousand Oaks: Sage.

Bluthenthal, R. N., Heinzerling, K. G., Anderson, R., Flynn, N. M., & Kral, A. H. (2007). Approval of syringe exchange programs in California: Results from a local approach to HIV prevention. *American Journal of Public Health, 98*(2), 278–283.

Boehmer, T. K., Luke, D. A., Haire-Joshu, D. L., Bates, H. S., & Brownson, R. C. (2008). Preventing childhood obesity through state policy: Predictors of bill enactment. *American Journal of Preventive Medicine, 34*(4), 333–340.

Bogenschneider, K., & Corbett, T. J. (2010). Family policy: Becoming a field of inquiry and subfield of social policy. *Journal of Marriage and Family, 72*(3), 783–803.

Boix, C., & Stokes, S. (2003). Endogenous democratization. *World Politics, 55*(4), 517–549.

Bonilla-Silva, E. (1997). Rethinking racism: Toward a structural interpretation. *American Sociological Review, 62*(3), 465–480.

Borenstein, S. (2011). *After cutting value of life, EPA ditching the term*. Boston.com. *2011*. Retrieved from www.boston.com/news/science/articles/2011/01/20/after_cutting_value_of_life_epa_ditching_the_term/

Borgatti, S. P., Mehra, A., Brass, D. J., & Labianca, G. (2009). Network analysis in the social sciences. *Science, 323*(5916), 892–895.

Boruch, R. (2005). Preface: Better evaluation for evidence-based policy: Place randomized trials in education, criminology, welfare, and health. *Annals of the American Academy of Political and Social Science, 599*, 6–18.

Braithwaite, J. (1989). *Crime, shame, and reintegration*. Cambridge: Cambridge University Press.

Braithwaite, J. (2008). *Regulatory capitalism: How it works, ideas for making it work better*. Cheltenham, UK; Northampton, MA: Edward Elgar.

Braithwaite, J., Coglianese, C., & Levi-Faur, D. (2007). Can regulation and governance make a difference? *Regulation and Governance, 1*(1), 1–7.

Braithwaite, J., & Drahos, P. (2000). *Global business regulation*. Cambridge: Cambridge University Press.

Braithwaite, J., Healy, J., & Dwan, K. (2005). *The governance of health safety and quality*. Canberra, Australia: Commonwealth of Australia.

Brand, P. A., & Anastasio, P. A. (2006). Violence-related attitudes and beliefs. *Journal of Interpersonal Violence, 21*(7), 856–868.

Braun, J. M., Kahn, R. S., Froelich, T., Auinger, P., & Lamphear, B. P. (2006). Exposures to environmental toxicants and attention deficit hyperactivity disorder in U.S. children. *Environmental Health Perspectives, 114*(12), 1904–1909.

Braveman, P., Egerter, S., & Barclay, C. (2011). How social factors shape health: Income, wealth and health. *Robert Wood Johnson Foundation Issue Brief: Exploring the Social Determinants of Health*. Retrieved September 1, 2012, from www.rwjf.org/files/research/4%20Income%20and%20wealth%20health%20Issue%20brief%20.pdf

Brender, J. D., Maantay, J. A., & Chakraborty, J. (2011). Residential proximity to environmental hazards and adverse health outcomes. *American Journal of Public Health, 101*, S37–S52.

Brewer, J. (2004). Ethnography. In C. Cassell & G. Symon (Eds.), *Essential guide to qualitative methods in organizational research* (pp. 312–322). London; Thousand Oaks, CA: Sage.

Briss, P. A., Rodewald, L. E., Hinman, A. R., et al. (2000). Reviews of evidence regarding interventions to improve vaccination coverage in children, adolescents, and adults: The Task Force on Community Preventive Services. *American Journal of Preventive Medicine, 18*(1), 97–140.

Brody, H., Rip, M. R., Vinten-Johansen, P., Paneth, N., & Rachman, S. (2000). Map-making and myth-making in Broad Street: The London cholera epidemic, 1854. *Lancet, 356*, 64–68.

Bronfrenbrenner, U. (2005). *Making human beings human: Bioecological perspectives on human development*. Thousand Oaks, CA: Sage.

Browning, C. R., & Cagney, K. A. (2002). Neighborhood structural disadvantage, collective efficacy, and self-rated physical health in an urban setting. *Journal of Health and Social Behavior, 43*(4), 383–399.

Brownson, R. C., & Bright, F. S. (2004). Chronic disease control in public health practice: Looking back and moving forward. *Public Health Reports, 119*(3), 230–238.

Brownson, R. C., Colditz, G. A., & Proctor, E. K. (2012). *Dissemination and implementation research in health: Translating science to practice*. New York: Oxford University Press.

Brownson, R. C., Eriksen, M. P., Davis, R. M., & Warner, K. E. (1997). Environmental tobacco smoke: Health effects and policies to reduce exposure. *Annual Review of Public Health, 18*, 163–185.

Bryan, G., Chowdhury, S., & Mobarak, A. M. (2010). *The effect of seasonal migration on households during food shortages in Bangladesh*. Unpublished ongoing study. Yale University.

Brydon-Miller, M., Greenwood, D., & Maguire, P. (2003). Why Action Research? *Action Research, 1*(1), 9–28.

Buehler, J. W., Whitney, E. A., & Berkelman, R. L. (2006). Business and public health collaboration for emergency preparedness in Georgia: A case study. *BMC Public Health, 6*, 285.

Burris, S. (1998a). Gay marriage and public health. *Temple Political & Civil Rights Law Review, 7*(2), 417–427.

Burris, S. (1998b). Law and the social risk of health care: Lessons from HIV testing. *Albany Law Review, 61*, 831–895.

Burris, S. (2003). Legal aspects of regulating bathhouses: Cases from 1984 to 1995. *Journal of Homosexuality, 44*(3–4), 131–151.

Burris, S. (2006). From security to health. In J. Woods & B. Dupont (Eds.), *Democracy and the governance of security* (pp. 196–216). Cambridge: Cambridge University Press.

Burris, S. (2008). Regulatory innovation in the governance of human subjects research: A cautionary tale and some modest proposals. *Regulation and Governance, 2*, 1–20.

Burris, S. (2011a). From health care law to the social determinants of health: A public health law research perspective. *University of Pennsylvania Law Review, 159*(6), 1649–1667.

Burris, S. (2011b). Law in a social determinants strategy: A public health law research perspective. *Public Health Reports, 126* (Suppl. 3), 22–27.

Burris, S., Anderson, E. D., Craigg, A., Davis, C. S., & Case, P. (2010). Racial disparities in injection-related HIV: A case study of toxic law. *Temple Law Review, 82*(5), 1263–1302.

Burris, S., Blankenship, K. M., Donoghoe, M., et al. (2004). Addressing the "risk environment" for injection drug users: The mysterious case of the missing cop. *The Milbank Quarterly, 82*(1), 125–156.

Burris, S., & Cameron, E. (2008). The case against criminalization of HIV transmission. *Journal of the American Medical Association, 300*(5), 578–581.

Burris, S., Kawachi, I., & Sarat, A. (2002). Integrating law and social epidemiology. *Journal of Law, Medicine & Ethics, 30*, 510–521.

Burris, S., Kempa, M., & Shearing, C. (2008). Changes in governance: A cross-disciplinary review of current scholarship. *Akron Law Review, 41*(1), 1–66.

Burris, S., Wagenaar, A. C., Swanson, J., et al., (2010). Making the case for laws that improve health: A framework for public health law research. *The Milbank Quarterly, 88*(2), 169–210.

Burris, S. C., Beletsky, L., Burleson, J. A., Case, P., & Lazzarini, Z. (2007). Do criminal laws influence HIV risk behavior? An empirical trial. *Arizona State Law Journal, 39*, 467–517.

Burris, S. C., Swanson, J. W., Moss, K., Ullman, M. D., & Ranney, L. M. (2006). Justice disparities: Does the ADA enforcement system treat people with psychiatric disabilities fairly? *Maryland Law Review*, 94–139.

Buse, K., & Lee, K. (2005). *Business and global health governance.* London: London School of Hygiene & Tropical Medicine.

Butler, D. M., & Smith, D. M. (2007). Serosorting can potentially increase HIV transmissions. *AIDS, 21*(9), 1218–1220.

Cabanac, M. (1992). Pleasure: The common currency. *Journal of Theoretical Biology, 155* (2), 173–200.

Campbell Collaboration. (2009). *What helps? What harms? Based on what evidence? Systematic reviews of the effects of interventions in education, crime and justice, and social welfare, to promote evidence-based decision-making.* Retrieved October 16, 2009, from www.campbellcollaboration.org/artman2/uploads/1/C2_GeneralBrochure_low_May09.pdf

Cast, A. D., & Burke, P. (2002). A theory of self-esteem. *Social Forces, 80*(3), 1041–1068.

Caulkins, J., Pacula, R., Paddock, S., & Chiesa, J. R. (2002). *School-based drug prevention: What kind of drug use does it prevent?* (MR-1459-RWJ). Santa Monica, CA: RAND.

Cawley, J., & Liu, F. (2008). Correlates of state legislative action to prevent childhood obesity. *Obesity, 16*(1), 162–167.

Center for Law and the Public's Health. (2001). *Core legal competencies for public health professionals*. Retrieved September 15, 2011, from www.publichealthlaw.net/Training/TrainingPDFs/PHLCompetencies.pdf

Centers for Disease Control and Prevention. (1999a). Achievements in public health, 1900–1999: Decline in deaths from heart disease and stroke—United States, 1900–1999. *Morbidity and Mortality Weekly Report, 48*(30), 649–656.

Centers for Disease Control and Prevention. (1999b). Achievements in public health, 1900–1999: Impact of vaccines universally recommended for children—United States, 1990–1998. *Morbidity and Mortality Weekly Report, 48*(12), 243–248.

Centers for Disease Control and Prevention. (1999c). Achievements in public health, 1900–1999: Motor-vehicle safety: A 20th century public health achievement. *Morbidity and Mortality Weekly Report, 48*(18), 369–374.

Centers for Disease Control and Prevention. (1999d). Achievements in public health, 1900–1999: Tobacco use—United States, 1900–1999. *Morbidity and Mortality Weekly Report, 48*(43), 986–993.

Centers for Disease Control and Prevention. (1999e). Ten great public health achievements—United States, 1900–1999. *Morbidity and Mortality Weekly Report, 48* (12), 241–243. Retrieved September 1, 2012, from www.cdc.gov/about/history/tengpha.htm

Centers for Disease Control and Prevention. (1999f). *Backgrounder: State laws on tobacco Control*. Retrieved October 16, 2009, from www.cdc.gov/media/pressrel/r990625.htm

Centers for Disease Control and Prevention. (2008). Smoking-attributable mortality, years of potential life lost, and productivity losses—United States, 2000–2004. *Morbidity and Mortality Weekly Report, 57*(45), 1226–1228.

Centers for Disease Control and Prevention. (2010). State cigarette minimum price laws—United States, 2009. *Morbidity and Mortality Weekly Report, 59*(13), 389–392.

Centers for Disease Control and Prevention. (2011a). *National Public Health Performance Standards Program (NPHPSP)*. Retrieved April 1, 2011, from www.cdc.gov/nphpsp/index.html

Centers for Disease Control and Prevention. (2011b). Ten great public health achievements—United States, 2001–2010. *Journal of the American Medical Association, 306* (1), 36–38.

Chalkidou, K., Tunis, S., Lopert, R., et al. (2009). Comparative effectiveness research and evidence-based health policy: Experience from four countries. *The Milbank Quarterly, 87*(2), 339–367.

Chaloupka, F. J. (2004). The effects of price on alcohol use, abuse, and their consequences. In R. J. Bonnie & M. E. O'Connell (Eds.), *Reducing underage drinking: A collective responsibility*. Washington, DC: National Academies Press.

Chaloupka, F. J., Powell, L. M., & Chriqui, J. F. (2011). Sugar-sweetened beverages and obesity: The potential impact of public policies. *Journal of Policy Analysis and Management, 30*(3), 645–655.

Chaloupka, F. J., Tauras, J. A., and Grossman, M. (2000). The economics of addiction. In P. Jha & F. J. Chaloupka (Eds.), *Tobacco control in developing countries* (pp. 106–130). Oxford: Oxford University Press.

Chapman, S. (2006). Butt clean up campaigns: Wolves in sheep's clothing? *Tobacco Control, 15*, 273.

Chauncey, G. (1994). *Gay New York: Gender, urban culture, and the makings of the gay male world, 1890–1940*. New York: Basic Books.

Cheng, A. K., Rubin, H. R., Powe, N. R., et al. (2000). Cost-utility analysis of the cochlear implant in children. *Journal of the American Medical Association, 284*(7), 850–856.

Chetty, R., & Friedman, J. N. (2011). The long-term effects of early childhood education. *Communities & Banking, Summer*, 6–7.

Chin, A., Karkoviata, L., & Wilcox, N. (2010). Impact of bank accounts on migrant savings and remittances: Evidence from a field experiment. Unpublished working paper. University of Houston.

Chriqui, J. F., Frosh, M., Brownson, R. C., et al. (2002). Application of a rating system to state clean indoor air laws. *Tobacco Control, 11*(1), 26–34.

Chriqui, J. F., O'Connor, J. C., & Chaloupka, F. J. (2011). What gets measured, gets changed: Evaluating law and policy for maximum impact. *Journal of Law, Medicine & Ethics, 39* (Suppl. 1), 21–26.

Chriqui, J. F., Ribisl, K. M., Wallace, R. M., et al. (2008). A comprehensive review of state laws governing Internet and other delivery sales of cigarettes in the United States. *Nicotine & Tobacco Research, 10*(2), 253–265.

Clemens, M. (2010). How visas affect skilled labor: A randomized natural experiment. Unpublished working paper. Tufts University, Center for Global Development.

Cobigo, V., & Stuart, H. (2010). Social inclusion and mental health. *Current Opinion in Psychiatry, 23*, 453–457.

Cochrane Collaboration. (2009). *An introduction to Cochrane reviews and the Cochrane library*. Retrieved October 16, 2009, from www.cochrane.org/reviews/clibintro.htm

Cohen, D., & Crabtree, B. (2006). *Qualitative Research Guidelines Project*. Robert Wood Johnson Foundation. Retrieved November 1, 2011, from www.qualres.org/index.html

Cohen, J. (1988). *Statistical power analysis for the behavioral sciences* (2nd ed.). Hillsdale, NJ: Lawrence Erlbaum Associates.

Cohen, J., & Dupas, P. (2010). Free distribution or cost-sharing? Evidence from a randomized malaria prevention experiment. *The Quarterly Journal of Economics, 125*(1), 1–45.

Cohen, L., Manion, L., & Morrison, K. (2000). *Research methods in education* (5th ed.). New York: Routledge.

Cohen, M. A. (1998). The monetary value of saving a high risk youth. *Journal of Quantitative Criminology, 14*(1), 5–33.

Cohen, M. A. (2000). Measuring the costs and benefits of crime and justice. In D. Duffee (Ed.), *Criminal justice: Measurement and analysis of crime and justice* (Vol. 4, pp. 263–315). Washington, DC: National Institute of Justice.

Cohen, S., Kessler, R. C., & Underwood-Gordon, L. (1995). Strategies for measuring stress in studies of psychiatric and physical disorders. In S. Cohen, R. C. Kessler, & L. Underwood-Gordon (Eds.), *Measuring stress: A guide for health and social scientists* (Vol. 28, pp. 3–26). New York: Oxford University Press.

Collins, J., & Koplan, J. P. (2009). Health impact assessment: A step toward health in all policies. *Journal of the American Medical Association, 302*(3), 315–317.

Commission on Social Determinants of Health. (2008). *Closing the gap in a generation: Health equity through action on the social determinants of health*. Geneva: World Health Organization.

Concato, J., Shah, N., & Horwitz, R. I. (2000). Randomized, controlled trials, observational studies, and the hierarchy of research designs. *New England Journal of Medicine, 342*(25), 1887–1892.

Conners, C. K., Sitarenios, G., Parker, J.D.A., & Epstein, J. N. (1998). Revision and restandardization of the Conners Teacher Rating Scale (CTRS-R): Factor structure, reliability, and criterion validity. *Journal of Abnormal Child Psychology, 26*(4), 279–291.

Cook, P. J. (2007). *Paying the tab: The costs and benefits of alcohol control*. Princeton, NJ: Princeton University Press.

Cooper, D. (1995). Local government legal consciousness in the shadow of juridification. *Journal of Law and Society, 22*(4), 506–526.

Cooper, H., Moore, L., Gruskin, S., & Krieger, N. (2005). The impact of a police drug crackdown on drug injectors' ability to practice harm reduction: A qualitative study. *Social Science & Medicine, 61*(3), 673–684.

Corbin, J. M., & Strauss, A. L. (2008). *Basics of qualitative research: Techniques and procedures for developing grounded theory* (3rd ed.). Los Angeles: Sage.

Corral-Verdugo, V., & Frías-Armenta, M. (2006). Personal normative beliefs, antisocial behavior, and residential water conservation. *Environment and Behavior, 38*(3), 406–421.

Corrigan, P. W., Watson, A. C., Heyrman, M. L., et al. (2005). Structural stigma in state legislation. *Psychiatric Services, 56*(5), 557–563.

Coryn, C.L.S., & Scriven, M. (2008). The logic of research evaluation. In C.L.S. Coryn & M. M. Scriven (Eds.), *Reforming the evaluation of research* (*New Directions for Evaluation*, Vol. 118, pp. 89–105). San Francisco: Jossey-Bass and American Evaluation Association.

Cowen, T. (1992). Consequentialism implies a zero rate of discount. In P. Laslett & J. Fishkin (Eds.), *Philosophy, politics, and society* (pp. 162–168). New Haven, CT: Yale University Press.

Cowen, T. (2001). *What is the correct intergenerational discount rate?* Fairfax, VA: George Mason University.

Cowen, T., & Parfit, D. (1992). Against the social discount rate. In P. Laslett & J. Fishkin (Eds.), *Philosophy, politics, and society* (pp. 144–161). New Haven, CT: Yale University Press.

Creswell, J. W. (2007). *Qualitative inquiry & research design: Choosing among five approaches* (2nd ed.). Thousand Oaks, CA: Sage.

Creswell, J. W., Klassen, A. C., Plano Clark, V. L., Smith, K. C., & The Office of Behavioral and Social Sciences Research. (2011). *Best practices for mixed methods research in the health sciences*. Retrieved September 14, 2011, from obssr.od.nih.gov/scientific_areas/methodology/mixed_methods_research/index.aspx

Creswell, J. W., & Plano Clark, V. L. (2007). *Designing and conducting mixed methods research*. Thousand Oaks, CA: Sage.

Croley, S. (2008). *Regulation and public interests: The possibility of good regulatory government*. Princeton, NJ: Princeton University Press.

Crowder, K., & Downey, L. (2010). Inter-neighborhood migration, race, and environmental hazards: Modeling micro-level processes of environmental inequality. *American Journal of Sociology, 115*(4), 1110–1149.

Csete, J., Pearshouse, R., & Symington, A. (2009). Vertical HIV transmission should be excluded from criminal prosecution. *Reproductive Health Matters, 17*(24), 1–9.

Cullen, F. T., Pratt, T. C., Miceli, S. L., & Moon, M. M. (2002). Dangerous liason? Rational choice theory as the basis for correctional intervention. In A. R. Piquero & S. Tibbetts (Eds.), *Rational choice and criminal behavior: Recent research and future challenges* (pp. 279–298). New York: Routledge.

Cullen, F. T., Wright, J. P., & Applegate, B. K. (1996). Control in the community: The limits of reform? In A. T. Harland (Ed.), *Choosing correctional options that work: Defining the demand and evaluating the supply* (pp. 69–116). Thousand Oaks, CA: Sage.

Curtis, V., Cairncross, S., & Yonli, R. (2000). Review: Domestic hygiene and diarrhea—pinpointing the problem. *Tropical Medicine & International Health, 5*(1), 22–32.

Cutler, D. M., & Lleras-Muney, A. (2006). *Education and health: Evaluating theories and evidence* (NBER Working Paper 12352). Cambridge, MA.: National Bureau of Economic Research.

Cutler, D. M., & Miller, G. (2004). *The role of public health improvements in health advances: The 20th century United States*. Cambridge, MA: National Bureau of Economic Research.

Dahl, R. A. (1956). *A preface to democratic theory*. Chicago: University of Chicago Press.

Dannenberg, A. L., Bhatia, R., Cole, B. L., et al. (2008). Use of health impact assessment in the U.S.: 27 case studies, 1999–2007. *American Journal of Preventive Medicine, 34*, 241–256.

Dansereau, D. F., & Simpson, D. D. (2009). A picture is worth a thousand words: The case for graphic representations. *Professional Psychology: Research and Practice, 40* (1), 104–110.

Darley, J. M., Tyler, T. R., & Bilz, K. (2003). The Sage handbook of social psychology. In M. A. Hogg & J. Cooper (Eds.), *Enacting justice: The interplay of individual and institutional perspectives.* Thousand Oaks, CA: Sage.

Daudel, P., & Daudel, R. (1948). The molecular diagram method. *The Journal of Chemical Physics, 16*(7), 639–643.

Dausey, D. J., Buehler, J. W., & Lurie, N. (2007). Designing and conducting tabletop exercises to assess public health preparedness for manmade and naturally occurring biological threats. *BMC Public Health, 7,* 92.

Davis, C. S., Burris, S., Kraut-Becher, J., Lynch, K. G., & Metzger, D. (2005). Effects of an intensive street-level police intervention on syringe exchange program use in Philadelphia, PA. *American Journal of Public Health, 95*(2), 233–236.

Davis, F. D., & Warshaw, P. R. (1992). What do intention scales measure? *The Journal of General Psychology, 119*(4), 391–407.

De Cremer, D., & Tyler, T. R. (2005). Managing group behavior: The interplay between procedural justice, sense of self, and cooperation. *Advances in Experimental Social Psychology, 37,* 151–218.

De La O, A., & Wantchekon, L. (2010). Experimental research on democracy and development. In J. N. Druckman, D. P. Green, J. H. Kuklinski, & A. Lupia (Eds.), *Cambridge handbook of experimental political science* (pp. 384–399). Cambridge, U.K.: Cambridge University Press.

Deal, L. W., Gomby, D. S., Zippiroli, L., & Behrman, R. E. (2000). Unintentional injuries in childhood: Analysis and recommendations. *The Future of Children, 10*(1), 4–22.

Dean, K. (1996). Using theory to guide policy relevant health promotion research. *Health Promotion International, 11*(1), 19–26.

Dearlove, J. V., & Glantz, S. A. (2002). Boards of health as venues for clean indoor air policy making. *American Journal of Public Health, 92*(2), 257–265.

Deci, E. L., & Ryan, R. M. (1985). *Intrinsic motivation and self-determination in human behavior.* New York: Plenum Press.

Deflem, M. (2004). Social control and the policing of terrorism: Foundations for a sociology of counterterrorism. *The American Sociologist, 35*(2), 75–92.

Delavande, A., Goldman, D. P., & Sood, N. (2007). *Criminal prosecution and HIV-related risky behavior* (NBER Working Paper No. W12903). Washington, DC: National Bureau of Economic Research.

Denzin, N. K., & Lincoln, Y. S. (2005). *The Sage handbook of qualitative research* (3rd ed.). Thousand Oaks, CA: Sage.

Detweiler, J. B., Bedell, B. T., Salovey, P., Pronin, E., & Rothman, A. J. (1999). Message framing and sunscreen use: Gain-framed messages motivate beach-goers. *Health Psychology, 18*(2), 189–196.

Deutermann, W. (2004). *Motorcycle helmet effectiveness revisited report* (Technical Report DOT HS 809 715). Washington, DC: National Highway Traffic Safety Adminstration.

DeVille, K. (2009). The Turning Point Model State Public Health Act and responsible public health advocacy. *Journal of Public Health Management and Practice, 15*(4), 281–283.

Devoto, F., Duflo, E., Dupas, P., Parienté, W., & Pons, V. (2011). *Happiness on tap: The demand for and impact of piped water in urban Morocco* (NBER Working Paper 16933). Cambridge, MA: National Bureau of Economic Research.

Dillman, D. A. (1991). The design and administration of mail surveys. *Annual Review of Sociology, 17*, 225–249.

Dillman, D. A. (2007). *Mail and Internet surveys: The tailored design method.* New York: John Wiley & Sons.

Dinh-Zarr, T. B., Sleet, D. A., Shults, R. A., et al. (2001). Reviews of evidence regarding interventions to increase the use of safety belts. *American Journal of Preventive Medicine, 21* (Suppl. 4), 48–65.

Dobbin, F. (2009). *Inventing equal opportunity.* Princeton, NJ: Princeton University Press.

Dobbin, F., & Sutton, J. R. (1998). The strength of a weak state: The rights revolution and the rise of human resources management divisions. *American Journal of Sociology, 104*(2), 441–476.

Dodds, C., Bourne, A., & Weait, M. (2009). Responses to criminal prosecutions for HIV transmission among gay men with HIV in England and Wales. *Reproductive Health Matters, 17*(34), 135–145.

Dodson, E. A., Fleming, C., Boehmer, T. K., et al. (2009). Preventing childhood obesity through state policy: Qualitative assessment of enablers and barriers. *Journal of Public Health Policy, 30* (Suppl. 1), S161–S176.

Downing, P. B. (1981). Policy consequences of indirect regulatory costs. *Public Policy, 29* (4), 507–526.

Drummond, M. F., Sculpher, M., Torrance, G. W., O'Brien, B., & Stoddart, G. L. (2005). *Methods for the economic evaluation of health care programmes* (3rd ed.). Oxford: Oxford University Press.

DuBois, D. L., Flay, B. R., & Fagen, M. C. (2009). Self-esteem enhancement theory: An emerging framework for promoting health across the life-span. In R. J. DiClement, M. C. Kegler, & R. A. Crosby (Eds.), *Emerging theories in health promotion practice and research* (2nd ed.). San Francisco: Jossey-Bass.

Duflo, E., Hanna, R., & Ryan, S. (2008). *Monitoring works: Getting teachers to come to school.* Cambridge, MA: National Bureau of Economic Research.

Duflo, E., & Saez, E. (2003). The role of information and social interactions in retirement plan decisions: Evidence from a randomized experiment. *The Quarterly Journal of Economics, 118*(3), 815–842.

Duncan, O. D. (1966). *Path analysis: Sociological examples*. Indianapolis: Bobbs-Merrill.

Durkheim, E. (1951). *Suicide: A study in sociology*. Glencoe, IL: Free Press.

Durlauf, S. N., & Nagin, D. S. (2011). Imprisonment and crime: Can both be reduced? *Criminology & Public Policy, 10*(1), 13–54.

Easton, D. (1965). *A systems analysis of political life*. New York: John Wiley & Sons.

Easton, D. (1975). A re-assessment of the concept of political support. *British Journal of Political Science, 5*(4), 435–457.

Edelman, L., & Suchman, M. C. (1997). Legal ambiguity and symbolic structures: Organizational mediation of civil rights law. *American Journal of Sociology, 97*, 1531–1576.

Edelman, L. B. (1992). Legal ambiguity and symbolic structures: Organizational mediation of civil rights law. *American Journal of Sociology, 97*(6), 199–205.

Edelman, L. B. (2005). Law at work: The endogenous construction of civil rights law. In L. B. Nielsen & R. L. Nelson (Eds.), *Handbook of employment discrimination research: Rights and realities* (pp. 337–352). Dordrecht: Springer.

Edelman, L. B., Erlanger, H. S., & Lande, J. (1993). Internal dispute resolution: The transformation of civil rights in the workplace. *Law & Society Review, 27*(3), 497–534.

Edelman, L. B., Krieger, L. H., Eliason, S. R., Albiston, C. R., & Mellema, V. (2011). When organizations rule: Judicial deference to institutionalized employment structures. *American Journal of Sociology, 117*(3), 888–954.

Edelman, L. B., & Stryker, R. (2005). A sociological approach to law and the economy. In N. Smelser & R. Swedberg (Eds.), *Handbook of economic sociology* (pp. 527–551). Princeton, NJ: Princeton University Press.

Edwards, J. R., & Lambert, L. S. (2007). Methods for integrating moderation and mediation: A general analytical framework using moderated path analysis. *Psychological Methods, 12*(1), 1–22.

Egerter, S., Braveman, P., Sadegh-Nobari, T., Grossman-Kahn, R., & Dekker, M. (2009). *Education matters for health*. Princeton, NJ: Robert Wood Johnson Foundation.

Eissa, N., & Hoynes, H. W. (2006). Behavioral responses to taxes: Lessons from the EITC and labor supply. In J. Poterba (Ed.), *Tax policy and the economy* (Vol. 20, pp. 73–110). Cambridge, MA: MIT Press.

Ellermann, C. R., Kataoka-Yahiro, M. R., & Wong, L. C. (2006). Logic models used to enhance critical thinking. *The Journal of Nursing Education, 45*(6), 220–227.

Elovainio, M., Kivimäki, M., Eccles, M., & Sinervo, T. (2002). Team climate and procedural justice as predictors of occupational strain. *Journal of Applied Social Psychology, 32*(2), 359–372.

Elvik, R. (1994). The external costs of traffic injury: Definition, estimation, and possibilities for internalization. *Accident Analysis & Prevention, 26*(6), 719–732.

Eman, K. E., Mercer, J., Moreau, M., et al. (2011). Physician privacy concerns when disclosing patient data for public health purposes during a pandemic influenza outbreak. *BMC Public Health, 11*, 454.

Emerson, R. M., Fretz, R. I., & Shaw, L. L. (1995). *Writing ethnographic fieldnotes.* Chicago: University of Chicago Press.

Engel, D. M., & Munger, F. W. (1996). Rights, remembrance, and the reconciliation of difference. *Law and Society Review, 30*(1), 7–54.

Engel, D. M., & Munger, F. W. (2003). *Rights of inclusion: Law and identity in the life stories of Americans with disabilities.* Chicago: University of Chicago Press.

Epstein, F. H. (1996). Cardiovascular disease epidemiology: A journey from the past into the future. *Circulation, 93*, 1755–1764.

Epstein, L., & King, G. (2002). The rules of inference. *University of Chicago Law Review, 69*(1), 1.

Epstein, L. H., Dearing, K. K., Roba, L. G., & Finkelstein, E. (2010). The influence of taxes and subsidies on energy purchased in an experimental purchasing study. *Psychological Science, 21*(3), 406–414.

Epstein, R. A. (2003). Let the shoemaker stick to his last: A defense of the "old" public health. *Perspectives in Biology & Medicine, 46* (Suppl. 3), S138–S159.

Erickson, D. L., Gostin, L. O., Street, J., & Mills, S. P. (2002). The power to act: Two model state statutes. *The Journal of Law, Medicine & Ethics, 30*(3), 57–62.

Eriksson, P., & Kovalainen, A. (2008). *Qualitative methods in business research.* Los Angeles; London: Sage.

Erwin, P. C. (2008). The performance of local health departments: A review of the literature. *Journal of Public Health Management and Practice, 14*(2), E9–E18.

Esrey, S. A. (1996). Water, waste, and well-being: A multicountry study. *American Journal of Epidemiology, 143*(6), 608–623.

Estin, A. L. (2010). Sharing governance: Family law in Congress and the states. *Cornell Journal of Law and Public Policy, 18*(2), 267–335.

Evans, W. N., & Garthwaite, C. L. (2010). *Giving mom a break: The impact of higher EITC payments on maternal health.* Cambridge, MA: National Bureau of Economic Research.

Ewick, P., & Silbey, S. (1998). *The common place of law: Stories from everyday life.* Chicago: University of Chicago Press.

Facione, P., & Facione, N. (1992). *The California critical thinking dispositions inventory test manual.* Millbrae, CA: California Academic Press.

Fearon, J. D., Weinstein, J. M., & Humphreys, M. (2009). Can development aid contribute to social cohesion after civil war? Evidence from a field experiment in post-conflict Liberia. *American Economic Review, 99*(2), 287–291.

Feather, N. T. (1982). *Expectations and actions: Expectancy-value models in psychology.* Hillsdale, NJ: Lawrence Erlbaum Associates.

Feldman, Y., & Tyler, T. R. (2010). Mandated justice: The potential promise and possible pitfalls of mandating procedural justice in the workplace. Unpublished manuscript. Bar-Ilan University.

Fell, J. C., Fisher, D. A., Voas, R. B., Blackman, K., & Tippetts, A. S. (2009). Changes in alcohol-involved fatal crashes associated with tougher state alcohol legislation. *Alcoholism—Clinical and Experimental Research, 33*(7), 1208–1219.

Fichtenberg, C. M., & Glantz, S. A. (2002). Effect of smoke-free workplaces on smoking behaviour: Systematic review. *British Medical Journal, 325*(7357), 188–190.

Fidler, D. (2004). Constitutional outlines of public health's "new world order." *Temple Law Review, 77*, 247–289.

Finkelstein, A., Taubman, S., Wright, B., et al. (2011). *The Oregon health insurance experiment: Evidence from the first year* (NBER Working Paper 17190). Stanford, CA: National Bureau of Economic Research.

Fishbein, M., & Ajzen, I. (1975). *Belief, attitude, intention, and behavior: An introduction to theory and research.* Reading, MA: Addison-Wesley.

Fishbein, M., Triandis, H. C., Kanfer, F. H., et al. (2001). Factors influencing behavior and behavior change. In A. Baum, T. A. Revison, & J. E. Singer (Eds.), *Handbook of health psychology* (pp. 3–17). Mahwah, NJ: Lawrence Erlbaum Associates.

Fishburn, P. C. (1981). Subjective expected utility: A review of normative theories. *Theory and Decision, 13*(2), 139–199.

Fisher, R. A. (1935). *The design of experiments.* Edinburgh, London: Oliver and Boyde.

Fishman, J. A., Allison, H., Knowles, S. B., et al. (1999). State laws on tobacco control—United States, 1998. *MMWR CDC Surveill Summ, 48*(3), 21–40.

Fitzpatrick, B. (2007). *National cultural values survey: America—a nation in moral and spiritual confusion.* Alexandria, VA: Culture and Media Institute.

Fitzpatrick, P., & Hunt, A. (1987). Critical legal studies: Introduction. *Journal of Law and Society, 14*(1), 1–3.

Fixsen, D. L., Naoom, S. F., Blase, K. A., Friedman, R. M., & Wallace, F. (2005). *Implementation research: A synthesis of the literature* (FMHI Publication #231). Tampa, FL: University of South Florida, Louis de La Parte Florida Mental Health Institute.

Flay, B. R., & Petraitis, J. (1994). The theory of triadic influence: A new theory of health behavior with implications for preventive interventions. *Advances in Medical Sociology, 4*, 19–44.

Flay, B. R., Snyder, F. J., & Petraitis, J. (2009). The theory of triadic influence. In R. J. DiClemente, M. C. Kegler, & R. A. Crosby (Eds.), *Emerging theories in health promotion practice and research* (2nd ed., pp. 451–510). San Francisco: Jossey-Bass.

Fong, G. T., Cummings, K. M., Borland, R., et al. (2006). The conceptual framework of the international tobacco control (itc) policy evaluation project. *Tobacco Control, 15* (Suppl. 3), iii3–iii11.

Fong, G. T., Hammond, D., Laux, F. L., et al. (2004). The near-universal experience of regret among smokers in four countries: Findings from the International Tobacco Control Policy Evaluation Survey. *Nicotine & Tobacco Research, 6*, 341–351.

Forster, J. L., Murray, D. M., Wolfson, M., et al. (1998). The effects of community policies to reduce youth access to tobacco. *American Journal of Public Health, 88*(8), 1193–1198.

Foss, R. D., Feaganes, J. R., & Rodgman, E. A. (2001). Initial effects of graduated driver licensing on 16-year-old driver crashes in North Carolina. *Journal of the American Medical Association, 286*(13), 1588–1592.

Frattaroli, S., & Teret, S. P. (2006). Understanding and informing policy implementation: A case study of the domestic violence provisions of the Maryland Gun Violence Act. *Evaluation Review, 30*(3), 347–360.

Freeman, J., & Watson, B. (2006). An application of Stafford and Warr's reconceptualization of deterrence to a group of recidivist drink drivers. *Accident Analysis and Prevention, 38*(3), 462–471.

Frey, B. S. (1997). *Not just for the money: An economic theory of personal motivation.* Cheltenham, UK: Edward Elgar.

Frey, B. S. (1998). Institutions and morale: The crowding-out effect. In A. B. Ner & L. Putterman (Eds.), *Economics, values, and organization.* Cambridge, UK: Cambridge University Press.

Frey, B. S., & Oberholzer-Gee, F. (1997). The cost of price incentives: An empirical analysis of motivation crowding-out. *The American Economic Review, 87*(4), 746–755.

Frick, K. D., Carlson, M. C., Glass, T. A., et al. (2004). Modeled cost-effectiveness of the Experience Corps Baltimore based on a pilot randomized trial. *Journal of Urban Health, 81*(1), 106–117.

Friedman, B. (2006). Taking law seriously. *Perspectives on Politics, 4*(2), 261–276.

Friedman, L. M. (1989). Law, lawyers, and popular culture. *Yale Law Journal, 98*(8), 1579–1606.

Friedman, L. M. (2005). Coming of age: Law and society enters an exclusive club. *Annual Review of Law and Social Science, 1*(1), 1–16.

Friedman, S. R., Cooper, H. L., Tempalski, B., et al. (2006). Relationships of deterrence and law enforcement to drug-related harms among drug injectors in U.S. metropolitan areas. *AIDS, 20*(1), 93–99.

Fryer, R. G. (2011). *Teacher incentives and student achievement: Evidence from New York City public schools* (NBER Working Paper 16850). Cambridge, MA: National Bureau of Economic Research.

Gadzella, B. M., Stacks, J., Stephens, R. C., & Masten, W. G. (2005). Watson-Glaser Critical Thinking Appraisal, Form S for education majors. *Journal of Instructional Psychology, 32*(1), 9–12.

Galanter, M. (1974). Why the "haves" come out ahead: Speculations on the limits of legal change. *Law and Society Review, 9*(1), 95–160.

Galletly, C. L., DiFranceisco, W., & Pinkerton, S. D. (2008). HIV-positive persons' awareness and understanding of their state's criminal HIV disclosure law. *AIDS Behavior, 13*, 1262–1269.

Galletly, C. L., & Pinkerton, S. D. (2004). Toward rational criminal HIV exposure laws. *Journal of Law, Medicine & Ethics, 32* (Summer), 327–337.

Galletly, C. L., & Pinkerton, S. D. (2008). Preventing HIV transmission via HIV exposure laws: Applying logic and mathematical modeling to compare statutory approaches to penalizing undisclosed exposure to HIV. *Journal of Law, Medicine & Ethics, 36*(3), 577–584.

Gamper-Rabindran, S., Khan, S., & Timmins, C. (2010). The impact of piped water provision on infant mortality in Brazil: A quantile panel data approach. *Journal of Development Economics, 92*(2), 188–200.

Gebbie, K., Rosenstock, L., & Hernandez, L. M. (Eds.). (2003). *Who will keep the public healthy? Educating public health professionals for the 21st century*. Washington, DC.: National Academies Press.

Gebbie, K. M., Hodge, J. G. Jr., Meier, B. M., et al. (2008). Improving competencies for public health emergency legal preparedness. *Journal of Law, Medicine & Ethics, 36*(1 Suppl.), 52–56.

Gee, G., & Walsemann, K. (2009). Does health predict the reporting of racial discrimination or do reports of discrimination predict health? Findings from the National Longitudinal Study of Youth. *Social Science and Medicine, 68*(9), 1676–1684.

General Accounting Office. (1993). *Developing and using questionnaires* (GAO/PEMD-10.1.7). Washington, DC: Government Printing Office.

Genn, H. G., Partington, M., Wheeler, S., & Nuffield Foundation. (2006). Law in the real world improving our understanding of how law works: Final report and recommendations. *The Nuffield Inquiry on Empirical Legal Research*. Retrieved November 1, 2011, from www.ucl.ac.uk/laws/socio-legal/empirical/docs/inquiry_report.pdf

Gibbins, K., & Walker, I. (1993). Multiple interpretations of the Rokeach value survey. *The Journal of Social Psychology, 133*(6), 797–805.

Gibson, J., McKenzie, D., & Stillman, S. (2010). *Accounting for selectivity and duration-dependent heterogeneity when estimating the impact of emigration on incomes and poverty in sending areas* (Policy Research Working Paper 5268). Washington, DC: World Bank.

Givel, M. (2005). Oklahoma tobacco policy-making. [Comparative Study]. *Journal of the Oklahoma State Medical Assocation, 98*(3), 89–94.

Glanz, K., & Yarock, A. L. (2004). Strategies for increasing fruit and vegetable intake in grocery stores and communities: Policy, pricing and environmental change. *Preventive Medicine, 39* (Suppl. 2), 75–80.

Glaser, B. G., & Strauss, A. L. (1967). *The discovery of grounded theory: Strategies for qualitative research*. Chicago: Aldine.

Glass, T. A., & McAtee, M. J. (2006). Behavioral science at the crossroads in public health: Extending horizons, envisioning the future. *Social Science & Medicine, 62*(7), 1650–1671.

Glass, G. V., Wilson, V. L., & Gottman, J. M. (1975). *Design and analysis of time-series experiments*. Boulder: Colorado Associated University Press.

Global Smokefree Partnership. (2009). *The trend toward smokefree outdoor areas*. Retrieved from www.globalsmokefree.com/gsp/resources/ficheiros/SF_Outdoors.pdf

Godin, G., & Shephard, R. J. (1986). Psychosocial factors influencing intentions to exercise of young students from grades 7 to 9. *Research Quarterly for Exercise and Sport, 57*(1), 41–52.

Gold, M. R., Siegel, J. E., Russell, L. B., & Weinstein, M. C. (Eds.). (1996). *Cost-effectiveness in health and medicine: Report of the panel on cost-effectiveness in health and medicine.* New York: Oxford University Press.

Goldman, B. M., Gutek, B. A., Stein, J. H., & Lewis, K. (2006). Employment discrimination in organizations: Antecedents and consequences. *Journal of Management, 32*(6), 786–830.

Goldsmith, J., & Vermeule, A. (2002). Empirical methodology and legal scholarship. *The University of Chicago Law Review, 69*(1), 153–167.

Goode, W. J. (1970). *World revolution and family patterns* (2 ed.). New York: Free Press.

Goode, W. J. (Ed.). (1971). *The contemporary American family.* Chicago: Quadrangle Books.

Gostin, L. O. (2000). Public health law in a new century, part I: Law as a tool to advance the community's health. *Journal of the American Medical Association, 283*(21), 2837–2841.

Gostin, L. O. (2008). *Public health law: Power, duty, restraint* (2nd ed.). Berkeley: University of California Press.

Gostin, L. O., Burris, S., & Lazzarini, Z. (1999). The law and the public's health: A study of infectious disease law in the United States. *Columbia Law Review, 99*(1), 59–128.

Gostin, L. O., Lazzarini, Z., Neslund, V. S., & Osterholm, M. T. (1996). The public health information infrastructure: A national review of the law on health information privacy. *Journal of the American Medical Association, 275*(24), 1921–1927.

Gottfredson, D. C., Najaka, S. S., & Kearley, B. (2003). Effectiveness of drug treatment courts: Evidence from a randomized trial. *Criminology and Public Policy, 2*(2), 171–196.

Gottfredson, M. R., & Hirschi, T. (1990). *A general theory of crime.* Stanford, CA: Stanford University Press.

Grad, F. P. (2005). *Public health law manual* (3rd ed.). Washington, DC: American Public Health Association.

Graham, H. (2004). Social determinants and their unequal distribution: Clarifying policy understandings. *The Milbank Quarterly, 82*(1), 101–124.

Gramlich, E. M. (1981). *Benefit-cost analysis of government programs.* Englewood Cliffs, NJ: Prentice-Hall.

Granovetter, M. (1978). Threshold models of collective behavior. *American Journal of Sociology, 83*(6), 1420–1443.

Gray, V. (1973). Innovation in the States: A diffusion study. *American Political Science Review, 67*(4), 1174–1185.

Greenbaum, R. T., & Landers, J. (2009). Why are state policy-makers still proponents of enterprise zones? What explains their action in the face of a preponderance of the research? *International Regional Science Review, 32*(4), 466–479.

Greenland, S., & Brumback, B. (2002). An overview of relations among causal modelling methods. *International Journal of Epidemiology, 31*(5), 1030–1037.

Grosse, S. D., Krueger, K. V., & Mvundura, M. (2009). Economic productivity by age and sex: 2007 estimates for the United States. *Medical Care, 47*(7 Suppl. 1), S94–S103.

Gruber, J., & Kőszegi, B. (2008). *A modern economic view of tobacco taxation.* Paris: International Union Against Tuberculosis and Lung Disease.

Guilfoyle, J. (2011, February 16). *Toll of tobacco in the United States of America.* Fact sheet. Washington DC: Campaign for Tobacco-Free Kids.

Gunningham, N. (2007). Corporate environmental responsibility: Law and the limits of voluntarism. In D. J. McBarnet, A. Voiculescu, & T. Campbell (Eds.), *The new corporate accountability: Corporate social responsibility and the law.* New York: Cambridge University Press.

Gunningham, N. (2009a). Environment law, regulation and governance: Shifting architectures. *Journal of Environmental Law, 21*(2), 179–212.

Gunningham, N. (2009b). The new collaborative environmental governance: The localization of regulation. *Journal of Law and Society, 36*(1), 145–166.

Guyatt, G. H., DiCenso, A., Farewell, V., Willan, A., & Griffith, L. (2000). Randomized trials versus observational studies in adolescent pregnancy prevention. *Journal of Clinical Epidemiology, 53*(2), 167–174.

Haar, C. M., Sawyer, J. P. Jr., & Cummings, S. J. (1977). Computer power and legal reasoning: A case study of judicial decision prediction in zoning amendment cases. *American Bar Foundation Research Journal, 2*(3), 651–768.

Hall, J. R. (2010). *The smoking-material fire problem.* Quincy, MA: National Fire Protection Association.

Hall, M. A. (2003). The scope and limits of public health law. *Perspectives in Biology & Medicine, 46* (Suppl. 3), S199–S209.

Hall, M. A., Rust Smith, T., Naughton, M., & Ebbers, A. (1996). Judicial protection of managed care consumers: An empirical study of insurance coverage disputes. *Seton Hall Law Review, 26*, 1055–1068.

Hall, M. A., & Wright, R. F. (2008). Systematic content analysis of judicial opinions. *California Law Review, 96*, 63–122.

Hallfors, D., Cho, H., Rusakaniko, S., et al. (2011). Supporting adolescent orphan girls to stay in school as HIV risk prevention: Evidence from a randomized controlled trial in Zimbabwe. *American Journal of Public Health, 101*(6), 1082–1088.

Hamilton, J., Bronte-Tinkew, J., & Child Trends Inc. (2007). *Logic models in out-of-school time programs: What are they and why are they important?* (#2007-01). Washington, DC: Child Trends.

Harbison, P. A., & Whitman, M. V. (2008). Barriers associated with implementing a campus-wide smoke-free policy. *Health Education, 108*(4), 321–331.

Harrell, A., & Smith, B. E. (1996). Effects of restraining orders on domestic violence victims. In E. S. Buzawa & C. G. Buzawa (Eds.), *Do arrests and restraining orders work?* (pp. 214–242). Thousand Oaks, CA: Sage.

Harris, K. J., Stearns, J. N., Kovach, R. G., & Harrar, S. W. (2009). Enforcing an outdoor smoking ban on a college campus: Effects of a multicomponent approach. *Journal of American College Health, 58*(2), 121–126.

Harris, R. P., Helfand, M., Woolf, S. H., et al. (2001). Current methods of the US Preventive Services Task Force: A review of the process. *American Journal of Preventive Medicine, 20*(3 Suppl.), 21–35.

Hartsfield, D., Moulton, A. D., & McKie, K. L. (2007). A review of model public health laws. *American Journal of Public Health, 97* (Suppl. 1), S56–S61.

Haynes, L., Service, O., Goldacre, G., & Torgerson, D. (2012). *Test, learn, adapt: Developing public policy with randomized controlled trials.* Report for the Cabinet Office of the United Kingdom. Retrieved August 30, 2012, from www.cabinetoffice.gov.uk/sites/default/files/resources/TLA-1906126.pdf

Healton, C. G., Cummings, M., O'Connor, R. J., & Novotny, T. E. (2011). Butt really? The environmental impact of cigarettes. *Tobacco Control, 20,* i1.

Heath, G. W., Brownson, R. C., Kruger, J., et al. (2006). The effectiveness of urban design and land use policies and practices to increase physical activity: A systematic review. *Journal of Physical Activity and Health, 3* (Suppl. 1), S55–S76.

Hecht, F. M., Chesney, M. A., Lehman, J. S., et al. (2000). Does HIV reporting by name deter testing? MESH Study Group. *AIDS, 14*(12), 1801–1808.

Heckathorn, D. D. (1997). Respondent-driven sampling: A new approach to the study of hidden populations. *Social Problems, 44*(2), 174–199.

Heckathorn, D. D. (2007). Extensions of respondent-driven sampling: Analyzing continuous variables and controlling for differential recruitment. *Sociological Methodology, 37*(1), 151–207.

Heckathorn, D. D. (2008). Respondent-driven sampling (RDS). In P. J. Lavrakas (Ed.), *Encyclopedia of survey research methods* (pp. 741–743). Thousand Oaks, CA: Sage.

Hedstrom, P., & Ylikoski, P. (2010). Causal mechanisms in the social sciences. *Annual Review of Sociology, 36*(1), 49–67.

Heimer, C. A. (1999). Competing institutions: Law, medicine, and family in neonatal intensive care. *Law & Society Review, 33*(1), 17–66.

Hein, W., Burris, S., & Shearing, C. (2009). Conceptual models for global health governance. In K. Buse, W. Hein, & N. Drager (Eds.), *Making sense of global health governance: A policy perspective* (pp. 72–98). Houndsmills, UK: Palgrave MacMillan.

Heloma, A., & Jaakkola, M. S. (2003). Four-year follow-up of smoke exposure, attittudes and smoking behaviour following enactment of Finland's national smoke-free workplace law. *Addiction, 98,* 1111–1117.

Hemenway, D. (2009). *While we were sleeping: Success stories in injury and violence prevention.* Berkeley: University of California Press.

Heponiemi, T., Kouvonen, A., Vèanskèa, J., et al. (2008). Health, psychosocial factors and retirement intentions among Finnish physicians. *Occupational Medicine, 58*(6), 406–412.

Herbert, S. (2000). For ethnography. *Progress in Human Geography, 24*(4), 550–568.

Herek, G. M. (1988). An epidemic of stigma: Public reactions to AIDS. *American Psychologist, 43*(11), 886–891.

Herek, G. M. (1993). Public reactions to AIDS in the United States: A second decade of stigma. *American Journal of Public Health, 83*(4), 574–577.

Herek, G. M., Capitanio, J., & Widaman, K. (2002). HIV-related stigma and knowledge in the United States: Prevalence and trends, 1991–1999. *American Journal of Public Health, 92*(3), 371–377.

Hesse-Biber, S. N., & Leavy, P. (2006). *The practice of qualitative research*. Thousand Oaks, CA: Sage.

Hill, A. B. (1965). The environment and disease: Association or causation? *Proceedings of the Royal Society of Medicine, 58*, 295–300.

Hillestad, R., Bigelow, J., Bower, A., et al. (2005). Can electronic medical record systems transform health care? Potential health benefits, savings, and costs. *Health Affairs, 24*(5), 1103–1117.

Hirano, K., & Hahn, J. (2010). Design of randomized experiments to measure social interaction effects. *Economics Letters, 48*(1), 51–53.

Hirsch, B. T. (2008). Sluggish institutions in a dynamic world: Can unions and industrial competion co-exist? *Journal of Economic Perspectives, 22*(1), 153–176.

Hirschi, T. (2002). *Causes of delinquency*. New Brunswick, NJ: Transaction.

Ho, D. E., & Rubin, D. B. (2011). Credible causal inference for empirical legal studies. *Annual Review of Law and Social Science, 7*(1), 17–40.

Hodge, J. G. Jr., Lant, T., Arias, J., & Jehn, M. (2011). Building evidence for legal decision making in real time: Legal triage in public health emergencies. *Disaster Medicine and Public Health Preparedness, 5* (Suppl. 2), S242–S251.

Hodge, J. G. Jr., Pulver, A., Hogben, M., Bhattacharya, D., & Brown, E. F. (2008). Expedited partner therapy for sexually transmitted diseases: Assessing the legal environment. *American Journal of Public Health, 98*(2), 238–243.

Hoffman, D. A., Izenman, A. J., & Lidicker, J. R. (2007). Docketology, district courts, and doctrine. *Washington University Law Review, 85*(4), 681–752.

Holla, A., Kremer, M., & Center for Global Development. (2009). *Pricing and access: Lessons from randomized evaluations in education and health* (Working Paper 158). Washington, DC: Center for Global Development.

Homans, G. C. (1958). Social behavior as exchange. *American Journal of Sociology, 63*(6), 597–606.

Horlick, G. A., Beeler, S. F., & Linkins, R. W. (2001). A review of state legislation related to immunization registries. *American Journal of Preventive Medicine, 20*(3), 208–213.

Horton, H., Birkhead, G. S., Bump, C., et al. (2002). The dimensions of public health law research. *The Journal of Law, Medicine & Ethics, 30*(3), 197–201.

Horvath, K. J., Weinmeyer, R., & Rosser, S. (2010). Should it be illegal for HIV-positive persons to have unprotected sex without disclosure? An examination of attitudes among U.S. men who have sex with men and the impact of state law. *AIDS Care, 22* (10), 1221–1228.

Hotz, V. J. (2003). The Earned Income Tax Credit. In R. A. Moffit (Ed.), *Means-tested transfer programs in the United States*. Chicago: University of Chicago Press.

House, J. S., Kessler, R. C., & Herzog, A. R. (1990). Age, socioeconomic status, and health. *The Milbank Quarterly, 68*(3), 383–411.

Houston, A. (1997). *Survey handbook* (TQLO Publication Number 97-06). Washington, DC: Department of the Navy.

Houston, D. J., & Richardson, L. E. Jr. (2005). Getting Americans to buckle up: The efficacy of state seat belt laws. [Evaluation Studies]. *Accident Analysis & Prevention, 37*(6), 1114–1120.

Howard, K. A., Ribisl, K. M., Howard-Pitney, B., Norman, G. J., & Rohrbach, L. A. (2001). What factors are associated with local enforcement of laws banning illegal tobacco sales to minors? A study of 182 law enforcement agencies in California. [Research Support, Non-U.S. Gov't]. *Preventive Medicine, 33*(2 Pt. 1), 63–70.

Howe, E. S., & Brandau, C. J. (1988). Additive effects of certainty, severity, and celerity of punishment on judgments of crime deterrence scale value. *Journal of Applied Social Psychology, 18*(9), 796–812.

Howe, E. S., & Loftus, T. C. (1996). Integration of certainty, severity, and celerity information in judged deterrence value: Further evidence and methodological equivalence. *Journal of Applied Social Psychology, 26*(3), 226–242.

Howell, W. G., & Peterson, P. E. (2002). *The education gap: Vouchers and urban schools.* Washington, DC: Brookings Institution Press.

Huesmann, L. R., & Guerra, N. G. (1997). Children's normative beliefs about aggression and aggressive behavior. *Journal of Personality and Social Psychology, 72*, 408–419.

Hull, K. E. (2003). The cultural power of law and the cultural enactment of legality: The case of same-sex marriage. *Law & Social Inquiry, 28*(3), 629–657.

Humphreys, M., and Weinstein, J. M. (2009). Field experiments and the political economy of development. *Annual Review of Political Science, 12*, 367–378.

Hung, D. Y., Rundall, T. G., Tallia, A. F., et al. (2007). Rethinking prevention in primary care: Applying the chronic care model to address health risk behaviors. *The Milbank Quarterly, 85*(1), 69–91.

Hupert, N., Mushlin, A. I., & Callahan, M. A. (2002). Modeling the public health response to bioterrorism: Using discrete event simulation to design antibiotic distribution centers. *Medical Decision Making, 22* (Suppl. 5), S17–S25.

Hyde, J. K., & Shortell, S. M. (2012). The structure and organization of local and state public health agencies in the U.S.: A systematic review. *American Journal of Preventive Medicine, 42*(5 Suppl. 1), S29–S41.

Ibrahim, J. K., Anderson, E. D., Burris, S. C., & Wagenaar, A. C. (2011). State laws restricting driver use of mobile communications devices: "Distracted-driving" provisions, 1992–2010. *American Journal of Preventive Medicine, 40*(6), 659–665.

Ibrahim, J. K., Tsoukalas, T. H., & Glantz, S. A. (2004). Public health foundations and the tobacco industry: Lessons from Minnesota. *Tobacco Control, 13*(3), 228–236.

Innvaer, S., Vist, G., Trommald, M., & Oxman, A. (2002). Health policy-makers' perceptions of their use of evidence: A systematic review. *Journal of Health Services Research & Policy, 7,* 239–244.

Institute of Medicine. (1988). *The future of public health.* Washington, DC: National Academies Press.

Institute of Medicine. (2002). *The future of the public's health in the 21st century.* Retrieved from www.nap.edu/openbook.php?record_id=10548&page=1

Institute of Medicine. (2011). *For the public's health: Revitalizing law and policy to meet new challenges.* Washington, DC: The National Academies Press.

Institute of Medicine Committee on the Assessment of the U.S. Drug Safety System, Baciu, A., Stratton, K. R., & Burke, S. P. (2007). *The future of drug safety promoting and protecting the health of the public.* Washington, DC: National Academies Press.

Insurance Institute for Highway Safety. (2011). *Q & A: Motorcycle helmet use laws.* Retrieved September 5, 2011, from www.iihs.org/research/qanda/helmet_use.html

International Agency for Research on Cancer [IARC] & World Health Organization. (2009). *IARC handbooks of cancer prevention tobacco control: Evaluating the effectiveness of smoke-free policies* (Vol. 13). Lyon, France: International Agency for Research on Cancer.

International Agency for Research on Cancer [IARC] & World Health Organization. (2011). *IARC handbooks of cancer prevention tobacco control: Effectiveness of tax and price policies in tobacco control* (Vol. 14). Lyon, France: International Agency for Research on Cancer.

International Tobacco Control Policy Evaluation Project [ITCPEP]. (2009). *FTC Article 11 tobacco warning labels: Evidence and recommendations from the ITC.* Waterloo: University of Waterloo.

Jabbari, D. (1998). Is there a proper subject matter for "socio-legal studies"? *Oxford Journal of Legal Studies, 18*(4), 707–728.

Jacobson, N., Butterill, D., & Goering, P. (2005). Consulting as a strategy for knowledge transfer. *The Milbank Quarterly, 83*(2), 299–321.

Jacobson, P. D., & Soliman, S. (2002). Litigation as public health policy: Theory or reality? *Journal of Law, Medicine & Ethics, 30*(2), 224–238.

Jacobson, P. D., & Warner, K. E. (1999). Litigation and public health policy making: The case of tobacco control. *Journal of Health Politics, Policy & Law, 24*(4), 769–804.

Jacobson, P. D., & Wasserman, J. (1999). The implementation and enforcement of tobacco control laws: Policy implications for activists and the industry. *Journal of Health Politics, Policy & Law, 24*(3), 567–598.

Jacobson, P. D., Wasserman, J., Botoseneanu, A., Silverstein, A., & Wu, H. W. (2012). The role of law in public health preparedness: Opportunities and challenges. *Journal of Health Politics, Policy & Law, 37*(2), 297–328.

Jalan, J., & Somanathan, E. (2008). The importance of being informed: Experimental evidence on demand for environmental quality. *Journal of Development Economics, 87*(1), 14–28.

Janesick, V. J. (2004). *"Stretching" exercises for qualitative researchers* (2nd ed.). Thousand Oaks, CA: Sage.

Jenkins, P. H. (1997). School delinquency and the school social bond. *Journal of Research in Crime and Delinquency, 34*(3), 337–367.

Jewell, C. A., & Bero, L. A. (2008). Developing good taste in evidence: Facilitators of and hindrances to evidence-informed health policymaking in state government. *The Milbank Quarterly, 86*(2), 177–208.

Jha, P., Musgrove, P., Chaloupka, F. J., & Yurekli, A. (2000). The economic rationale for intervention in the tobacco market. In P. Jha & F. J. Chaloupka (Eds.), *Tobacco control in developing countries*. Oxford; New York: Oxford University Press.

Johansson-Stenman, O., & Martinsson, P. (2008). Are some lives more valuable? An ethical preferences approach. *Journal of Health Economics, 27*(3), 739–752.

Johnson, C. A. (1987). Law, politics, and judicial decision making: Lower federal court uses of supreme court decisions. *Law & Society Review, 21*(2), 325–340.

Johnson, R. B., & Onwuegbuzie, A. J. (2004). Mixed methods research: A research paradigm whose time has come. *Educational Researcher, 33*(7), 14–26.

Johnson, S. W., & Walker, J. (1996). *The Crash Outcome Data Evaluation System (CODES)*. Washington, DC: National Highway Traffic Safety Adminstration.

Johnston, L. D., O'Malley, P. M., Bachman, J. G., & Schulenberg, J. E. (2011). *Monitoring the future national survey results on drug use, 1975–2010. Volume II: College students and adults ages 19–50*. Ann Arbor, MI: Institute for Social Research, University of Michigan.

Jolls, C. (2006). *Behavioral law and economics*. Yale Law School, Public Law working paper no. 130; Yale Law & Economics research paper no. 342. Retrieved from Social Sciences Research Network at papers.ssrn.com/sol3/papers.cfm?abstract_id=959177

Jolls, C., Sunstein, C. R., & Thaler, R. (1998). A behavioral approach to law and economics. *Stanford Law Review, 50*, 1471–1550.

Jones, B. T., Corbin, W., & Fromme, K. (2001). A review of expectancy theory and alcohol consumption. *Addiction, 96*(1), 57–72.

Jones, S. J., Jahns, L., Laraia, B. A., & Haughton, B. (2003). Lower risk of overweight in school-aged food insecure girls who participate in food assistance. *Archives of Pediatrics and Adolescent Medicine, 157*(8), 780–784.

Jordan, G. B. (2010). A theory-based logic model for innovation policy and evaluation. *Research Evaluation, 19*(4), 263–273.

Joseph, J. G., Emmons, C. A., Kessler, R. C., et al. (1984). Coping with the threat of AIDS: An approach to psychosocial assessment. *The American Psychologist, 39*(11), 1297–1302.

Jost, J. T., & Major, B. (2001). *The psychology of legitimacy: Emerging perspectives on ideology, justice, and intergroup relations*. New York: Cambridge University Press.

Kagan, R. A., & Skolnick, J. H. (1993). Banning smoking: Compliance without enforcement. In R. L. Rabin & S. D. Sugerman (Eds.), *Smoking policy: Law, politics and culture* (pp. 69–94). New York: Oxford University Press.

Kahn, L. M. (2000). Wage inequality, collective bargaining, and relative employment from 1985 to 1994: Evidence from fifteen OECD countries. *The Review of Economics and Statistics, 82*(4), 564–579.

Kahneman, D. (1999). Objective happiness in well being: The foundations of hedonic psychology. In D. Kahneman, E. Diener, & N. Schwarz (Eds.), *Well-being: Foundations of hedonic psychology*. New York: Russell Sage Foundation.

Kahneman, D., Fredrickson, B. L., Schreiber, C. A., & Redelmeier, D. A. (1993). When more pain is preferred to less. *Psychological Science, 4*(6), 401–405.

Kahnemann, D., Slovic, P., & Tversky, A. (Eds.). (1982). *Judgment under uncertainty: Heuristics and biases*. Cambridge: Cambridge University Press.

Kalev, A., Dobbin, F., & Kelly, E. (2006). Best practices or best guesses? Assessing the efficacy of corporate affirmative action and diversity policies. *American Sociological Review, 71*(4), 589–617.

Kellogg, K. C. (2011). *Challenging operations: Medical reform and resistance in surgery*. Chicago: University of Chicago Press.

Kelly, E. L., Moen, P., & Tranby, E. (2011). Changing workplaces to reduce work-family conflict: Schedule control in a white-collar organization. *American Sociological Review, 76*(2), 265–290.

Khan, M., Wohl, D., Weir, S., et al. (2008). Incarceration and risky sexual partnerships in a southern U.S. city. *Journal of Urban Health, 85*(1), 100–113.

Kidd, P. S., & Parshall, M. B. (2000). Getting the focus and the group: Enhancing analytical rigor in focus group research. *Qualitative Health Research, 10*(3), 293–308.

Kim, S., LeBlanc, A., & Michalopoulos, C. (2009). *Working toward wellness: Early results from a telephone care management program for Medicaid recipients with depression* (Working paper). New York: MDRC.

Kimball, A. M., Moore, M., French, H. M., et al. (2008). Regional infectious disease surveillance networks and their potential to facilitate the implementation of the international health regulations. *Medical Clinics of North America, 92*(6), 1459–1471.

King, E. B., Dawson, J. F., Kravitz, D. A., & Gulick, L. M. (2012). A multilevel study of the relationships between diversity training, ethnic discrimination and satisfaction in organizations. *Journal of Organizational Behavior, 33*(1), 5–20.

King, G., Gakidou, E., Ravishankar, N., et al. (2007). A "politically robust" experimental design for public policy evaluation with application to the Mexican universal health insurance program. *Journal of Policy Analysis and Management, 26*(3), 479–509.

Kinney, E. D. (2002). Administrative law and the public's health. *The Journal of Law, Medicine & Ethics, 30*(2), 212–223.

Kitzinger, J. (1994). The methodology of focus groups: The importance of interaction between research participants. *Sociology of Health & Illness, 16*(1), 103–121.

Kivimäki, M., Elovainio, M., Vahtera, J., Virtanen, M., & Stansfeld, S. A. (2003). Association between organizational inequity and incidence of psychiatric disorders in female employees. *Psychological Medicine, 33*(2), 319–326.

Kivimäki, M., Ferrie, J. E., Brunner, E., et al. (2005). Justice at work and reduced risk of coronary heart disease among employees. *Archives of Internal Medicine, 165*(19), 2245–2251.

Kivimäki, M., Ferrie, J. E., Head, J., et al. (2004). Organisational justice and change in justice as predictors of employee health. *Journal of Epidemiology and Community Health, 58*(11), 931–937.

Klepeis, N. E., Ott, W. R., & Switzer P. (2007). Real-time measurement of outdoor tobacco smoke particles. *Journal of the Air & Waste Management Association, 57,* 522–534.

Klepper, S., & Nagin, D. S. (1989). Certainty and severity of punishment revisited. *Criminology, 27*(4), 721–746.

Kling, J., & Liebman, J. (2005). *Experimental analysis of neighborhood effects on youth* (NBER Working Paper 11577). Cambridge, MA: National Bureau of Economic Research.

Klitzman, R., Kirshenbaum, S., Kittel, L., et al. (2004). Naming names: Perceptions of name-based HIV reporting, partner notification, and criminalization of non-disclosure among persons living with HIV. *Sexuality Research and Social Policy, 1*(3), 38–57.

Ko, N. Y., Lee, H. C., Hung, C. C., et al. (2009). Effects of structural intervention on increasing condom availability and reducing risky sexual behaviours in gay bathhouse attendees. *AIDS Care, 21*(12), 1499–1507.

Komro, K. A., Flay, B. R., Biglan, A., & the Promise Neighborhoods Research Consortium. (2011). Creating nurturing environments: A science-based framework for promoting child health and development within high-poverty neighborhoods. *Clinical Child and Family Psychology Review, 14*(2), 111–134.

Koopmanschapp, M. A., Rutten, F.F.H., van Ineveld, B. M., & van Roijen, L. (1995). The friction cost method for estimating the indirect costs of disease. *Journal of Health Economics, 14*(2), 171–189.

Kouvonen, A., Kivimäki, M., Elovainio, M., et al. (2008). Low organisational justice and heavy drinking: A prospective cohort study. *Occupational and Environmental Medicine, 65*(1), 44–50.

Kouvonen, A., Vahtera, J., Elovainio, M., et al. (2007). Organisational justice and smoking: The Finnish public sector study. *Journal of Epidemiology and Community Health, 61*(5), 427–433.

Kratochwill, T. R., Hitchcock, J., Horner, R. H., et al. (2010). *Single-case designs technical documentation.* Washington, DC: U.S. Department of Education, Institute of Education Sciences, National Center for Education Evaluation and Regional Assistance, What Works Clearinghouse. Retrieved from What Works Clearinghouse website at ies.ed.gov/ncee/wwc/pdf/wwc_scd.pdf

Kremer, M., & Miguel, E. (2007). The illusion of sustainability. *Quarterly Journal of Economics, 122*(3), 1007–1065.

Kremer, M., Miguel, E., Mullainathan, S., Null, C., & Zwane, A. P. (2009). Making water safe: Price, persuasion, peers, promoters, or product design? Unpublished working paper. Harvard University.

Kremer, M., Miguel, E., & Thornton, R. (2009). Incentives to learn. *Review of Economics and Statistics, 91*(3), 437–456.

Kremer, M., Moulin, S., & Namanyu, R. (2003). *Decentralization: A cautionary tale* (Paper no. 10). Cambridge, MA: Poverty Action Lab.

Kremer, M., & Vermeersch, C. (2004). *School meals, educational attainment, and school competition: Evidence from a randomized evaluation* (World Bank Policy Research Working Paper 2523). Washington, DC: World Bank.

Krieger, N., Chen, J. T., Waterman, P. D., Rehkopf, D. H., & Subramanian, S. V. (2005). Painting a truer picture of U.S. socioeconomic and racial/ethnic health inequalities: The public health disparities geocoding project. *American Journal of Public Health, 95*(2), 312–323.

Krippendorff, K. (1980). *Content analysis: An introduction to its methodology*. London: Sage.

Krippendorff, K. (2004). *Content analysis: An introduction to its methodology* (2nd ed.). Thousand Oaks, CA: Sage.

Krislov, S., Boyum, K. O., Clark, J. N., Shaefer, R. C., & White, S. O. (1966). *Compliance and the law: A multi-disciplinary approach*. Beverly Hills, CA: Sage.

Kromm, J. N., Frattaroli, S., Vernick, J. S., & Teret, S. P. (2009). Public health advocacy in the courts: Opportunities for public health professionals. *Public Health Reports, 124*(6), 889–894.

Krueger, A. B., & Zhu, P. (2004). Another look at the New York City school voucher experiment. *American Behavioral Scientist, 47*(5), 658–698.

Kruesi, F. E. (1997). *The value of saving travel time: Departmental guidance for conducting economic evaluations*. Washington, DC: Office of the Secretary of Transportation.

Lacey, A., & Luff, D. (2001). *Trent focus for research and development in primary health care: An introduction to qualitative data analysis*. Nottingham, UK: Trent Focus.

LaFond, C., Toomey, T. L., Rothstein, C., Wagenaar, A. C., & Manning, W. (2000). Policy evaluation research: Measuring the independent variables. *Evaluation Review, 24*(1), 92–101.

Lakey, B. (2010). Social support: Basic research and new strategies for intervention. In J. E. Maddux & J. P. Tangney (Eds.), *Social psychological foundations of clinical psychology* (pp. 177–194). New York: Guildford.

Lalive, R., & Cattaneo, M. A. (2009). Social interactions and schooling decisions. *Review of Economics and Statistics, 91*(3), 457–477.

Lamberty, G., Pachter, L. M., & Crnic, K. (2000). *Social stratification: Implications for understanding racial, ethnic and class disparities in child health and development*. Paper presented at the Role of Partnerships: Second Annual Meeting of Child Health Services Researchers, Rockville, Maryland, June 27, 2000.

Lamont, M., & White, P. (2005). *Workshop on interdisciplinary standards for systematic qualitative research*. National Science Foundation supported workshop. Retrieved September 13, 2011, from www.nsf.gov/sbe/ses/soc/ISSQR_workshop_rpt.pdf

Land, K. C. (1969). Principles of path analysis. *Sociological Methodology, 1*, 3–37.

Larkin, M. A., & McGowan, A. K. (2008). Introduction: Strengthening public health. *Journal of Law, Medicine & Ethics, 36* (Suppl. 3), 4–5.

Larsen, L. L., & Berry, J. A. (2003). The regulation of dietary supplements. *Journal of the American Academy of Nurse Practitioners, 15*(9), 410–414.

Larson, N. I., Story, M., & Nelson, M. C. (2009). Neighborhood environments: Disparities in access to healthy foods in the U.S. *American Journal of Preventive Medicine, 36*(1), 74–81.

Lave, L. B. (1987). Injury as externality: An economic perspective of trauma. *Accident Analysis and Prevention, 19*(1), 29–37.

Lavis, J., Oxman, A., Moynihan, R., & Paulsen, E. (2008). Evidence-informed health policy 1—Synthesis of findings from a multi-method study of organizations that support the use of research evidence. *Implementation Science, 3*(1), 53.

Law, D. S. (2005). Strategic judicial lawmaking: Ideology, publication, and asylum law in the Ninth Circuit. *University of Cincinnati Law Review, 73*(3), 817–866.

Lawson, J., & Xu, F. (2007). SARS in Canada and China: Two approaches to emergency health policy. *Governance, 20*(2), 209–232.

Lazzarini, Z., Bray, S., & Burris, S. (2002). Evaluating the impact of criminal laws on HIV risk behavior. *Journal of Law, Medicine & Ethics, 30*(2), 239–253.

Lazzarini, Z., & Rosales, L. (2002). Legal issues concerning public health efforts to reduce perinatal HIV transmission. *Yale Journal of Health Law, Policy, and Ethics, 3*(1), 67–98.

Lee, K., Ingram, A., Lock, K., & McInnes, C. (2007). Bridging health and foreign policy: The role of health impact assessments. *Bull World Health Organ, 85*(3), 207–211.

Lehmkuhl, D. (2008). Control modes in the age of transnational governance. *Law & Policy, 30*(3), 336–363.

Leischow, S. J., Best, A., Trochim, W. M., et al. (2008). Systems thinking to improve the public's health. *American Journal of Preventive Medicine, 35*(2), S196–S203.

Lemert, E. M. (1951). *Social pathology*. New York: McGraw-Hill.

Lemert, E. M. (1967). *Human deviance, social problems, and social control*. Englewood Cliffs, NJ: Prentice-Hall.

Lenaway, D., Halverson, P., Sotnikov, S., et al. (2006). Public health systems research: Setting a national agenda. *American Journal of Public Health, 96*(3), 410–413.

Lewin, K. (1952). *Field theory in social science: Selected theoretical papers*. New York: Harper & Brothers.

Lewis, J. (1985). Lead poisoning: A historical perspective. *EPA Journal, 11*(4), 15–18.

Libbey, H. P. (2004). Measuring student relationships to school: Attachment, bonding, connectedness, and engagement. *Journal of School Health, 74*(7), 274–283.

Libbey, P., & Miyahara, B. (2011). *Cross-jurisdictional relationships in local public health: Preliminary summary of an environmental scan.* Princeton, NJ: The Robert Wood Johnson Foundation.

Lichtveld, M., Hodge, J. G., Jr., Gebbie, K., Thompson, F. E. Jr., & Loos, D. I. (2002). Preparedness on the frontline: What's law got to do with it? *Journal of Law, Medicine & Ethics, 30*(3 Suppl.), 184–188.

Liebman, J. B, Katz, L. F., & Kling, J. R. (2004). *Beyond treatment effects: Estimating the relationship between neighborhood poverty and individual outcomes in the MTO Experiment* (NBER Working Paper 493). Cambridge, MA: National Bureau of Economic Research.

Liljegren, M., & Ekberg, K. (2009). The associations between perceived distributive, procedural, and interactional organizational justice, self-rated health and burnout. *Work, 33*(1), 43–51.

Lincoln, Y. S., & Guba, E. G. (1985). *Naturalistic inquiry.* Beverly Hills, CA: Sage.

Lind, E. A., & Tyler, T. R. (1988). *The social psychology of procedural justice.* New York: Plenum Press.

Link, B. G., & Phelan, J. (1995). Social conditions as fundamental causes of disease. *Journal of Health and Social Behavior, 35*, 80–94.

Liu, B. C., Ivers, R., Norton, R., et al. (2008). Helmets for preventing injury in motorcycle riders. *Cochrane Database of Systematic Reviews* (1), CD004333.

Lobel, O. (2004). The renew deal: The fall of regulation and the rise of governance in contemporary legal thought. *Minnesota Law Review, 89*, 342–471.

Lobel, O., & Amir, O. (2009). Stumble, predict, nudge: How behavioral economics informs law and policy. *Columbia Law Review*, 108; San Diego Legal Studies paper no. 09-006. Retrieved from Social Science Research Network at papers.ssrn.com/sol3/papers.cfm?abstract_id=1327077

Lochner, K. A., Kawachi, I., Brennan, R. T., & Buka, S. L. (2003). Social capital and neighborhood mortality rates in Chicago. *Social Science & Medicine, 56*, 1797–1805.

Loevinger, L. (1961). Jurimetrics: Science and prediction in the field of law. *Minnesota Law Review, 46*, 255–275.

Lofland, J. H., Pizzi, L., & Frick, K. D. (2004). A review of health-related workplace productivity loss instruments. *Pharmacoeconomics, 22*(3), 165–184.

Logan, W. A. (2009). *Knowledge as power: Criminal registration and community notification laws in America.* Palo Alto, CA: Stanford University Press.

Lombard, M., Snyder-Duch, J., & Campanella Bracken, C. (2005). *Practical resources for assessing and reporting intercoder reliability in content analysis research projects.* Retrieved July 1, 2011, from www.temple.edu/mmc/reliability/

Ludwig, J., & Cook, P. J. (2000). Homicide and suicide rates associated with implementation of the Brady Handgun Violence Prevention Act. *Journal of the American Medical Association, 284*(5), 585–591.

Ludwig, J., Kling, J. R., & Mullainathan, S. (2011). Mechanism experiments and policy evaluations. *Journal of Economic Perspectives, 25*(3), 17–38.

Ludwig, J., Sanbonmatsu, L., Gennetian, L., et al. (2011). Neighborhoods, obesity, and diabetes: A randomized social experiment. *New England Journal of Medicine, 365*(16), 1509–1519.

Lurie, N., Wasserman, J., Stoto, M., et al. (2004). Local variation in public health preparedness: Lessons from California. *Health Affairs, Web Exclusive*, W4341–W4353.

Lutfey, K., & Freese, J. (2005). Toward some fundamentals of fundamental causality: Socioeconomic status and health in the routine clinic visit for diabetes. *American Journal of Sociology, 110*(5), 1326–1372.

Maantay, J. (2002). Zoning law, health, and environmental justice: What's the connection? *Journal of Law, Medicine & Ethics, 30*(4), 572–593.

MacCoun, R. J. (1993). Drugs and the law: A psychological analysis of drug prohibition. *Psychological Bulletin, 113*(3), 497–512.

Macdonald, H. R., & Glantz, S. A. (1997). Political realities of statewide smoking legislation: The passage of California's Assembly Bill 13. *Tobacco Control, 6*(1), 41–54.

MacKinnon, D. P. (2008). *Introduction to statistical mediation analysis*. New York: Taylor & Francis Group.

Magnusson, R. S. (2007). Mapping the scope and opportunities for public health law in liberal democracies. *The Journal of Law, Medicine & Ethics, 35*(4), 571–587.

Magnusson, R. S. (2009). Rethinking global health challenges: Towards a "global compact" for reducing the burden of chronic disease. *Public Health, 123*(3), 265–274.

Mamudu, H. M., & Glantz, S. A. (2009). Civil society and the negotiation of the Framework Convention on Tobacco Control. *Global Public Heatlh, 4*(2), 150–168.

Manning, W. G. (1991). *The costs of poor health habits*. Cambridge, MA: Harvard University Press.

Mariner, W. K. (2009). Toward an architecture of health law. *American Journal of Law and Medicine, 35*(1), 67–87.

Marks, M., Wood, J., Ali, F., Walsh, T., & Witbooi, A. (2010). Worlds apart? On the possibilities of police/academic collaborations. *Policing: A Journal of Policy and Practice, 4*(2), 112–118.

Marmot, M. (2005). Social determinants of health inequalities. *Lancet, 365*, 1099–1104.

Martin, R., Conseil, A., Longstaff, A., et al. (2010). Pandemic influenza control in Europe and the constraints resulting from incoherent public health laws. *BMC Public Health, 10*(1), 532.

Matthews, G., & Markiewicz, M. (2011). *Legal frameworks supporting public health department accreditation: Key findings and lessons learned from ten states*. Chapel Hill, NC: UNC Gillings School of Global Public Health.

Mayer, D. P., Peterson, P. E., Myers, D. E., Tuttle, C. C., & Howell, W. G. (2002). *School choice in New York City after three years: An evaluation of the School Choice Scholarships Program*. (Report No. 8404-045). Cambridge, MA: Mathematica Policy Research.

Mays, G., Beitsch, L. M., Corso, L., Chang, C., & Brewer, R. (2007). States gathering momentum: Promising strategies for accreditation and assessment activities in multistate learning collaborative applicant States. *Journal of Public Health Management & Practice, 13*(4), 364–373.

Mays, G. P. (2011). Leading improvement through inquiry: Practice-based research networks in public health. *Public Health Leadership, 9*(3), 1–3.

Mays, G. P., Halverson, P. K., & Scutchfield, F. D. (2004). Making public health improvement real: The vital role of systems research. *Journal of Public Health Management and Practice, 10*(3), 183–185.

Mays, G. P., Scutchfield, F. D., Bhandari, M. W., & Smith, S. A. (2010). Understanding the organization of public health delivery systems: An empirical typology. *Milbank Quarterly, 88*(1), 81–111.

McAlinden, A. M. (2006). Managing risk: From regulation to the reintegration of sex offenders. *Criminology and Criminal Justice, 6*(2), 197–218.

McBarnet, D. J., Voiculescu, A., & Campbell, T. (Eds.). (2007). *The new corporate accountability: Corporate social responsibility and the law*. Cambridge, UK: Cambridge University Press.

McCann, M. W. (1994). *Rights at work: Pay equity reform and the politics of legal mobilization*. Chicago: University of Chicago Press.

McCann, P.J.C. (2009). Agency discretion and public health service delivery. *Health Services Research, 44*(5), 1897–1908.

McChesney, F. S. (1993). Doctrinal analysis and statistical modeling in law: The case of defective incorporation. *Washington University Law Quarterly, 71*(3), 493–534.

McCleary, R., & Hay, R. A. (1980). *Applied time series analysis for the social sciences*. Beverly Hills, CA: Sage.

McCluskey, J. D. (2003). *Police requests for compliance: Coercive and procedurally just tactics*. New York: LFB Scholarly.

McCormick, W. B. Jr., & Shane, J. N. (1993). *Treatment of valuing life and injuries in preparing economic evaluations*. Washington, DC: Office of the Secretary of Transportation.

McCoy, D., & Hilson, M. (2009). Civil society, its organizations, and global health governance. In K. Buse, W. Hein, & N. Drager (Eds.), *Making sense of global health governance* (pp. 209–231). London: Palgrave MacMillan.

McDougall, G. (1997). Direct legislation: Determinants of legislator support for voter initiatives. *Public Finance Review, 25*(3), 327–343.

McDowell, I. (2006). *Measuring health: A guide to rating scales and questionnaires*. (3rd ed.). New York: Oxford University Press.

McGuire, K. T., Vanberg, G., Smith, C. E., & Caldeira, G. A. (2009). Measuring policy content on the U.S. Supreme Court. *The Journal of Politics, 71*(04), 1305–1321.

McKenzie, D., Gibson, J., & Stillman, S. (2010). How important is selection? Experimental vs. non-experimental measures of the income gains from migration. *Journal of the European Economic Association, 8*(4), 913–945.

McKenzie, D., & Yang, D. (2010). *Experimental approaches in migration studies* (World Bank Policy Research Working Paper No. 5395). Washington, DC: World Bank.

McMillen, R. C., Winickoff, J. P., Klein, J. D., & Weitzman, M. (2003). U.S. adult attitudes and practices regarding smoking restrictions and child exposure to environmental tobacco smoke: Changes in the social climate from 2000–2001. *Pediatrics, 112*(1), e55–60.

McNeill, L. H., Kreuter, M. W., & Subramanian, S. V. (2006). Social environment and physical activity: A review of concepts and evidence. *Social Science and Medicine, 63*(4), 1011–1022.

McNeill, W. (1977). *Plagues and peoples*. Garden City, NJ: Anchor Press.

Mead, G. H. (1934). *Mind, self, & society: From the standpoint of a social behaviorist* (Vol. 1). Chicago: University of Chicago Press.

Meier, B. M., Hodge, J. G. Jr., & Gebbie, K. M. (2009). Transitions in state public health law: Comparative analysis of state public health law reform following the Turning Point Model State Public Health Act. *American Journal of Public Health, 99*(3), 423–430.

Meier, B. M., Merrill, J., & Gebbie, K. M. (2009). Modernizing state public health enabling statutes to reflect the mission and essential services of public health. *Journal of Public Health Management and Practice, 15*(4), 284–291.

Meier, L. L., Semmer, N. K., & Hupfeld, J. (2009). The impact of unfair treatment on depressive mood: The moderating role of self-esteem level and self-esteem instability. *Personality and Social Psychology Bulletin, 35*(5), 643–655.

Mello, M., & Brennan, T. (2002). Deterrence of medical errors: Theory and evidence for malpractice reform. *Texas Law Review, 80*, 1595–1638.

Mello, M. M., Pomeranz, J., & Moran, P. (2008). The interplay of public health law and industry self-regulation: The case of sugar-sweetened beverage sales in schools. *American Journal of Public Health, 98*(4), 595–604.

Mello, M. M., Powlowski, M., Nañagas, J.M.P., & Bossert, T. (2006). The role of law in public health: The case of family planning in the Philippines. *Social Science & Medicine, 63*(2), 384–396.

Mello, M. M., & Zeiler, K. (2008). Empirical health law scholarship: The state of the field. *Georgetown Law Journal, 96*(2), 649–702.

Melnick, R. S. (1983). *Regulation and the courts: The case of the Clean Air Act*. Washington, DC: Brookings Institution.

Melton, G. B. (Ed.) (1986). *The law as a behavioral instrument: Nebraska Symposium on Motivation, 1985*. Volume 33 in the series *Current Theory and Research in Motivation*. Lincoln: University of Nebraska Press.

Merrill, J., Keeling, J., Meier, B. M., Gebbie, K. M., & Jia, H. (2009). Examination of the relationship between public health statute modernization and local public health system performance. *Journal of Public Health Management and Practice, 15*(4), 292–298.

Merry, S. E. (1990). *Getting justice and getting even: Legal consciousness among working-class Americans*. Chicago: University of Chicago Press.

Mertz, K. J., & Weiss, H. B. (2008). Changes in motorcycle-related head injury deaths, hospitalizations, and hospital charges following repeal of Pennsylvania's mandatory motorcycle helmet law. *American Journal of Public Health, 98*(8), 1464–1467.

Meyer, P. (2010, December 15). Marijuana use is rising; ecstasy use is beginning to rise; and alcohol use is declining among U.S. teens. *University of Michigan, University Record Online.* Retrieved from www.ur.umich.edu/update/archives/101215/mtfdrugs15

Meyers, D. G., Neuberger, J. S., & He, J. (2009). Cardiovascular effect of bans on smoking in public places. *Journal of the American College of Cardiology, 54*(15), 1249–1255.

Miguel, E., & Kremer, M. (2004). Worms: Identifying impacts on education and health in the presence of treatment externalities. *Econometrica, 72*(1), 159–217.

Miller Brewing Company. (2000). *Beer is volume with profit 2000.* Milwaukee, WI: Miller Brewing.

Miller, M., Azrael, D., & Hemenway, D. (2002). Rates of household firearm ownership and homicide across U.S. regions and states. *American Journal of Public Health, 92*(12), 1988–1993.

Miller, T. R. (1994). *Costs of safety belt and motorcycle helmet nonuse—Testimony to Subcommittee on Surface Transportation.* Paper presented at the House Committee on Public Works and Transportation, Washington, DC, March 3.

Miller, T. R. (2001). *Computing and presenting injury costs.* Conference report from the 1st Safe Community-Conference on Cost Calculation and Cost-Effectiveness in Injury Prevention and Safety Promotion. Viborg County, Denmark, Sept. 30–Oct. 3, 2001. Retrieved from www.phs.ki.se/csp/pdf/rapport-net.pdf

Miller, T. R., Bhattacharya, S., Zaloshnja, E., et al. (2011). Costs of crashes to government, United States, 2008. *Annals of Advances in Automotive Medicine, 55,* 347–356.

Miller, T. R., & Blewden, M. (2001). Costs of alcohol-related crashes: New Zealand estimates and suggested measures for use internationally. *Accident Analysis and Prevention, 33*(6), 783–791.

Miller T. R., Cohen M. A., & Wiersema, B. (1996). *Victim costs and consequences: A new look.* Research report. Washington DC: National Institute of Justice.

Miller, T. R., & Hendrie, D. (2009). *Cost and benefit analysis of substance abuse prevention interventions.* Rockville, MD: Substance Abuse and Mental Health Services Administration.

Miller, T. R., & Hendrie, D. (2012). Economic evaluation of interventions. In G. Li & S. P. Baker (Eds.), *Injury research: Theories, methods and approaches* (pp. 641–666). New York: Springer.

Miller, T. R., Hunter, W., Waller, P., Whiting, B., & Whitman, R. (1985). *Development of a value criteria methodology for assessing highway systems cost-effectiveness* (# FHWA/RD-83/078). Washington, DC: The Granville Corp.

Miller, T. R., & Levy, D. T. (1997). Cost-outcome analysis in injury prevention and control: A primer on methods. *Injury Prevention, 3*(4), 288–293.

Miller, T. R., Zaloshnja, E., & Hendrie, D. (2009). Cost of traumatic brain injuries in the United States and the return to helmet investments. In J. Jallo & C. Loftus (Eds.), *Neurotrauma and critical care of the brain* (pp. 445–459). New York: Thieme.

Miller, W. L., & Crabtree, B. F. (2004). Depth interviewing. In S. N. Hesse-Biber & P. Leavy (Eds.), *Approaches to qualitative research: A reader on theory and practice* (pp. 185–202). New York: Oxford University Press.

Mindell, J., Sheridan, L., Joffe, M., Samson-Barry, H., & Atkinson, S. (2004). Health impact assessment as an agent of policy change: Improving the health impacts of the mayor of London's draft transport strategy. *Journal of Epidemiology and Community Health, 58*(3), 169–174.

Misue, K., Eades, P., Lai, W., & Sugiyama, K. (1995). Layout adjustment and the mental map. *Journal of Visual Languages & Computing, 6*(2), 183–210.

Moehler, D. C. (2010). Democracy, governance, and randomized development assistance. *Annals of the American Academy of Political and Social Science, 628*(1), 30–46.

Moen, P., Kelly, E. L., Huang, Q., & Tranby, E. (2011). Changing work, changing health: Can real work-time flexibility promote health behaviors and well-being? *Journal of Health and Social Behavior, 52*(4), 404–429.

Moerman, J. W., & Potts, G. E. (2011). Analysis of metals leached from smoked cigarette litter. *Tobacco Control, 20,* i30–i35.

Mokdad, A. H., Marks, J. S., Stroup, D. F., & Gerberding, J. L. (2004). Actual causes of death in the United States, 2000. *Journal of the American Medical Association, 291*(10), 1238–1245.

Mokdad, A. H., Marks, J. S., Stroup, D. F., & Gerberding, J. L. (2005). Correction: Actual causes of death in the United States, 2000. *Journal of the American Medical Association, 293*(3), 293–294.

Montini, T., & Bero, L. (2008). Implementation of a workplace smoking ban in bars: The limits of local discretion. *BMC Public Health, 8*(1), 402.

Moran, M. (2002). Review article: Understanding the regulatory state. *British Journal of Political Science, 32*(2), 391–413.

Moreau, S. (2010). What is discrimination? *Philosophy and Public Affairs, 38*(2), 143–179.

Morgan, D. L. (2004). Focus groups. In S. N. Hesse-Biber & P. Leavy (Eds.), *Approaches to qualitative research: A reader on theory and practice* (pp. 263–285). New York: Oxford University Press.

Morrisey, M. A., Grabowski, D. C., Dee, T. S., & Campbell, C. (2006). The strength of graduated drivers license programs and fatalities among teen drivers and passengers. *Accident Analysis and Prevention, 38*(1), 135–141.

Motorcycle Industry Council. (2009, May 21). *Motorcycling in America goes mainstream says 2008 Motorcycle Industry Council owner survey* [Press release]. Retrieved September 4, 2001, from www.mic.org/news052109.cfm

Moulton, A., Gottfried, R., Goodman, R., Murphy, A., & Rawson, R. (2003). What is public health legal preparedness? *Journal of Law, Medicine & Ethics, 31*(4), 672–683.

Moulton, A. D., Mercer, S. L., Popovic, T., et al. (2009). The scientific basis for law as a public health tool. *American Journal of Public Health, 99*(1), 17–24.

Murray, D. M. (1998). *Design and analysis of group-randomized trials*. New York: Oxford University Press.

Musheno, M. (1997). Legal consciousness on the margins of society: Struggles against stigmatization in the AIDS crisis. *Identities, 2*(1/2), 101.

Myers, T., Orr, K. W., Locker, D., & Jackson, E. A. (1993). Factors affecting gay and bisexual men's decisions and intentions to seek HIV testing. *American Journal of Public Health, 83*(5), 701–704.

Mykhalovskiy, E. (2011). The problem of "significant risk": Exploring the public health impact of criminalizing HIV non-disclosure. *Social Science & Medicine, 73*(5), 668–675.

Nagin, D. S. (1998). Criminal deterrence research at the outset of the twenty-first century. In M. Tonry (Ed.), *Crime and justice: A review of research* (Vol. 23, pp. 1–42). Chicago: University of Chicago Press.

Nagin, D. S. (2010). Imprisonment and crime control: Building evidence-based policy. In R. Rosenfeld, K. Quinet, & C. Garcia (Eds.), *Contemporary issues in criminological theory and research: The role of social institutions*. Belmont, CA: Wadsworth.

Nagin, D. S., & Pogarsky, G. (2001). Integrating celerity, impulsivity, and extralegal sanction threats into a model of general deterrence: Theory and evidence. *Criminology, 39*(4), 865–891.

Nakkash, R., & Lee, K. (2009). The tobacco industry's thwarting of marketing restrictions and health warnings in Lebanon. *Tobacco Control, 18*(4), 310–316.

National Association of Local Boards of Health. (2011). *Profile of local boards of health launched*. Retrieved May 5, 2011, from www.nalboh.org/Profile.htm

National Cancer Institute [NCI]. (2008). *The role of the media in promoting and reducing tobacco use* (NIH Publication No. 07–6242). Bethesda, MD: National Cancer Institute.

National Highway Traffic Safety Administration. (2010). *Motorcycle helmet use in 2010— Overall results* (DOT HS-811–419). Washington, DC: U.S. Department of Transportation, National Highway Traffic Safety Administration.

National Highway Traffic Safety Administration. (2011). *Fatality Analysis Reporting System (FARS) encyclopedia*. Retrieved December 16, 2011, from www-fars.nhtsa .dot.gov/Main/index.aspx

National Institute on Alcohol Abuse and Alcoholism. (2011a). *Alcohol Policy Information System (APIS)*. Retrieved August 18, 2011, from www.alcoholpolicy.niaaa.nih.gov

National Institute on Alcohol Abuse and Alcoholism. (2011b). Underage drinking: Underage purchase of alcohol. *Alcohol Policy Information System (APIS) Web Site*. Retrieved November 1, 2012, from alcoholpolicy.niaaa.nih.gov/Underage_Purchase_ of_Alcohol.html

National Research Council & Institute of Medicine. (2002). Executive summary. *Health insurance is a family matter*. Washington, DC: The National Academies Press.

Neuendorf, K. A. (2002). *The content analysis guidebook*. Thousand Oaks, CA: Sage.

Neuendorf, K. A. (2007). *The content analysis guidebook online.* Retrieved from academic.csuohio.edu/kneuendorf/content/

Neumark, D., & Wascher, W. (2001). Using the EITC to help poor families: New evidence and a comparison with the minimum wage. *National Tax Journal, 54*(2), 281–317.

New State Ice Co. v. Liebmann, 285 U.S. 262 (1932).

New York State Office of Mental Health. (2011). *Implementation of assisted outpatient treatment.* Retrieved October 1, 2011, from www.omh.ny.gov/omhweb/Kendra _web/interimreport/implementation.htm

Nixon, M. L., Mahmoud, L., & Glantz, S. A. (2004). Tobacco industry litigation to deter local public health ordinances: The industry usually loses in court. *Tobacco Control, 13*(1), 65–73.

Novak, J. D., & Cañas, A. J. (2008). *The theory underlying concept maps and how to construct and use them.* Ponta Grossa, Puerto Rico: Universidade Estadual de Ponta Grossa.

Novick, L., Morrow, C., & Mays, G. (Eds.). (2008). *Public health administration: Principles for population-based management.* Sudbury, MA: Jones and Bartlett.

Novotny, T. E., Lum, K., Smith, E., Wang, V., & Barnes, R. (2009). Cigarette butts and the case for an environmental policy on hazardous cigarette waste. *International Journal of Environmental Research and Public Health, 6*(5), 1691–1705.

Nunez-Smith, M., Pilgrim, N., Wynia, M., et al. (2009). Health care workplace discrimination and physician turnover. *Journal of the National Medical Association, 101*(12), 1274–1282.

Obama, B. (2009, January 20). *President Barack Obama's inaugural address.* Retrieved November 3, 2009, from www.whitehouse.gov/blog/inaugural-address/

Oetting, E. R., & Beauvais, F. (1986). Peer cluster theory: Drugs and the adolescent. *Journal of Counseling and Development, 65,* 17–65.

Office of Disease Prevention and Health Promotion & U.S. Department of Health and Human Services. (2010). *Healthy people 2010.* Retrieved March 14, 2011, from www. healthypeople.gov/2010/default.htm

Office of Disease Prevention and Health Promotion & U.S. Department of Health and Human Services. (2011). *Healthy people 2020.* Retrieved March 14, 2011, from www. healthypeople.gov/2020/topicsobjectives2020/objectiveslist.aspx?topicid=35

Olds, D. L. (2006). The nurse-family partnership: An evidence-based preventive intervention. *Infant Mental Health Journal, 27*(1), 5–25.

Olken, B. A. (2010). Direct democracy and local public goods: Evidence from a field experiment in Indonesia. *American Political Science Review, 104*(2), 243–267.

Omran, A. R. (1971). The epidemiologic transition: A theory of the epidemiology of population change. *Milbank Memorial Fund Quarterly, 49*(4), 509–538.

Orphanides, A., & Zervos, D. (1995). Rational addiction with learning and regret. *Journal of Political Economy, 103*(4), 739–758.

Osborne, D., & Gaebler, T. (1993). *Reinventing government.* New York: Plume.

Ostrom, E. (2005). *Understanding institutional diversity*. Princeton: Princeton University Press.

Outterson, K. (2005). The vanishing public domain: Antibiotic resistance, pharmaceutical innovation and global public health. *University of Pittsburgh Law Review, 67*, 67–123.

Pachter, L. M., & Coll, C. G. (2009). Racism and child health: A review of the literature and future directions. *Journal of Developmental and Behavioral Pediatrics, 30*(3), 255–263.

Paradies, Y. (2006). A systematic review of empirical research on self-reported racism and health. *International Journal of Epidemiology, 35*(4), 888–901.

Park, R. E., Fink, A., Brook, R. H., et al. (1986). Physician ratings of appropriate indications for six medical and surgical procedures. *American Journal of Public Health, 76*(7), 766–772.

Parker, C. (2002). *The open corporation: Effective self-regulation and democracy*. Cambridge: Cambridge University Press.

Parker, C., & Braithwaite, J. (2003). Regulation. In P. Cane & M. Tushnet (Eds.), *Oxford handbook of legal studies* (pp. 119–145). Oxford: Oxford University Press.

Parmet, W. (2009). *Populations, public health, and the law*. Washington, DC: Georgetown University Press.

Parmet, W. E., & Daynard, R. A. (2000). The new public health litigation. *Annual Review of Public Health, 21*, 437–454.

Parrott, S., Godfrey, C., & Raw, M. (2000). Costs of employee smoking in the workplace in Scotland. *Tobacco Control, 9*(2), 187–192.

Parsons, T. (1967). *Sociological theory and modern society*. New York: Free Press.

Pascoe, E. A., & Richman, L. S. (2009). Perceived discrimination and health: A meta-analytic review. *Psychological Bulletin, 135*(4), 531–554.

Pataki, G. E., & Carpinello, S. E. (2005). *Kendra's Law: Final report on the status of assisted outpatient treatment*. Albany: New York State Office of Mental Health. Retrieved from www.omh.ny.gov/omhweb/kendra_web/finalreport/

Paternoster, R., & Piquero, A. R. (1995). Reconceptualizing deterrence: An empirical test of personal and vicarious experiences. *Journal of Research in Crime and Delinquency, 32*(3), 251–286.

Patton, C. (1990). *Inventing AIDS*. New York: Routledge.

Pawson, R. (2006). *Evidence-based policy: A realist perspective*. London; Thousand Oaks, CA: Sage.

Pedriana, N., & Abraham, A. (2006). Now you see them, now you don't: The legal field and newspaper desegregation of sex-segregated help wanted ads 1965–75. *Law & Social Inquiry, 31*(4), 905–938.

Pedriana, N., & Stryker, R. (2004). The strength of a weak agency: Enforcement of Title VII of the 1964 Civil Rights Act and the expansion of state capacity, 1965–1971. *American Journal of Sociology, 110*(3), 709–760.

Pell, J. P., Haw, S., Cobbe, S., et al. (2008). Smoke-free legislation and hospitalizations for acute coronary syndrome. *New England Journal of Medicine, 359*(5), 482–491.

Percy, S. L. (1989). *Disability, civil rights, and public policy: The politics of implementation.* Tuscaloosa, AL: University of Alabama Press.

Percy, S. L. (2001). Challenges and dilemmas in implementing the Americans with Disabilities Act: Lessons from the first decade. *Policy Studies Journal, 29*(4), 633–640.

Perdue, W. C., Gostin, L. O., & Stone, L. A. (2003). Public health and the built environment: Historical, empirical, and theoretical foundations for an expanded role. *The Journal of Law, Medicine & Ethics, 31*(4), 557–566.

Pérez, D. J., & Larkin, M. A. (2009). Commentary: Partnership for the future of public health services and systems research. *Health Services Research, 44*(5p2), 1788–1795.

Persky, J. (1995). Retrospectives: The ethology of homo economicus. *The Journal of Economic Perspectives, 9*(2), 221–231.

Petraitis, J., Flay, B. R., & Miller, T. Q. (1995). Reviewing theories of adolescent substance use: Organizing pieces in the puzzle. *Psychological Bulletin, 117*(1), 67–86.

Pigou, A. C. (1962). *A study in public finance* (3rd revised ed.). London: Macmillan.

Piquero, A. R., & Paternoster, R. (1998). An application of Stafford and Warr's reconceptualization of deterrence to drinking and driving. *Journal of Research in Crime and Delinquency, 35*(1), 3–39.

Piquero, A. R., & Pogarsky, G. (2003). Can punishment encourage offending? Investigating the "resetting" effect. *Journal of Research in Crime and Delinquency, 40*(1), 95–120.

Plano, J. C., Riggs, R. E., & Robin, H. S. (1982). *The dictionary of political analysis.* Santa Barbara, CA: ABC-CLIO.

Poland, M. L., Dombrowski, M. P., Ager, J. W., & Sokol, R. J. (1993). Punishing pregnant drug users: Enhancing the flight from care. *Drug and Alcohol Dependence, 31*(3), 199–203.

Polaschek, D.L.L., Collie, R. M., & Walkey, F. H. (2004). Criminal attitudes to violence: Development and preliminary validation of a scale for male prisoners. *Aggressive Behavior, 30*(6), 484–503.

Polinsky, A. M., & Shavell, S. (2007). The theory of public enforcement of law. In A. M. Polinsky & S. Shavell (Eds.), *Handbook of law and economics* (Vol. 1, pp. 403–454). Amsterdam: Elsevier.

Popova, S., Giesbrecht, N., Bekmuradov, D., & Patra, J. (2009). Hours and days of sale and density of alcohol outlets: Impacts on alcohol consumption and damage: A systematic review. *Alcohol and Alcoholism, 44*(5), 500–516.

Population Services International. (2003). *What Is Social Marketing?* Washington, DC: Population Services International.

Powell, L. M., Chaloupka, F. J., & Bao, Y. (2007). The availability of fast food and full-service restaurants in the United States: Associations with neighborhood characteristics. *American Journal of Preventive Medicine, 33*(Suppl. 4), S240–S245.

Powell, L. M., & Chriqui, J. F. (2011). Food taxes and subsidies: Evidence and policies for obesity prevention. In J. Crawley (Ed.), *The Oxford handbook of the social science of obesity*. New York: Oxford University Press.

Powell, L. M., Schermbeck, R. M., Szczypka, G., Chaloupka, F. J., & Braunschweig, C. L. (2011). Trends in the nutritional content of television food advertisements seen by children in the United States: Analysis by age, food categories, and companies. *Archives of Pediatrics & Adolescent Medicine, 165*(12), 1078–1086.

Power, M. (1997). *The audit society: Rituals of verification*. Oxford; New York: Oxford University Press.

Pratt, T. C., & Cullen, F. T. (2005). Assessing macro-level predictors and theories of crime: A meta-analysis. In M. Tonry (Ed.), *Crime and justice: A review of research* (Vol. 32, pp. 373–450). Chicago: University of Chicago Press.

Pratt, T. C., Cullen, F. T., Blevins, K. R., Daigle, L. E., & Madensen, T. D. (2006). The empirical status of deterrence theory: A meta-analysis. In F. T. Cullen, J. P. Wright, & K. R. Blevins (Eds.), *Taking stock: The empirical status of criminological theory: Advances in criminological theory* (Vol. 15, pp. 367–395). New Brunswick, NJ: Transaction.

Preusser, D., & Tison, J. (2007). GDL then and now. *Journal of Safety Research, 38*(2), 159–163.

Przeworski, A., & Limongi, F. (1997). Modernization: Theories and facts. *World Politics, 49*(2), 155–183.

Public Health Accreditation Board. (2009). *Draft national voluntary accreditation standards for public health accreditation*. Retrieved May 5, 2011, from www.phaboard .org/index.php/beta_test/standards/

Public Health Functions Steering Committee Office of Disease Prevention and Health Promotion. (1994). *Public health in America*. Washington, DC: United States Public Health Service.

Public Health Law Research. (2012). *LawAtlas*. Retrieved September 26, 2012, from http://www.lawatlas.org

Quadagno, J. S. (2005). *One nation, uninsured: Why the U.S. has no national health insurance*. New York: Oxford University Press.

Rabin, B. A., Brownson, R. C., Haire-Joshu, D., Kreuter, M. W., & Weaver, N. (2008). A glossary for dissemination and implementation research in health. *Journal of Public Health Management and Practice, 14*(2), 117–123.

Rajkumar, A., & French, M. (1997). Drug abuse, crime costs, and the economic benefits of treatment. *Journal of Quantitative Criminology, 13*(3), 291–333.

Ratcliffe, J. H., Taniguchi, T., Groff, E. R., & Wood, J. D. (2011). The Philadelphia foot patrol experiment: A randomized controlled trial of police patrol effectiveness in violent crime hotspots. *Criminology, 49*(3), 795–831.

Reason, P., & Bradbury, H. (2008). *The Sage handbook of action research: Participative inquiry and practice*. Los Angeles, CA; London: Sage.

Recker, J., Rosemann, M., Indulska, M., & Green, P. (2009). Business process modeling: A comparative analysis. *Journal of the Association of Information Systems, 10*(4), 333–363.

Retting, R., & Cheung, I. (2008). Traffic speeds associated with implementation of 80 MPH speed limits on West Texas rural interstates. *Journal of Safety Research, 39*(5), 529–534.

Revesz, R. L. (1997). Environmental regulation, ideology, and the D.C. Circuit. *Virginia Law Review, 83*(8), 1717–1772.

Revesz, R. L. (2001). Congressional influence on judicial behavior? An empirical examination of challenges to agency action in the D.C. Circuit. *New York University Law Review, 76,* 1100–1137.

Rhodes, R.A.W. (1997). *Understanding governance: Policy networks, governance, reflexivity and accountability.* Buckingham; Philaldephia: Open University Press.

Richards, E. P., & Rathbun, K. C. (2003). *Legislative alternatives to the Model State Emergency Health Powers Act (MSEHPA)* (White Paper #2). Baton Rouge, LA: LSU Program in Law, Science, and Public Health.

Robinson, D. L. (2006). No clear evidence from countries that have enforced the wearing of helmets. *British Medical Journal, 322*(7543), 722–725.

Robson, L. S. (2007). The effectiveness of occupational health and safety management system interventions: A systematic review. *Safety Science, 45*(3), 329–353.

Rodgers, G. B., & Leland, E. W. (2008). A retrospective benefit-cost analysis of the 1997 stair-fall requirements for baby walkers. *Accident Analysis and Prevention, 40*(1), 61–68.

Rogers, E. M. (1962). *Diffusion of innovations.* New York: Free Press.

Rokeach, M. (1973). *The nature of human values*: New York: Free Press.

Rokeach, M., & Ball-Rokeach, S. J. (1989). Stability and change in American value priorities, 1968–1981. *American Psychologist, 44*(5), 775–784.

Rose, G. (1985). Sick individuals and sick populations. *International Journal of Epidemiology, 14*(1), 32–38.

Rosenbaum, M. (1980). A schedule for assessing self-control behaviors: Preliminary findings. *Behavior Therapy, 11*(1), 109–121.

Rosenberg, G. N. (1991). *The hollow hope: Can courts bring about social change?* Chicago: University of Chicago Press.

Rosenfeld, M. J. (2005). A critique of exchange theory in mate selection. *American Journal of Sociology, 110*(5), 1284–1325.

Ross, H. L. (1982). Interrupted time series studies of deterrence and drinking and driving. In J. Hagan (Ed.), *Deterrence reconsidered: Methodological innovations* (pp. 89–100). Beverly Hills, CA: Sage.

Rothman, K. J., & Greenland, S. (2005). Causation and causal inference in epidemiology. *American Journal of Public Health, 95,* S144–S150.

Rothstein, M. A. (2002). Rethinking the meaning of public health. *Journal of Law, Medicine & Ethics, 30*(2), 144–149.

Rubin, D. (1974). Estimating causal effects of treatments in randomized and non-randomized studies. *Journal of Educational Psychology, 66*(5), 688–701.

Rubin, D. B. (1990). Comment: Neyman (1923) and causal inference in experiments and observational studies. *Statistical Science, 5*(4), 472–480.

Ruger, J. P. (2006). Toward a theory of a right to health: Capability and incompletely theorized agreements. *Yale Journal of Law & the Humanities, 18*, 273–326.

Ruhl, S., Stephens, M., & Locke, P. (2003). The role of non-governmental organizations (NGOs) in public health law. *Journal of Law, Medicine & Ethics, 31* (Suppl. 4), 76–77.

Rutkow, L., & Teret, S. P. (2010). Role of state attorneys general in health policy. *Journal of the American Medical Association, 304*(12), 1377–1378.

Ryan, R. M., & Deci, E. L. (2000). Self-determination theory and the facilitation of intrinsic motivation, social development, and well-being. *American Psychologist, 55*(1), 68–78.

Sage, W. M. (2008). Relationship duties, regulatory duties, and the widening gap between health law and collective health policy. *Georgetown Law Journal, 96*(2), 497–522.

Salganik, M. J., & Heckathorn, D. D. (2004). Sampling and estimation in hidden populations using respondent-driven sampling. *Sociological Methodology, 34*(1), 193–240.

Sampson, R. J., Morenoff, J., & Gannon-Rowley, T. (2002). Assessing "neighborhood effects": Social processes and new directions in research. *Annual Review of Sociology, 28*, 443–478.

Sampson, R. J., Raudenbush, S. W., & Earles, F. (1997). Neighborhoods and violent crime: A multilevel study of collective efficacy. *Science, 277*, 918–924.

Sandler, J. C., Freeman, N. J., & Socia, K. M. (2008). Does a watched pot boil? A time series analysis of New York State's sex offender registration and notification law. *Psychology, Public Policy and Law, 14*(4), 284–302.

Sarat, A. (1990). ". . . The law is all over": Power, resistance and the legal consciousness of the welfare poor. *Yale Journal of Law & the Humanities, 2*, 343–379.

Saunders, R. P., Pate, R. R., Felton, G., et al. (1997). Development of questionnaires to measure psychosocial influences on children's physical activity. *Preventive Medicine, 26*(2), 241–247.

Savage, L. J. (1954). *Foundations of statistics*. New York: John Wiley & Sons.

Scheingold, S. A. (2004). *The politics of rights: Lawyers, public policy, and political change* (2nd ed.). Ann Arbor, MI: University of Michigan Press.

Schelling, T. C. (1995). Intergenerational discounting. *Energy Policy, 23*(4/5), 395–401.

Schensul, J. J. (1999). Organizing community research partnerships in the struggle against AIDS. *Health Education & Behavior, 26*(2), 266–283.

Schilling, J., & Linton, L. S. (2005). The public health roots of zoning: In search of active living's legal genealogy. *American Journal of Preventive Medicine, 28*(2 Suppl. 2), 96–104.

Schmitt, M., & Dorfel, M. (1999). Procedural injustice at work, justice sensitivity, job satisfaction and psychosomatic well-being. *European Journal of Social Psychology, 29*(4), 443–453.

Schneider, J. E., Peterson, N. A., Kiss, N., Ebeid, O., & Doyle, A. S. (2011). Tobacco litter costs and public policy: A framework and methodology for considering the use of fees to offset abatement costs. *Tobacco Control, 20* (Suppl. 1), i36–i41.

Schneider, T. R., Salovey, P., Pallonen, U., et al. (2001). Visual and auditory message framing effects on tobacco smoking. *Journal of Applied Social Psychology, 31*(4), 667–682.

Schnittker, J., & McLeod, J. D. (2005). The social psychology of health disparities. *Annual Review of Sociology, 31*, 75.

Schramm, D. D., & Milloy, C. D. (1995). *Community notification: A study of offender characteristics and recidivism* (95-10-1101). Seattle: Urban Policy Research.

Schultz, P. (2004). School subsidies for the poor: Evaluating the Mexican PROGRESA poverty program. *Journal of Development Economics, 74*(1), 199–250.

Schure, M. B., Lewis, K. M., Bavarian, N., et al. (2011). *Effects of the Positive Action program on problem behaviors in middle school students: A matched-pair randomized control trial in Chicago*. Unpublished manuscript.

Scollo, M., Lal, A., Hyland, A., & Glantz, S. A. (2003). Review of the quality of studies on the economic effects of smoke-free policies on the hospitality industry. *Tobacco Control, 12*(1), 13–20.

Scott, C. (2001). Analysing regulatory space: Fragmented resources and institutional design. *Public Law, 2001* (Summer), 329–353.

Scott, C. (2002). Private regulation of the public sector: A neglected facet of contemporary governance. *Journal of Law and Society, 29*(1), 56–76.

Scott, W. R., Ruef, M., Mendel, P. J., & Caronna, C. A. (Eds.). (2000). *Institutional change and healthcare organizations: From professional dominance to managed care*. Chicago: University of Chicago Press.

Scutchfield, F. D. (2009). Foreword. *Health Services Research, 44*(5p2), 1773–1774.

Scutchfield, F. D., Lawhorn, N., Ingram, R., et al. (2009). Public health systems and services research: Dataset development, dissemination, and use. *Public Health Reports, 124*(3), 372–377.

Scutchfield, F. D., Marks, J. S., Perez, D. J., & Mays, G. P. (2007). Public health services and systems research. *American Journal of Preventive Medicine, 33*(2), 169–171.

Scutchfield, F. D., Mays, G. P., & Lurie, N. (2009). Applying health services research to public health practice: An emerging priority. *Health Services Research, 44*(5p2), 1775–1187.

Scutchfield, F. D., & Patrick, K. (2007). Public health systems research: The new kid on the block. *American Journal of Preventive Medicine, 32*(2), 173–174.

Seelye, K. Q. (2003, May 9). EPA drops policy that values young lives over elderly. *Deseret News*. Retrieved from findarticles.com/p/articles/mi_qn4188/is_20030509/ai_n11387650/

Seeman, T. E., & Crimmins, E. (2001). Social environment effects on health and aging: Integrating epidemiologic and demographic approaches and perspectives. *Annals of the New York Academy of Sciences, 954*, 88–117.

Selznick, P., Nonet, P., & Vollmer, H. M. (1969). *Law, society, and industrial justice*. New York: Russell Sage Foundation.

Shadish, W. R. (2010). Campbell and Rubin: A primer and comparison of their approaches to causal inference in field settings. *Psychological Methods, 15*, 3–17.

Shadish, W. R., Cook, T. D., & Campbell, D. T. (2002). *Experimental and quasi-experimental designs for generalized causal inference*. Boston: Houghton–Mifflin.

Shadish, W. R., & Sullivan K. (2012). Theories of causation in psychological science. In H. Cooper (Ed.), *APA handbook of research methods in psychology* (Vol. 1, pp. 23–52). Washington, DC: American Psychological Association.

Shamir, R. (2008). Corporate social responsibility: Towards a new market-embedded morality? *Theoretical Inquiries in Law, 9*(2), 371–394.

Shattuck, L., Massachusetts Sanitary Commission, Banks, N. P., & Abbott, J. (1850). *Report of a general plan for the promotion of public and personal health*. Boston: Dutton & Wentworth.

Shaw, F. E., McKie, K. L., Liveoak, C. A., & Goodman, R. A. (2007). Legal tools for preparedness and response: Variation in quarantine powers among the 10 most populous U.S. states in 2004. *American Journal of Public Health, 97*(Suppl. 1), S38–S43.

Sheffer, C., Stitzer, M., & Wheeler, G. J. (2009). Smoke-free medical facility campus legislation: Support, resistance, difficulties and cost. *International Journal of Environmental Research and Public Health, 6*(1), 246–258.

Shekelle, P. G., Kahan, J. P., Bernstein, S. J., et al. (1998). The reproducibility of a method to identify the overuse and underuse of medical procedures. *New England Journal of Medicine, 338*(26), 1888–1895.

Sherman, L. W., & Strang, H. (2004). Experimental ethnography: The marriage of qualitative and quantitative research. *Annals of the American Academy of Political and Social Science, 595*(1), 204–222.

Silbey, S. (2002). The law and society movement. In H. Kritzer (Ed.), *Legal systems of the world: A political social and cultural encyclopedia* (Vol. 2, pp. 860–863). Santa Barbara, CA: ABC-CLIO.

Silbey, S. S. (2005). After legal consciousness. *Annual Review of Law and Social Science, 1*(1), 323–368.

Simester, D., Hu, Y. U., Brynjolfsson, E., & Anderson, E. T. (2009). Dynamics of retail advertising: Evidence from a field experiment. *Economic Inquiry, 47*(3), 482–499.

Simon, H. A. (1959). Theories of decision-making in economics and behavioral science. *The American Economic Review, 49*(3), 253–283.

Singer, J. W. (1984). The player and the cards: Nihilism and legal theory. *Yale Law Journal, 94*(1), 1–70.

Slaughter, E., Gersberg, R. M., Watanabe, K., et al. (2011). Toxicity of cigarette butts, and their chemical components, to marine and freshwater fish. *Tobacco Control, 20* (Suppl. 1), i25–i29.

Smith, A. (1776). *An inquiry into the nature and causes of the wealth of nations.* Dublin: Whitestone.

Smith, T. A. (2005). *The web of law.* San Diego Legal Studies research paper no. 06-11. Retrieved from Social Science Research Network at papers.ssrn.com/sol3/papers .cfm?abstract_id=642863

Snowdon, C. (2010). *The spirit level delusion: Fact-checking the Left's new theory of everything.* Ripton, North Yorkshire: Little Dice.

Sobeyko, J., Leszczyszyn-Pynka, M., Duklas, T., et al. (2006). *Bridging the gaps between needs and services in the health and criminal justice systems: Szczecin RPAR final report and recommendations.* Szczecin, Poland: RPAR.

Sonfield, A., & Gold, R. B. (2001). States' implementation of the Section 510 abstinence education program, FY 1999. *Family Planning Perspective, 33*(4), 166–171.

Sosin, D. M., & Sacks, J. J. (1992). Motorcycle helmet-use laws and head injury prevention. *Journal of the American Medical Association, 267*(12), 1649–1651.

Sox, H. C., & Greenfield, S. (2009). Comparative effectiveness research: A report from the Institute of Medicine. *Annals of Internal Medicine, 151*(3), 203–205.

Spencer, J. H. (2007). Neighborhood economic development effects of the earned income tax credit in Los Angeles. *Urban Affairs Review, 42*(6), 851–873.

Sperling, D. (2010). Food law, ethics, and food safety regulation: Roles, justifications, and expected limits. *Journal of Agricultural and Environmental Ethics, 23*(3), 267–278.

Splawa-Neyman, J. (1923). On the application of probability theory to agricultural experiments: Essay on principles, section 9. *Roczniki Nauk Rolniczynch Tom X*, 1–51.

Stafford, M., & Warr, M. (1993). A reconceptualization of general and specific deterrence. *Journal of Research in Crime and Delinquency, 30*(2), 123–135.

Stake, R. E. (2005). Qualitative case studies. In N. K. Denzin & Y. S. Lincoln (Eds.), *The Sage handbook of qualitative research* (3rd ed., pp. 443–466). Thousand Oaks, CA: Sage.

Starmer, C. (2000). Developments in non-expected utility theory: The hunt for a descriptive theory of choice under risk. *Journal of Economic Literature, 38*(2), 332–382.

Stein, M. A. (2004). Under the empirical radar: An initial expressive law analysis of the ADA. *Virginia Law Review, 90*(4), 1151–1191.

Sterman, J. D. (2006). Learning from evidence in a complex world. *American Journal of Public Health, 96*(3), 505–514.

Stern, A. M., & Markel, H. (2005). The history of vaccines and immunization: Familiar patterns, new challenges. *Health Affairs, 24*(3), 611–621.

Stigler, G. J. (1950). The development of utility theory. *The Journal of Political Economy, 58*(4), 307–327.

Stillman, S., McKenzie, D., & Gibson, J. (2009). Migration and mental health: Evidence from a natural experiment. *Journal of Health Economics, 28*(3), 677–687.

Stringer, E. T. (2007). *Action research* (3rd ed.). Thousand Oaks, CA: Sage.

Strully, K. W., Rehkopf, D. H., & Xuan, Z. (2010). Effects of prenatal poverty on infant health: State earned income tax credits and birth weight. *American Sociological Review, 75*(4), 534–562.

Stryker, R. (1994). Rules, resources, and legitimacy processes: Some implications for social conflict, order, and change. *American Journal of Sociology, 99*(4), 847–910.

Stryker, R. (2000). Legitimacy processes as institutional politics: Implications for theory and research in the sociology of organizations. In M. Lounsbury (Ed.), *Research in the sociology of organizations* (Vol. 17, pp. 179–223). Bingley, UK: Emerald Group.

Stryker, R. (2007). Half empty, half full, or neither: Law, inequality, and social change in capitalist democracies. *Annual Review of Law and Social Science, 3*(1), 69–97.

Stryker, R., Docka-Filipek, D., & Wald, P. (2011). Employment discrimination law and industrial psychology: Social science as social authority and the co-production of law and science. *Law & Social Inquiry.* doi:10.1111/j.1747-4469.2011.01277.x.

Stryker, S., & Serpe, R. T. (1982). Commitment, identity salience and role behavior. In W. Ickes & E. S. Knowles (Eds.), *Personality, roles and social behavior* (pp. 199–218). New York: Springer-Verlag.

Studdert, D. M., Mello, M. M., Gawande, A. A., Brennan, T. A., & Wang, Y. C. (2007). Disclosure of medical injury to patients: An improbable risk management strategy. *Health Affairs, 26*(1), 215–226.

Suchman, M. (2010). *Sharing is (s)caring on the digital frontier: The challenges of IT governance in health care organizations.* Paper presented at the Center for the Study of Law and Society at the University of California-Berkeley, October 11, 2010. Retrieved from www.law.berkeley.edu/files/SuchmanPaper11Oct2010(1).pdf

Sunshine, J., & Tyler, T. R. (2003a). The role of procedural justice and legitimacy in shaping public support for policing. *Law & Society Review, 37*(3), 513–548.

Sunshine, J., & Tyler, T. R. (2003b). Moral solidarity, identification with the community, and the importance of procedural justice: The police as prototypical representatives of a group's moral values. *Social Psychology Quarterly, 66*(2), 153–165.

Sunstein, C. (2004). *Are poor people worth less than rich people? Disaggregating the value of statistical lives.* Chicago: University of Chicago Law and Economics.

Sunstein, C., & Thaler, R. (2008). *Nudge: Improving decisions about health, wealth, and happiness.* New Haven, CT: Yale University Press.

Sutherland, E. H. (1942). Development of the theory. In K. Schuessier & H. Edwin (Eds.), *On analyzing crime* (pp. 13–29). Chicago: University of Chicago Press.

Sutton, J. R., Dobbin, F., Meyer, J. W., & Scott, W. R. (1994). The legalization of the workplace. *American Journal of Sociology, 99*(4), 944–971.

Suurd, C. D. (2009). *A test of the relationships among justice facets, overall justice, strain and turnover intention in a military context*. Ottawa, Canada: Defence Research & Development Canada.

Swanson, J. W., Burris, S. C., Moss, K., Ullman, M. D., & Ranney, L. M. (2006). Justice disparities: Does the ADA enforcement system treat people with psychiatric disabilities fairly? *Maryland Law Review, 66*, 94–139.

Swanson, J. W., McCrary, S. V., Swartz, M. S., Elbogen, E. B., & Van Dorn, R. A. (2006). Superseding psychiatric advance directives: Ethical and legal considerations. *Journal of the American Academy of Psychiatry and the Law, 34*(3), 385–394.

Swartz, M. S., Swanson, J. W., Kim, M., & Petrila, J. (2006). Use of outpatient commitment or related civil court treatment orders in five U.S. communities. *Psychiatric Services, 57*(3), 343–349.

Syme, S. L. (2004). Social determinants of health: The community as an empowered partner. *Preventing Chronic Disease, 1*(1), 1–5.

Tapp, J. L., & Levine, F. J. (1977). *Law, justice, and the individual in society: Psychological and legal issues*. New York: Holt, Rinehart and Winston.

Temple University, Beasley School of Law. (2004). *Rapid Policy Assessment and Response: Module 1: Project Planning and Community Action Boards*. Retrieved November 1, 2011, from www.temple.edu/lawschool/phrhcs/rpar/index.html

Teret, S. P., Wells, J. K., Williams, A. F., & Jones, A. S. (1986). Child restraint laws: An analysis of gaps in coverage. *American Journal of Public Health, 76*(1), 31–34.

Terry, K. J., & Ackerman, A. R. (2009). A brief history of major sex offender laws. In R. G. Wright (Ed.), *Sex offender laws: Failed policies, new directions* (pp. 65–98). New York: Springer.

Tesoriero, J. M., Battles, H. B., Heavner, K., et al. (2008). The effect of name-based reporting and partner notification on HIV testing in New York State. *American Journal of Public Health, 98*(4), 728–735.

Teubner, G. (1987). Juridification: Concepts, aspects, limits, solutions. In G. Teubner (Ed.) *Juridification of social spheres: A comparative analysis in the areas of labor, corporate, antitrust and social and welfare law* (pp. 3–48). Berlin: De Gruyter.

Tewksbury, R. (2005). Collateral consequences of sex offender registration. *Journal of Contemporary Criminal Justice, 21*(1), 67–81.

Tewksbury, R., & Jennings, W. G. (2010). Assessing the impact of sex offender registration and community notification on sex offending trajectories. *Criminal Justice and Behavior, 37*(5), 570–582.

Thaler, R. H., & Sunstein, C. R. (2008). *Nudge: Improving decisions about health, wealth, and happiness*. New Haven, CT: Yale University Press.

The Community Guide. (2009). *Community guide 101: Using evidence for public health decision making*. Retrieved October 16, 2009, from www.thecommunityguide.org/about/cg_101.html

Thoits, P. A. (1986). Multiple identities: Examining gender and marital status differences in distress. *American Sociological Review, 51*(2), 259–272.

Thomas, R., & Perera, R. (2006). Are school-based programmes effective in the long term in preventing uptake of smoking? *Cochrane Database of Systematic Reviews, 3* (CD001293).

Thomas, W. I., & Thomas, D. S. (1928). *The child in America: Behavior problems and programs*. New York: Alfred A. Knopf.

Thornton, R. (2005). The demand for and impact of HIV testing: Evidence from a field experiment. Unpublished working paper. Harvard University.

Tidwell, J. E., & Doyle, D. (1995). Driver and pedestrian comprehension of pedestrian law and traffic control devices. *Transportation Research Record*, (1502), 119–128.

Tobey, J. (1939). *Public health law: A manual of law for sanitarians* (2d ed.). New York: Commonwealth Press.

Tremper, C., Thomas, S., & Wagenaar, A. C. (2010). Measuring law for evaluation research. *Evaluation Review, 34*(3), 242–266.

Trochim, W.M.K. (2005). *Research methods: The concise knowledge base*. Cincinnati: Atomic Dog.

Trubek, L. (2006). New governance and soft law in health care reform. *Indiana Health Law Review, 2006*(4), 139–169.

Trumbull, W. N. (1990). Who has standing in cost-benefit analysis? *Journal of Policy Analysis and Management, 9*(2), 201–218.

Tsoukalas, T., & Glantz, S. A. (2003). The Duluth clean indoor air ordinance: Problems and success in fighting the tobacco industry at the local level in the 21st century. *American Journal of Public Health, 93*(8), 1214–1221.

Tversky, A., & Kahneman, D. (1974). Judgment under uncertainty: Heuristics and biases. *Science, 185*(4157), 1124–1131.

Tyler, T. R. (1990). *Why people obey the law*. New Haven, CT: Yale University Press.

Tyler, T. R. (1999). Why people cooperate with organizations: An identity-based perspective. *Research in Organizational Behavior, 21*, 201–246.

Tyler, T. R. (2000). Social justice: Outcome and procedure. *International Journal of Psychology, 35*(2), 117–125.

Tyler, T. R. (2003). Procedural justice, legitimacy, and the effective rule of law. In M. H. Tonry (Ed.), *Crime and justice: A review of research* (Vol. 30, pp. 431–505). Chicago; London: University of Chicago Press.

Tyler, T. R. (2006a). *Why people obey the law*. Princeton, NJ: Princeton University Press.

Tyler, T. R. (2006b). Psychological perspectives on legitimacy and legitimation. *Annual Review of Psychology, 57*(1), 375–400.

Tyler, T. R. (2007). *Psychology and the design of legal institutions*. Nijmegen, The Netherlands: Wolf Legal Publishers.

Tyler, T. R. (2008). Psychology and institutional design. *Review of Law & Economics, 4*(3), 801–887.

Tyler, T. R. (2009). Tom Tyler and why people obey the law. In S. Halliday & P. D. Schmidt (Eds.), *Conducting law and society research: Reflections on methods and practices* (pp. 141–151). Cambridge; New York: Cambridge University Press.

Tyler, T. R., & Blader, S. L. (2000). *Cooperation in groups: Procedural justice, social identity, and behavioral engagement*. Philadelphia: Psychology Press.

Tyler, T. R., & Fagan, J. (2008). Legitimacy and cooperation: Why do people help the police fight crime in their communities? *Ohio State Journal of Criminal Law, 6*(1), 231–275.

Tyler, T. R., & Huo, Y. J. (2002). *Trust in the law: Encouraging public cooperation with the police and courts*. New York: Russell Sage Foundation.

Tyler, T. R., & Markell, D. L. (2008). Using empirical research to explore ways to enhance citizen roles in environmental compliance and enforcement. *University of Kansas Law Review, 57*, 1–38.

Tyler, T. R., Mentovich, T., & Satyavada, S. (2011). Accepting health care recommendations: Assessing the role of procedural justice. Unpublished manuscript. New York University.

Tyler, T. R., Sherman, L., Strang, H., Barnes, G. C., & Woods, D. (2007). Reintegrative shaming, procedural justice, and recidivism: The engagement of offenders' psychological mechanisms in the Canberra RISE drinking-and-driving experiment. *Law & Society Review, 41*(3), 553–586.

U.S. Bureau of Justice. (2011). *Criminal justice system flowchart*. Retrieved October 1, 2011, from bjs.ojp.usdoj.gov/content/largechart.cfm#prosecution

U.S. Department of Health and Human Services. (2004). *The health consequences of smoking: A report of the Surgeon General*. Washington, DC: U.S. DHHS, Centers for Disease Control and Prevention, National Center for Chronic Disease Prevention and Health Promotion, Office on Smoking and Health.

U.S. Department of Health and Human Services. (2006). *Healthy People 2010 midcourse review*. Washington, DC: U.S. DHHS.

U.S. Interagency Working Group on Social Cost of Carbon & Government. (2010). Technical support document: *Social cost of carbon for regulatory impact analysis under executive order 12866*. Retrieved September 8, 2011, from www.epa.gov/otaq/climate/regulations/scc-tsd.pdf

Uchino, B. (2009). Understanding the links between social support and physical health: A life-span perspective with emphasis on the separability of perceived and received support. *Perspectives on Psychological Science, 4*(3), 236–255.

Ulmer, R. G., & Preusser, D. F. (2003). *Evaluation of the repeal of motorcycle helmet laws in Kentucky and Louisiana* (HS-809 530). Washington, DC: U.S. Department of Transportation.

Unger, J. B., Cruz, T., Baezconde-Garbanati, L., et al. (2003). Exploring the cultural context of tobacco use: A transdisciplinary framework. *Nicotine & Tobacco Research, 5*(Suppl. 1), S101–S117.

Unger, R. M. (1983). The critical legal studies movement. *Harvard Law Review, 96*(3), 561–675.

Vasquez, B. E., Maddan, S., & Walker, J. T. (2008). The influence of sex offender registration and notification laws in the United States: A time-series analysis. *Crime & Delinquency, 54*(2), 175–192.

Vermunt, R., & Steensma, H. (2003). Physiological relaxation: Stress reduction through fair treatment. *Social Justice Research, 16*(2), 135–149.

Vernick, J. S., & Teret, S. P. (2000). A public health approach to regulating firearms as consumer products. *University of Pennsylvania Law Review, 148*(4), 1193–1211.

Vining, A., & Weimer, D. L. (2010). An assessment of important issues concerning the application of benefit-cost analysis to social policy. *Journal of Benefit-Cost Analysis, 1*(1), Article 6.

Viscusi, W. K. (1994). Equivalent frames of reference for judging risk regulation policies. *New York University Environmental Law Journal, 431,* 431–468.

Viscusi, W. K. (2009). The devaluation of life. *Regulation and Governance, 3*(2), 103–127.

Voas, R., Tippetts, A. S., & Fell, J. C. (2003). Assessing the effectiveness of minimum legal drinking age and zero tolerance laws in the United States. *Accident Analysis and Prevention, 35*(4), 579–587.

Voas, R. B., & Kelley-Baker, T. (2008). Licensing teenagers: Nontraffic risks and benefits in the transition to driving status. *Traffic Injury Prevention, 9*(2), 88–97.

von Tigerstrom, B., Larre, T., & Sauder, J. (2011). Using the tax system to promote physical activity: Critical analysis of Canadian initiatives. *American Journal of Public Health, 101*(8), e10–e16.

Vyshemirskaya, I., Osipenko, V., Koss, A., et al. (2008). *HIV and drug policy in Kaliningrad: Risk, silence and the gap between human needs and health services.* Kaliningrad, Russia: RPAR.

W. K. Kellogg Foundation. (2004). *Logic model development guide: Using logic models to bring together planning, evaluation.* Battle Creek, MI: W.K. Kellogg Foundation.

Waddington, H., & Snilstveit, B. (2009). Effectiveness and sustainability of water, sanitation, and hygiene interventions in combating diarrhoea. *Journal of Development Effectiveness, 1*(3), 295–335.

Wagenaar, A. C. (1983a). *Alcohol, young drivers, and traffic accidents: Effects of minimum age laws.* Lexington, MA: Lexington Books.

Wagenaar, A. C. (1983b). Raising the legal drinking age in Maine: Impact on traffic accidents among young drivers. *International Journal of the Addictions, 18*(3), 365–377.

Wagenaar, A. C. (2007). Deterring sales and marketing of alcohol to youth: The role of litigation. In J. E. Henningfield, P. B. Santora, & W. K. Bickel (Eds.), *Addiction treatment: Science and the policy for the twenty-first century* (pp. 177–183). Baltimore: Johns Hopkins University Press.

Wagenaar, A. C., Erickson, D. J., Harwood, E. M., & O'Malley, P. M. (2006). Effects of state coalitions to reduce underage drinking: A national evaluation. *American Journal of Preventive Medicine, 31*(4), 307–315.

Wagenaar, A. C., Finnegan, J. R., Wolfson, M., et al. (1993). Where and how adolescents obtain alcoholic beverages. *Public Health Reports, 108*(4), 459–464.

Wagenaar, A. C., Maldonado-Molina, M. M., Erickson, D. J., et al. (2007). General deterrence effects of U.S. statutory DUI fine and jail penalties: Long-term follow-up in 32 states. *Accident Analysis & Prevention, 39*(5), 982–994.

Wagenaar, A. C., & Perry, C. L. (1994). Community strategies for the reduction of youth drinking: Theory and application. *Journal of Research on Adolescence, 4*(2), 319–345.

Wagenaar, A. C., Salois, M. J., & Komro, K. A. (2009). Effects of beverage alcohol price and tax levels on drinking: A meta-analysis of 1003 estimates from 112 studies. *Addiction, 104*(2), 179–190.

Wagenaar, A. C., Tobler, A. L., & Komro, K. A. (2010). Effects of alcohol tax and price policies on morbidity and mortality: A systematic review. *American Journal of Public Health, 100*(11), 2270–2278.

Wagenaar, A. C., & Wolfson, M. (1994). Enforcement of the legal minimum drinking age in the United States. *Journal of Public Health Policy, 15*(1), 37–53.

Wahlbeck, P. J., Spriggs, J. F., & Sigelman, L. (2002). Ghostwriters on the court? *American Politics Research, 30*(2), 166–192.

Wansink, B. (2006). *Mindless eating: Why we eat more than we think*. New York: Bantam.

Ward, A. (2009). Causal criteria and the problem of complex causation. *Medicine, Health Care and Philosophy, 12*(3), 333–343.

Ward, H. (2007). Prevention strategies for sexually transmitted infections: Importance of sexual network structure and epidemic phase. *Sexually Transmitted Infections, 83*(Suppl. 1), i43–i49.

Waters, I., & William, G. (1996). Values of travel time savings in road transport project evaluation, volume 3: Transport policy. Paper presented at the 7th World Conference on Transport Research, Sydney, July 16–21, 1995. Published in monograph *World transport research: Proceedings of the 7th World Conference on Transport*. Washington, DC: National Academy of Sciences, Transportation Research Board.

Waters, M., & Moore, W. J. (1990). The theory of economic regulation and public choice and the determinants of public sector bargaining legislation. *Public Choice, 66*(2), 161–175.

Watson, G., & Glaser, E. M. (1980). *Manual for the Watson Glaser critical thinking appraisal*. Cleveland: Psychological Corporation.

Watson, T. (2006). Public health investments and the infant mortality gap: Evidence from federal sanitation interventions on U.S. Indian reservations. *Journal of Public Economics, 90*(8–9), 1537–1560.

Weait, M. (2007). *Intimacy and responsibility: The criminalisation of HIV transmission*. Abingdon: Routledge-Cavendish.

Weber, M. (1968). *Economy and society*. Berkeley: University of California Press.

Webster, M., & Sell, J. (2007). *Laboratory experiments in the social sciences*. Boston: Academic Press.

Wells, J. K., Williams, A. F., & Fields, M. (1989). Coverage gaps in seat belt use laws. *American Journal of Public Health, 79*(3), 332–333.

Whitman, M. V., & Harbison, P. A. (2010). Examining general hospitals' smoke-free policies. *Health Education, 110*(2), 98–108.

Wiese, S. L., Vallacher, R. R., & Strawinska, U. (2010). Dynamical social psychology: Complexity and coherence in human experience. *Social and Personality Psychology Compass, 4*(11), 1018–1030.

Wigfield, A. (1994). Expectancy-value theory of achievement motivation: A developmental perspective. *Educational Psychology Review, 6*(1), 49–78.

Wigfield, A., & Eccles, J. S. (2000). Expectancy-value theory of achievement motivation. *Contemporary Educational Psychology, 25*(1), 68–81.

Wilkinson, R., & Pickett, K. (2009). *The spirit level: Why greater equality makes societies stronger*. London: Bloomsbury Press.

Williams-Piehota, P., Cox, A., Silvera, S. N., et al. (2004). Casting health messages in terms of responsibility for dietary change: Increasing fruit and vegetable consumption. *Journal of Nutrition Education and Behavior, 36*(3), 114–120.

Williams, D. R., & Collins, C. (1995). U.S. socioeconomic and racial differences in health: Patterns and explanations. *Annual Review of Sociology, 21*, 349–386.

Williams, D. R., & Collins, C. (2001). Racial residential segregation: A fundamental cause of racial disparities in health. *Public Health Reports, 116*, 404–416.

Williams, D. R., Costa, M. V., Odunlami, A. O., & Mohammed, S. A. (2008). Moving upstream: How interventions that address the social determinants of health can improve health and reduce disparities. *Journal of Public Health Management and Practice, 14*(6 Suppl.), S8–S17.

Williams, D. R., & Mohammed, S. A. (2009). Discrimination and racial disparities in health: Evidence and needed research. *Journal of Behavioral Medicine, 32*(1), 20–47.

Williams, D. R., Neighbors, H. W., & Jackson, J. S. (2003). Racial/ethnic discrimination and health: Findings from community studies. *American Journal of Public Health, 93*(2), 200–208.

Williams, K., & Hawkins, R. (1986). Perceptual research on general deterrence: A critical overview. *Law & Society Review, 20*(4), 545–572.

Willis, J. W. (2007). *Foundations of qualitative research: Interpretive and critical approaches*. Thousand Oaks, CA: Sage.

Wilson, J. W. (2009). Toward a framework for understanding forces that contribute to or reinforce racial inequality. *Race and Social Problems, 1*, 3–11.

Winston, G. C. (1980). Addiction and backsliding: A theory of compulsive consumption. *Journal of Economic Behavior & Organization, 1*(4), 295–324.

Wisdom, J. P., Michael, Y. L., Ramsey, K., & Berline, M. (2008). Women's health policies associated with obesity, diabetes, high blood pressure, and smoking: A follow-up on the Women's Health Report Card. *Women and Health, 48*(4), 103–122.

Wolf, L. E., & Vezina, R. (2004). Crime and punishment: Is there a role for criminal law in HIV prevention policy? *Whittier Law Review, 25*(Summer), 821–887.

Wolf, P. J., Silverberg, M., Institute of Education Sciences, & National Center for Education Evaluations and Regional Assistance. (2010). *Evaluation of the D.C. Opportunity Scholarship program: Final report*. Washington, DC: Institute of Education Sciences and National Center for Education Evaluation and Regional Assistance.

Wood, J. (2004). Cultural change in the governance of security. *Policing & Society, 14*(1), 31–48.

Woodruff, S. I., Pichon, L. C., Hoerster, K. D., et al. (2007). Measuring the stringency of states' indoor tanning regulations: Instrument development and outcomes. *Journal of the American Academy of Dermatology, 56*(5), 774–780.

Woods, W. J., Binson, D., Pollack, L. M., et al. (2003). Public policy regulating private and public space in gay bathhouses. *Journal of Acquired Immune Deficiency Syndromes, 32*, 417–423.

Woods, W. J., Euren, J., Pollack, L. M., & Binson, D. (2010). HIV prevention in gay bathhouses and sex clubs across the United States. *Journal of Acquired Immune Deficiency Syndromes, 55*(Suppl 2), S88–S90.

World Health Organization. (August 16, 2007). *WHO releases new guidance on insecticide-treated mosquito nets*. World Health Organization News Release. Retrieved from www.who.int/mediacentre/news/releases/2007/pr43/en/index.html

World Health Organization, United Nations Office on Drugs and Crime, & UNAIDS. (2007). *Interventions to address HIV in prisons: Comprehensive review*. Geneva: World Health Organization.

Wright, J., Parry, J., & Mathers, J. (2005). Participation in health impact assessment: Objectives, methods and core values. *Bulletin of the World Health Organization, 83*(1), 58–63.

Wright, R. F., & Huck, P. (2002). Counting cases about milk, our "most nearly perfect" food, 1860–1940. *Law & Society Review, 36*(1), 51–112.

Wright, S. (1934). The method of path coefficients. *Annals of Mathematical Statistics, 5*, 161–215.

Xu, X., & Chaloupka, F. J. (2011). The effects of prices on alcohol use and its consequences. *Alcohol Research and Health, 34*(2), 236–245.

Yeager, P. C. (1990). *The limits of law: The public regulation of private pollution*. Cambridge, England; New York: Cambridge University Press.

Yngvesson, B. (1988). Making law at the doorway: The clerk, the court, and the construction of community in a New England town. *Law and Society Review, 22*(3), 409–448.

Zaloshnja, E., & Miller, T. R. (2007). The economic benefits of child safety seat misuse reduction programs and design improvements for children in rear seats. *Annual*

Proceedings of the Association for the Advancement of Automotive Medicine, 51, 197–206.

Zelditch, M. Jr. (2001). Theories of legitimacy. In J. T. Jost & B. Major (Eds.), *The psychology of legitimacy* (pp. 33–53). Cambridge: Cambridge University Press.

Zerbe, R. O. Jr. (1991). Comment: Does benefit-cost analysis stand alone? Rights and standing. *Journal of Policy Analysis and Management, 10*(1), 96–105.

Zgoba, K., Veysey, B., & Dalessandro, M. (2010). An analysis of the effectiveness of community notification and registration: Do the best intentions predict the best practices? *Justice Quarterly, 27*(5), 667–691.

Zimring, F., Jennings, W. G., Piquero, A. R., & Hays, S. (2009). Investigating the continuity of sex offending: Evidence from the second Philadelphia birth cohort. *Justice Quarterly, 26*(1), 58–76.

Zimring, F., Piquero, A. R., & Jennings, W. G. (2007). Sexual delinquency in Racine: Does early sex offending predict later sex offending in youth and adulthood? *Criminology and Public Policy, 6*(3), 507–534.

Name Index

f represents figure; t represents table.

Subject Index

f represents figure; t represents table.

A

A + Opportunity Scholarship Program, 299

ABAB designs, 318

Academic disciplines, 218

AcademyHealth, 8

Access to health care. *See* Health care, access to

Accreditation, 38–39

ACGME. *See* American Council for Graduate Medical Education

Action research, 337–338

Addiction: effect of taxes on, 158; market failures related to, 152; public education campaigns and, 162

Administrative hearings, 99

Advanced Legislative Service (ALS), 249

Advertising, 162, 166

Advocacy: influence of, 12; lack of research in, 36

Affirmative action, 92–93

Africa, 299

Against the law legal consciousness, 89

Agency staff, 255

Aggression, 187

AHS. *See* American Housing Survey

Airbag technology, 198

Alcohol Policy Information System dataset, 246, 255

Alcohol sales, 163–164, 246, 364

Alcohol use: access to, effects of, 57, 58; causal diagram for, 224, 226f; drinking age for, 54, 171, 246, 320–321; effect of taxes on, 156; expectancy-value theory and, 173; joy of intoxication and, 364–365; legal costs associated with, 163; market failures regarding, 151; pricing strategies for, 160; procedural justice and, 140; prohibition of, 163; public education campaigns and, 162; soft laws and, 172; by youths, 224, 226f

All Stars substance abuse education program, 360

ALS. *See* Advanced Legislative Service

Alternative opinions, 352

Amendments, 254–255

American Community Survey, 67, 68t

American Council for Graduate Medical Education (ACGME), 95

American Housing Survey (AHS), 68t

Americans for Nonsmokers' Rights, 66

Americans with Disabilities Act of 1990 (ADA), 62; effects of, 90–91; interdisciplinary studies of, 380–381

Ancillary information, 250

Antecedents, in causal diagrams, 220

Anti-discrimination policies, 54

Antiquated statutes, 32

Antitrust laws, 149–150

Appellate courts, 270, 273

Area Resource File (ARF), 68t

Arrows, 220

Assisted Outpatient Treatment Program (AOT), 223, 224f, 225f

Association of State and Territorial Health Officials (ASTHO), 38, 40

Atlas.ti (software), 343

Attitudes, toward behavior: measures of, 186, 187; predicting behaviors and, 178; in theory of reasoned action, 174; theory of triadic influence and, 182